S0-BNW-389

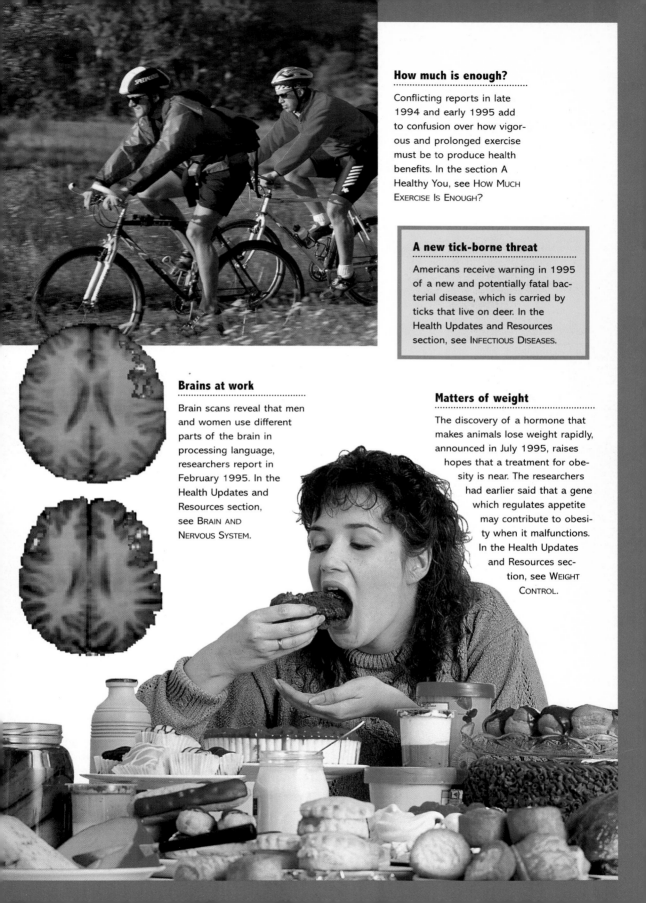

How much is enough?

Conflicting reports in late 1994 and early 1995 add to confusion over how vigorous and prolonged exercise must be to produce health benefits. In the section A Healthy You, see How Much Exercise Is Enough?

A new tick-borne threat

Americans receive warning in 1995 of a new and potentially fatal bacterial disease, which is carried by ticks that live on deer. In the Health Updates and Resources section, see Infectious Diseases.

Brains at work

Brain scans reveal that men and women use different parts of the brain in processing language, researchers report in February 1995. In the Health Updates and Resources section, see Brain and Nervous System.

Matters of weight

The discovery of a hormone that makes animals lose weight rapidly, announced in July 1995, raises hopes that a treatment for obesity is near. The researchers had earlier said that a gene which regulates appetite may contribute to obesity when it malfunctions. In the Health Updates and Resources section, see Weight Control.

See page 17.

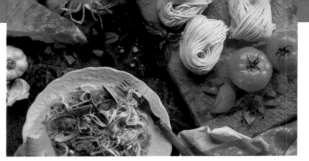

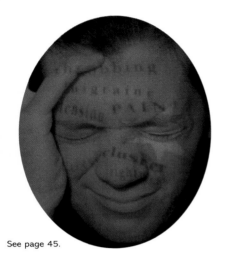

See page 45.

CONTENTS

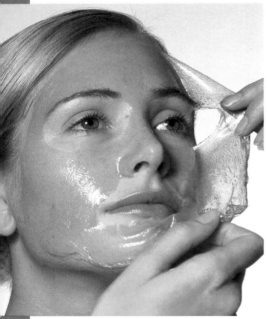

See page 74.

See page 117.

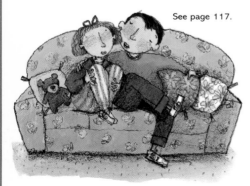

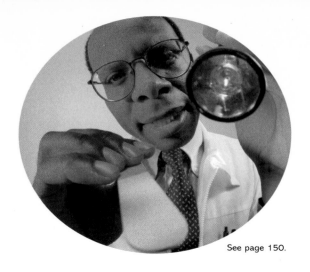

See page 150.

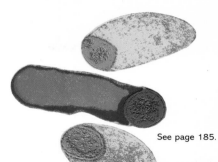

See page 185.

See page 205.

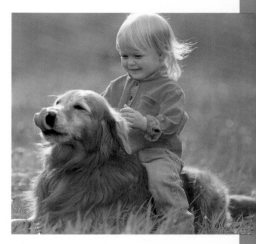

See page 343.

STAFF

EDITORIAL

Executive Editor
Darlene R. Stille

Managing Editor
Karin C. Rosenberg

Senior Editors
Mary Carvlin
David L. Dreier
Mark Dunbar
Carol L. Hanson
Patricia Ohlenroth

Contributing Editors
Jinger Hoop
Rod Such

Editorial Assistant
Ethel Matthews

Cartographic Services
H. George Stoll, Head
Wayne K. Pichler

Index Services
David Pofelski, Head

ART

Executive Director
Roberta Dimmer

**Senior Designer,
Health & Medical Annual**
Melanie J. Lawson

Senior Designers
Cari L. Biamonte
Brenda B. Tropinski

Senior Photographs Editor
Sandra M. Dyrlund

Art Production Assistant
Stephanie K. Tunney

RESEARCH SERVICES

Director
Mary Norton

Library Services
Mary Ann Urbashich, Head

PRODUCTION

Daniel N. Bach,
Vice President

Manufacturing/Pre-Press
Sandra Van den Broucke,
Director
Barbara Podczerwinski
Joann Seastrom

Proofreaders
Anne Dillon
Karen Lenburg

Text Processing
Curley Hunter
Gwendolyn Johnson

Permissions Editor
Janet Peterson

EDITOR IN CHIEF

W. Richard Dell

PUBLISHER EMERITUS

William H. Nault

PRESIDENT

John E. Frere

IMPORTANT NOTE: The information contained in *The World Book Health & Medical Annual* is not intended to take the place of the care and attention of a physician or other medical or health care professional. The information contained in *The World Book Health & Medical Annual* is believed to be accurate but cannot be warranted. On any matters related to health, always consult a physician or other appropriate health care professional.

EDITORIAL
ADVISORY BOARD

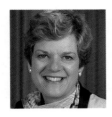

Linda H. Clever, M.D., is Chairman of the Department of Occupational Health at California Pacific Medical Center and Clinical Professor of Medicine at the University of California at San Francisco. She received the A.B. degree in 1962 and the M.D. degree in 1965, both from Stanford University. Dr. Clever served on the Board of Governors of the American College of Physicians from 1984 to 1989 and currently serves on its Board of Regents. Since 1990, she has been Editor of the *Western Journal of Medicine*. She is a member of the Institute of Medicine of the National Academy of Sciences.

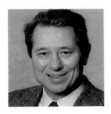

Jerome Kagan, Ph.D., is the Daniel and Amy Starch Professor of Psychology at Harvard University. He received the B.S. degree from Rutgers University in 1950 and the Ph.D. from Yale University in 1954. He received Distinguished Scientist awards from the American Psychological Association in 1987 and the Society for Research in Child Development in 1989 and was awarded the Hofheimer Prize for Research from the American Psychiatric Association in 1962. He is a fellow of the American Academy of Arts and Sciences and a member of the Institute of Medicine of the National Academy of Sciences.

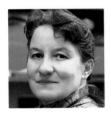

June E. Osborn, M.D., is on the faculty of the University of Michigan, where she is Professor of Epidemiology in the School of Public Health and Professor of Pediatrics and Communicable Diseases in the Medical School. Dr. Osborn received the B.A. degree from Oberlin College in 1957 and the M.D. degree from Case Western Reserve University in 1961. She was Chairman of the National Commission on AIDS from 1989 to 1993 and a member of the World Health Organization's Global Commission on AIDS from 1988 to 1992. She is a fellow of the American Academy of Pediatrics and a member of the Institute of Medicine of the National Academy of Sciences.

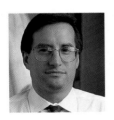

Mark W. Stolar, M.D., is on the faculties of Northwestern University Medical School and Rush University Medical School, where he is Associate Professor of Clinical Medicine. Dr. Stolar received the B.A. degree from Northwestern University in 1975 and the M.D. degree from the University of Illinois in 1979. He is on the board of the Endocrine Fellows Foundation and is a member of the American College of Physicians, the Endocrine Society, and the American Society of Clinical Endocrinologists.

CONTRIBUTORS

Balk, Robert A., M.D.
Director of Pulmonary Medicine,
Rush Medical College,
Rush-Presbyterian-St. Luke's
Medical Center.
[Health Updates and Resources:
Respiratory System]

Barone, Jeanine, M.S.
Nutritionist and Contributing
Editor, *University of California
at Berkeley Wellness Letter.*
[Spotlight on Eating Right: *Low-
Fat Diets; Ideal Weight: Science or
Fashion?; Restoring Family Meal-
time;* Health Updates and
Resources: *Nutrition and Food*]

Benowitz, Steven I., M.A.
Free-Lance Science Writer.
[On the Medical Frontier: *Are We
Winning the War on Cancer?*]

Berlfein, Judy Reiss, M.S.
Free-Lance Science and
Medical Writer.
[A Healthy You: *Drawing from
Your Own Blood Bank*]

Birnbaum, Gary, M.D.
Professor of Neurology,
University of Minnesota.
[Health Updates and Resources:
Brain and Nervous System]

Bowers, Kathryn E., M.D.
Clinical Instructor in
Dermatology,
Harvard Medical School.
[Health Updates and Resources:
Skin]

Clarkson, Priscilla M., Ph.D.
Associate Dean and Professor of
Exercise Science, School of Public
Health and Health Sciences,
University of Massachusetts
at Amherst.
[A Healthy You: *How Much
Exercise Is Enough?*]

Crawford, Michael H., M.D.
Chief, Division of Cardiology,
University of New Mexico
Health Sciences Center.
[Health Updates and Resources:
Heart and Blood Vessels]

Dudley, Ellen, B.A.
Free-Lance Writer.
[Medical and Safety Alerts:
Safe Hiking]

Foreman, Julie, M.S.
Program Administrator,
American Medical Association.
[Health Updates and Resources:
*Ear and Hearing; Eye and Vision;
Stroke; Surgery*]

Franklin, James L., M.D.
Associate Professor of Medicine,
Rush-Presbyterian-St. Luke's
Medical Center.
[A Healthy You: *Treating Hemor-
rhoids;* Health Updates and Re-
sources: *Digestive System*]

Friedman, Emily, B.A.
Health Policy Columnist,
*Journal of the American Medical
Association.*
[Health Updates and Resources:
Health-Care Issues]

Gartland, John J., M.D.
James Edwards Professor Emeritus
of Orthopedic Surgery,
Thomas Jefferson University.
[Health Updates and Resources:
Bone Disorders]

Gerber, Glenn S., M.D.
Assistant Professor,
Division of Urology,
University of Chicago.
[Health Updates and Resources:
Urology]

Glogau, Richard G., M.D.
Clinical Professor of Dermatology,
University of California at
San Francisco.
[A Healthy You: *Wrinkle Removal:
An Antidote to Aging Skin?*]

Golinkoff, Roberta Michnick,
Ph.D.
Professor of Educational
Psychology and Linguistics,
University of Delaware.
[A Healthy Family: *How
Children Learn to Talk*]

Hales, Dianne, M.S.
Free-Lance Writer.
[A Healthy Family: *Talking to
Your Child about Sex*]

Hamilton, Gayle, R., Ph.D.
Associate Research Professor,
George Mason University.
[Health Updates and Resources:
Alcohol and Drug Abuse; Smoking]

Hart, Benjamin, D.V.M., Ph.D.
Professor, School of
Veterinary Medicine,
University of California at Davis.
[Health Updates and Resources:
Veterinary Medicine]

Hirsh-Pasek, Kathy, Ph.D.
Associate Professor of Psychology,
Temple University.
[A Healthy Family: *How
Children Learn to Talk*]

Hussar, Daniel A., Ph.D.
Remington Professor of Pharmacy,
Philadelphia College of Pharmacy
and Science.
[Medical and Safety Alerts:
*Keeping the Wonder in Wonder
Drugs;* Health Updates and
Resources: *Drugs*]

Keefe, David, M.D.
Chief, Reproductive Aging Unit,
Yale University School of
Medicine.
[On the Medical Frontier:
Pregnancy Through Technology]

Levine, Carol, M.A.
Executive Director,
The Orphan Project,
Fund for the City of New York.
[Health Updates and Resources:
Medical Ethics]

Lewis, Ricki, Ph.D.
Adjunct Professor of Biology,
State University of New York
at Albany.
[Health Updates and Resources:
Weight Control]

Lockshin, Michael D., M.D.
Acting Director,
National Institute of Arthritis and
Musculoskeletal and Skin Diseases.
[Health Updates and Resources:
*Arthritis and Connective Tissue
Disorders*]

Maugh, Thomas H., II, Ph.D.
Science Writer,
Los Angeles Times.
[Health Updates and Resources:
Environmental Health]

McInerney, Joseph D., M.A., M.S.
Director, Biological Sciences
Curriculum Study,
Colorado College.
[Health Updates and Resources:
Genetics]

Minotti, Dominick, A.,
M.D., M.P.H.
Chief, Allergy Service, and
Clinical Professor of Medicine,
University of Washington
Medical Center.
[Health Updates and Resources:
Allergies and Asthma]

Moore, Margaret E.,
A.M.L.S., M.P.H.
Head, Education Services,
Health Sciences Library, University
of North Carolina at Chapel Hill.
[Health Updates and Resources:
Books of Health and Medicine]

Netherton, Robin, A.B., B.J.
Free-Lance Writer and Editor.
[Medical and Safety Alerts:
Poison on the Menu]

Rinehart, Rebecca D.
Associate Director, Publications,
American College of Obstetricians
and Gynecologists.
[Health Updates and Resources:
Pregnancy and Childbirth]

Rinzler, Carol Ann
Free-Lance Writer.
[Spotlight on Eating Right: *The
Mediterranean Diet; Deciphering
Food Labels*]

Roodman, G. David, M.D., Ph.D.
Professor of Medicine,
University of Texas
Health Science Center.
[Health Updates and Resources:
Blood]

Rosberger, Anne W.,
M.S.W., A.B.D.
Director,
Bereavement and Loss Center
of New York.
[A Healthy Family: *When a Parent
Dies*]

Seaborg, Eric, B.A.
Free-lance Writer.
[Medical and Safety Alerts:
Safe Hiking]

Siscovick, David S., M.D., M.P.H.
Associate Professor of Medicine
and Epidemiology,
University of Washington.
[Health Updates and Resources:
Exercise and Fitness]

Stephenson, Joan, Ph.D.
Associate News Editor,
*Journal of the American Medical
Association.*
[Medical and Safety Alerts:
*Germ Warfare: Battling the Strep A
"Bug"*; Health Updates and Re-
sources: *Cancer*]

Stone, Katherine M., M.D.
Medical Epidemiologist,
Centers for Disease Control.
[Health Updates and Resources:
Sexually Transmitted Diseases]

Terr, Lenore, M.D.
Clinical Professor of Psychiatry,
University of California at San
Francisco.
[Health Updates and Resources:
Child Development; Mental Health]

Thompson, Jeffrey R., M.D.
President,
Dallas Kidney Specialists.
[Health Updates and Resources:
Kidney]

Tideiksaar, Rein, Ph.D.
Assistant Professor,
Henry L. Schwartz Department
of Geriatrics,
Mount Sinai Medical Center.
[Health Updates and Resources:
Aging]

Trubo, Richard, M.A.
Free-Lance Medical Writer.
[Medical and Safety Alerts:
*Hypertension: A Ticking Time
Bomb*; Health Updates and
Resources: *AIDS; Diabetes*]

Turkington, Carol A., B.A.
Free-Lance Medical Writer.
[On the Medical Frontier:
*Cochlear Implants: Delivering
Sound to the Deaf*]

Van Herle, Andre J., M.D.
Professor of Medicine,
School of Medicine, University
of California at Los Angeles.
[Health Updates and Resources:
Glands and Hormones]

Voelker, Rebecca, M.S.J.
Associate News Editor,
*Journal of the American Medical
Association.*
[A Healthy You: *Headache: Complex
Pain with Origins in the Brain*;
Medical and Safety Alerts:
Which to Apply: Heat or Cold?]

Wardlaw, Gordon, Ph.D., R.D.
Associate Professor,
School of Allied Medical
Professions, Ohio State University.
[Spotlight on Eating Right:
*Following a Healthful Diet;
Changing Lifetime Nutrition Needs*]

Woods, Michael, B.S.
Science Editor,
The Toledo Blade.
[Medical and Safety Alerts: *The
Hazards of Carbon Monoxide*; Health
Updates and Resources: *Dentistry;
Infectious Diseases; Safety*]

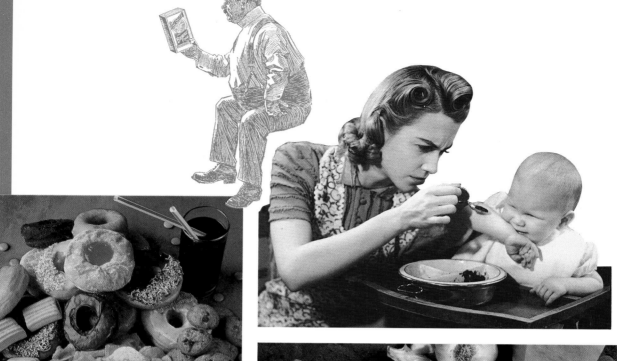
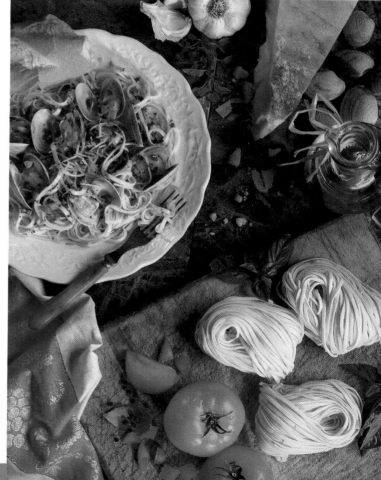

Spotlight on Eating Right

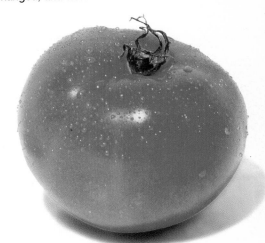

> Although it may seem as if nutrition advice changes constantly, the nutrition basics usually remain the same.

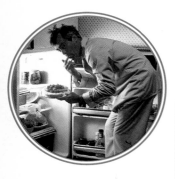

Following a Healthful Diet

By Gordon Wardlaw

The author:

Gordon Wardlaw is an associate professor of medical dietetics at Ohio State University and coauthor of *Contemporary Nutrition: Issues and Insights.*

I F CLAIMS ABOUT THE HEALTH BENEFITS OF VARIOUS FOODS leave you confused, you are not alone. The barrage of nutrition stories in newspapers, magazines, and television and radio news reports can create the impression that nutrition advice is changing constantly. A reader confronting yet another nutrition story—"Eat olive oil and oat bran to lower blood cholesterol" or "Beta-carotene may help reduce your risk for certain cancers"—may wonder how much fact backs up these words and whether tomorrow's findings will overturn this advice. The end result is to make nutrition seem an ever-deepening mystery rather than an expanding science.

Yet the basics of nutrition remain quite simple and rarely change. Health professionals generally agree that the average American diet provides excess calories, fat, salt, sugar, and alcohol and insufficient fruits, vegetables, and fiber. Eating habits out of balance with the body's nutrient needs contribute to a number of the diseases that commonly kill or disable Americans, including high blood pressure, heart disease, stroke, some cancers, adult-onset diabetes, and *osteoporosis* (diminished bone mass).

Getting all the nutrients essential for health is mainly a matter of eating a variety of well-chosen foods. Yet a 1994 survey by the American Dietetic Association, a national organization of dieticians, showed that two out of five Americans believe that following a healthful diet means giving up the foods they enjoy. But eliminating favorite foods is unlikely to improve nutrition because most people won't tolerate such a regimen for long. A healthful diet requires some careful planning and effort, rather than deprivation, misery, or vast expense.

The Food Guide Pyramid

The Food Guide Pyramid was developed by the U.S. Department of Agriculture on the basis of years of research on diet and health. It recommends eating more daily servings from the food groups near the base of the pyramid—grains, fruits, and vegetables—than from the food groups near the pyramid's top—dairy products and meat and meat substitutes.

Fats, oils, and sweets
Use sparingly

Milk, yogurt, and cheese group

2-3 servings

One serving equals:
- 1 cup skim or low-fat milk
- 1 cup low-fat yogurt
- 1½ oz. natural cheddar cheese
- 2 oz. processed cheese

Meat, poultry, fish, dry beans, eggs, and nuts group

2-3 servings

One serving equals:
- 1 egg
- 2-3 oz. cooked chicken or other lean meat
- 2 tbsp. peanut butter
- ½ cup cooked dried beans

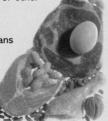

 Fruit group

2-4 servings

One serving equals:
- 1 apple, banana, or other whole fruit
- ½ cup canned fruit
- ¾ cup fruit juice
- ¼ cup raisins or other dried fruit

Vegetable group

3-5 servings

One serving equals:
- 1 cup salad greens
- ½ cup cooked vegetable
- ½ cup raw, nonleafy vegetable
- ¾ cup vegetable juice

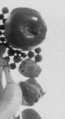

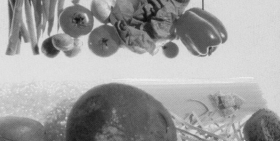

 Bread, cereal, rice, and pasta group

6-11 servings

One serving equals:
- 1 slice bread
- 1 oz. breakfast cereal
- ½ cup cooked rice or pasta
- 2 pancakes

The basics of nutrition

The best nutrition plans, according to dieticians, build on three principles: balance, variety, and moderation. Incorporating balance into the diet means choosing foods from the five food groups established by the U.S. Department of Agriculture (USDA). The five groups are breads, cereals and other grain products; fruits; vegetables; dairy products; and meat, poultry, fish, beans, eggs, and nuts.

To help Americans plan healthful diets, the USDA has designed a food guide pyramid that indicates how much we should eat daily from each group. People who eat the recommended number of servings from each food group are likely to get all the nutrients their bodies need. The pyramid recommends 6 to 11 servings of grains, 3 to 5 servings of vegetables, 2 to 4 servings of fruit, 2 to 3 servings of dairy products, and 2 to 3 servings from the group comprising meat, fish, beans, eggs, and nuts every day.

The second principle of nutrition, variety, means varying the selections within each food group. Carrots might be a woman's favorite food, but if she doesn't eat other vegetables, she might get too little of the B vitamin folic acid. This nutrient is important to women in their childbearing years because it lowers the risk of spinal birth defects. When we eat a variety of foods, we increase our chances of consuming the vitamins and minerals essential to health.

Moderation means not overdoing portion size. While 6 to 11 serv-

Fruits and vegetables, five times a day

The National Cancer Institute recommends eating at least five servings of fruits and vegetables every day, because studies suggest that these foods help protect against cancer. Five servings may seem like a lot, but these tips should help.

Breakfast	Lunch	Dinner	Snack	Dessert
• Drink a glass of juice.	• Eat a salad.	• Add vegetables to the main meal, such as raw onions to chili.	• Drink a glass of juice.	• Add chopped fruit to baked goods.
• Add sliced bananas or berries to your cereal.	• Choose vegetable soup.	• Add raw peppers, carrots, and cabbage to your salad.	• Try dried fruit, such as raisins.	• Top frozen yogurt with fresh fruit.
• Have a bowl of fruit, such as melon or peaches.	• Add lettuce, tomatoes, sprouts, and onions to sandwiches.	• Use fruit as a garnish.	• Nibble on fresh fruit.	• Try fruit-based desserts, such as baked apples.
• Top pancakes or French toast with fruit instead of syrup.	• Munch on carrot or celery sticks.	• When eating out, order extra vegetables.	• Keep raw, cut vegetables handy.	

Source: National Cancer Institute.

ings from the grains at the pyramid's base may sound like a lot, take note of the serving sizes. The two pieces of bread in a sandwich constitute two servings, for example, and a nine-ounce steak counts for three servings from the meat group.

The Food Guide Pyramid is designed to give adults the nutrients they need in approximately 1,800 calories. This is the minimum, in amount and variety, most adults should consume to obtain the nutrients they need. Dieters who try to cut calories by cutting back on the number of servings from each group frequently find that hunger prompts them to choose unplanned snacks that are high in fat and calories and low in nutrients.

Most active adults need more than 1,800 calories to meet their energy needs and stave off hunger pangs. Moderately active women and sedentary men should take in about 2,200 calories daily; moderately active men, about 2,800 calories. When adding calories to your diet, remember to look to the base of the pyramid first. In general, maintaining an appropriate weight is a good indication that calorie intake is about right.

Forming healthful habits

In making healthful diet changes, it's useful to keep a log for a few days, noting when, what, and how much you eat. Then, compare your log to the Food Guide Pyramid and see which food groups fall short in your diet and which you overemphasize. It's also a good idea to plan healthful eating habits around your lifestyle. Suppose, for example, that you never eat breakfast but read that people who do so function best. Rather than forcing yourself to eat a big meal first thing in the morning, think of something—fruit, bagel, cereal, or toast—that you could bear to eat in a small amount. Remember that most people need "refueling" every three to four hours, so plan several small snacks in between two or three larger meals consisting of foods from at least three food groups.

For a closer look at specific nutrient needs that occur if you avoid dairy products or meat, it would be helpful to contact a registered dietitian. Your doctor may refer you to a dietitian, or you can locate one through the American Dietetic Association's referral

OAT BRAN MIRACLE

Reading nutrition stories

Reading the headlines may suggest that nutrition advice is changing constantly as a result of new findings. But breakthroughs are rare, and most studies add only one more piece to the sum of previous knowledge. Readers can better judge the significance of a study's findings by keeping these questions in mind.

- Who wrote the story and how was it written? Science or medical writers may have a better understanding of a study's significance than general reporters do. Words like "breakthrough" and "proof" should arouse your suspicions because the findings of a single study are rarely definitive. A sense that the writer has an ax to grind should be another red flag.

- Who paid for the study? Study findings that appear to endorse the underwriter's product are not necessarily invalid, but they should arouse skepticism. If a particular report arouses your suspicion, see where it was published. Scientific journals publish studies only after review by other scientists.

- Does the reporting of the story appear to be even-handed? Balanced reports usually present both sides of an issue, state whether the evidence is preliminary or widely accepted, and mention conflicting research findings. One-sided reports often lack supporting evidence from other scientists, make exaggerated claims for a particular product, or tout miracle cures.

- How large was the study and how long did it last? The larger the number of subjects and the longer they were studied, the more meaningful the results are likely to be.

network at (800) 366-1655. Many local hospitals run clinics staffed by dietitians, and dietitians also are listed in the telephone directory. Or, you may wish to read some nutrition-related books addressing your particular needs.

If you are considering taking vitamin or mineral supplements, a dietitian can provide guidance. If you do take a supplement, make sure your intake of that nutrient never exceeds 150 percent of the Daily Allowance listed on the product's label, unless your physician recommends otherwise. Taking a larger amount of some nutrients, such as iron and calcium, can be harmful to some people. Studies have found that about 1 American in 10 has the ability to over-absorb iron, which can cause liver damage and may increase the risk of heart disease. And some people who eat excessive amounts of calcium may develop painful stones in their kidneys. People who are predisposed to kidney stones should not absorb more than 1,500 milligrams of calcium a day. Major medical trials underway in 1995 will determine to what extent large amounts of certain vitamins, such as C and E, can harm the body. Doctors already know that excess vitamin A can be harmful, especially in the young.

What to believe?

Sifting nutrition fact from fallacy—whether in news reports or on product labels—can be difficult. The following suggestions may help in distinguishing between important new findings and hype.

- When reading nutrition advice, check whether the information is consistent with the basic principles of nutrition: balance, variety, and moderation. Be especially wary of reports that cite personal testimonials rather than evidence from scientific studies.
- As you read, consider the background of the individual, organization, or publication making the claim. Reputable researchers are generally affiliated with a nationally recognized university or medical center and usually report study findings in scientific journals, which require every article to be reviewed by other scientists.
- When reading about a particular product, consider whether the report mentions the product's shortcomings as well as its advantages. Be suspicious of exaggerated claims, for example that the product can cure a serious disease or that it represents a scientific breakthrough. Other red flags include attacks on the medical community or traditional medical treatments, and claims that the product can treat a wide variety of diseases.
- Examine product labels carefully. Federal law requires that health products be truthfully labeled and carry adequate directions for use. A product is unlikely to achieve results that are not specifically claimed on its label or package insert.

It is food that fuels life. You can help make yours a healthy life by paying attention to your food choices. •••

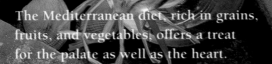

The Mediterranean diet, rich in grains, fruits, and vegetables, offers a treat for the palate as well as the heart.

The Mediterranean Diet

By Carol Ann Rinzler

THE MEDITERRANEAN DIET, its advocates say, is equally kind to the palate and the heart. This plan for healthful eating is based on the traditional cuisines of southern European and northern African countries bordering the Mediterranean Sea—regions with a low rate of heart disease. The diet was adapted for contemporary Americans and unveiled in 1994 by the Harvard School of Public Health in Boston, Massachusetts; the European regional office of the World Health Organization; and the Oldways Preservation & Exchange Trust, a private education group in Boston that has received some funds from the wine, olive oil, and nut industries.

What Mediterranean cuisines have in common is an abundance of grain; lots of fruits and vegetables; olive oil as the principal fat; moderate amounts of dairy products, such as cheese and yogurt; small quantities of fish, poultry, and red meat; and moderate amounts of wine, primarily at meals. The key components of the diet—grain, vegetables, and fruits—can be combined in various ways. Typical dishes include pasta tossed with tomatoes, eggplant, or other vegetables; couscous, steamed wheat with a vegetable sauce; tabouli, a salad of cracked wheat, raw vegetables, and herbs; and hummus, a spread for bread made of chickpeas and sesame-seed paste. Meals generally include bread and often finish with fruit.

The author:

Carol Ann Rinzler is the author of *The Complete Book of Food: A Nutritional, Medical, and Culinary Guide.*

17

In the 1960's, researchers at the University of Minnesota found that American men were nearly six times as likely to develop heart disease as were Greek men.

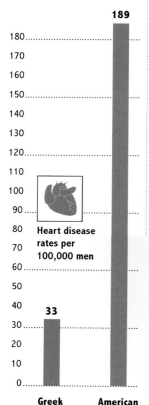

189

180..............................

170

160

150..............................

140

130

120..............................

110

100

90.....

80 **Heart disease**
70 **rates per**
    100,000 men
60..............................

50

40 **33**

30........

20

10

0......

Greek   American
men   men

Scientific support for the Mediterranean Diet goes back 30 years to the Seven Countries Study. Researchers from the University of Minnesota began this study in the late 1950's to evaluate the influence of eating habits on heart disease among more than 12,000 healthy, middle-aged men living in Finland, Greece, Italy, Japan, the Netherlands, the United States, and Yugoslavia. Researchers checked periodically to see how many of the men had developed or died of heart disease. After 10 years, they found the lowest rate of heart disease among Greek men who lived on the island of Crete. Of the 655 Cretans studied, only 2 percent had developed heart disease. The highest rate occurred among Finns: 28 percent of 755 Finns studied developed heart disease. The diets of both groups were high in fat, but the fat in the Cretans' diet came primarily from olive oil, while that in the Finns' diet came primarily from animal products.

Olive oil: Defense against disease?

Since the Seven Countries Study, nutrition researchers have learned more about olive oil. They believe that its protective effect comes from the oleic acid it is rich in. This fatty acid does not raise the level of so-called bad cholesterol, low-density-lipoprotein (LDL) cholesterol, which contributes to clogged arteries. And it may raise

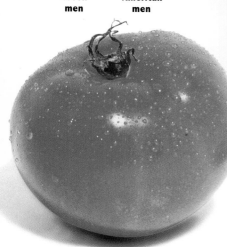

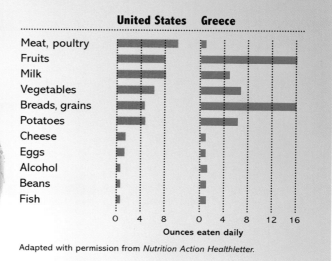

The Mediterranean diet and heart disease

Researchers suspected that the difference in disease rates among American men and Greek men stemmed from differences in diet. The Greek men in the study ate more fruit, vegetables, grains, beans, and fish than the American men. The Greeks also ate less meat, milk, cheese, and eggs.

Adapted with permission from *Nutrition Action Healthletter.*

health professionals, such as cardiologist Dean Ornish, go further. For heart patients, Ornish advocates a diet that obtains only 10 percent of calories from fat. Ornish directs the Preventive Medicine Research Center in Sausalito, California, where patients undergo a year of low-fat eating, stress management, meditation, and exercise.

Ornish claims that ultralow-fat eating can reverse heart disease in many patients. In 1990, he reported that of 22 cardiac patients who followed his program, 18 had some reversal of heart disease after a year. Angiograms showed that deposits in the arteries of these people lessened, on average by 10 percent, and many patients reported less chest pain. By contrast, a group of 19 cardiac patients who did not follow Ornish's program suffered more chest pain, and in 10 cases angiograms showed further narrowing of the arteries.

In a three-year follow-up study, 20 people took part in Ornish's

What's wrong with fat?

Diets high in fat have been linked with heart disease and with a higher risk for certain cancers. Fats are classified as saturated, polyunsaturated, or monounsaturated depending on their chemical structure. Some are less healthful than others.

- Saturated fat is found in animal products, such as meat, eggs, butter, and milk. Some vegetable oils, including coconut and palm oils, also are rich in saturated fat. Saturated fat is considered the least healthful fat.

- Polyunsaturated fat is found in many vegetable oils, including safflower, sunflower, corn, soy, and cottonseed oils. This fat was once considered the most healthful, but today nutritionists believe it lowers levels of artery-clearing HDL cholesterol as well as of artery-clogging LDL cholesterol.

- Monounsaturated fat is found in olive, canola, and peanut oils. This fat may be the most healthful of all, as it appears to lower LDL cholesterol but not HDL cholesterol.

How much fat is too much?

At most, 30 percent of the calories consumed each day should come from fat, according to the U.S. Department of Agriculture and the American Heart Association. Some health professionals say that fat should provide as few as 10 percent of total daily calories.

Calories eaten daily	Maximum fat intake (30% of calories)
1,200	36 grams
1,500	45 grams
1,800	54 grams
2,000	60 grams
2,400	72 grams

program and 28 followed an American Heart Association diet limiting fat to 30 percent of calories. In 16 of those following the Ornish regime, the clogged arteries opened up somewhat. The arteries of those following the 30-percent-fat diet became more blocked.

In the 1970's, Nathan Pritikin advocated a similar ultralow-fat diet to reduce cholesterol, weight, and the risk of heart disease. Pritikin was an inventor who was diagnosed with heart disease in 1955. He adopted a low-fat diet after he read data showing that, in countries where people normally ate fatty foods, the rate of heart disease dropped during World War II when such high-fat items as eggs, butter, and meat were rationed. Today, people suffering from chronic heart disease are treated with low-fat food, stress management, and exercise at the Pritikin Longevity Center in Santa Monica, California. Some followers of the Pritikin program have cut their cholesterol levels by 25 percent.

The Ornish nutrition plan revolves around fruits, vegetables, grains, and beans. Pritikin's plan allows minimal lean meat, chicken, and fish; little in the way of oils, nuts, avocados, or olives; only nonfat dairy foods; and no butter or margarine. What is left is a diet in which 70 to 75 percent of calories come from carbohydrates, such as bread, pasta, and rice.

Cutting down on fat

By making some simple substitutions for everyday foods, consumers can lower the amount of fat in their diets.

Instead of	Use	Fat savings
1 cup whole milk	1 cup skim milk	8 grams
1 cup cream	1 cup evaporated skim milk	60 grams
1 cup sour cream	1 cup nonfat sour cream	39 grams
1 egg	2 egg whites	6 grams
1 oz. baking chocolate	3 tbsp. cocoa and 2 tsp. oil	4 grams
1 cup cream cheese	1 cup soft-curd farmer's cheese	72 grams
1 cup whole-milk ricotta cheese	1 cup 1% fat cottage cheese	30 grams

Adapted with permission from *Tufts University Diet and Nutrition Letter*, December 1992.

The diet-disease connection

The link between heart disease and fatty diets has been documented in a number of scientific studies. High-fat diets, researchers believe, increase the risk of heart disease by raising the level of cholesterol in the blood, especially low-density-lipoprotein (LDL) cholesterol that can clog arteries.

Many nutrition researchers suspect that high-fat intake also plays a role in breast, ovarian, prostate, and colon cancers. A connection between fat and cancer, however, has been much harder to establish than that between fat and heart disease.

The earliest evidence for such a link was reported in 1981 by the American Health Foundation. A foundation study discovered higher rates of breast, colon, and prostate cancer in the United States and Western Europe, where diets are generally high in fat, than in Japan, China, and other regions where diets are lower in fat. Later studies also suggested a link. A 1992 study of 7,284 American men found that those whose diets were low in fat had less than one-third the risk of developing colon cancer as men whose diets were high in fat. Yet that same year, an ongoing Harvard University study of 89,494 women found no proof that a low-fat diet helps protect against breast cancer.

All fats were not created equal, though all are made up of fatty acids. The chemical structure of these fatty acids is critical to how they may affect health. Depending on that structure, fats are classified as saturated or unsaturated.

Saturated fat is a prime suspect in raising LDL cholesterol and hence the risk of heart disease. Fat that is solid at room temperature, such as lard and butter, is made up mostly of saturated fatty acids. Coconut and palm oils, which are highly saturated, are exceptions to this rule. Stick margarine acts as a saturated fat in the body as a result of hydrogenation, the process that solidifies it.

Liquid fat, such as oils and soft margarine, is mostly unsaturated. Corn, soy, safflower, and sunflower oils—the least saturated fats— are called polyunsaturated. Less unsaturated olive and canola oils, as well as avocados and nuts, provide monounsaturated fat. Most fat sources are mixtures of saturated, polyunsaturated, and monounsaturated fat, but supply more of one type than others. Those richest in monounsaturated fats are considered the least unhealthy.

A diet too drab?

Clearly, the 10-percent-fat diet is not for everyone, though the rewards of losing weight, lowering cholesterol, and perhaps easing heart disease symptoms motivate some individuals to stick with the program. Those who practice ultralow-fat eating have to make major changes in the food they keep in the kitchen. Eating out requires much more health-conscious ordering. Many favorite foods must go.

The difficulty of sticking to an ultralow-fat diet is not its only drawback. High-carbohydrate diets can lower levels of high-density-lipoproteins (HDL) cholesterol, the "good" cholesterol that protects arteries, according to researchers. Moreover, women who combine a low-fat diet with a low-calorie diet can lower their levels of sex hormones to such an extent that menstrual cycles become irregular or cease, possibly increasing their risk for osteoporosis and infertility.

In addition, an estimated 10 to 25 percent of the population may be insulin resistant and sensitive to carbohydrates. Some nutritionists believe that a high-carbohydrate diet can contribute to weight gain in such people. A high-carbohydrate diet stimulates the release of the hormone insulin, and insulin contributes to fat storage by body cells. According to one theory, high levels of insulin in these susceptible people may contribute to weight gain or impair weight loss. Critics argue that no scientific studies support this theory.

If you eat a typical American diet, cutting fat to 20 percent or 25 percent of all calories should help lower your risk of heart disease. Such a diet means filling three-quarters of your plate with vegetables, fruit, and grains, and serving lean meat on the plate's remaining quarter. It also means eating few processed foods, such as cakes and cookies, and choosing low-fat or nonfat versions of favorite items. •••

Sample low-fat menu plan

Very low-fat diets are high in starches, grains fruits, and vegetables. People on these diets may need to eat six small meals a day to stave off hunger. A sample meal plan might include:

Early morning
- A bowl of cereal and fruit

Mid-morning
- A bagel and low-fat cottage cheese

Noon
- Salad and chicken strips

Mid-afternoon
- Whole wheat crackers and low-fat cheese

Early evening
- Pasta with vegetables

Mid-evening
- Yogurt and sliced pears

Adapted from *Nutrition Action Healthletter,* December 1994.

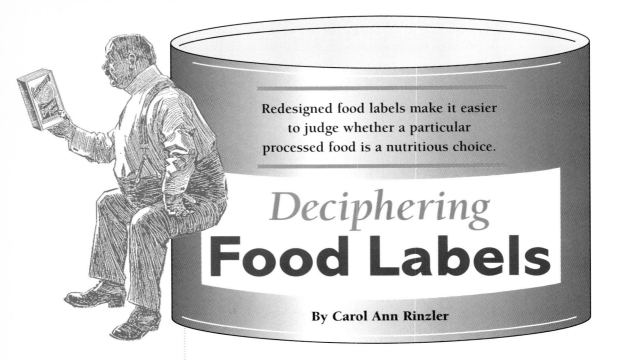

Redesigned food labels make it easier to judge whether a particular processed food is a nutritious choice.

Deciphering
Food Labels

By Carol Ann Rinzler

The author:

Carol Ann Rinzler is the author of *The Complete Book of Food: A Nutritional, Medical, and Culinary Guide.*

HAVE YOU READ A FOOD LABEL LATELY? If not, you are missing an easy-to-use source of nutrition information. Since May 1994, most processed foods have carried nutrition information showing how the food fits into your daily diet. This nutrition information is required under the Nutrition Labeling and Education Act passed by Congress in 1990. Under the labeling regulations, any health claim that appears on a food label must be scientifically sound. By mid-1995, the U.S. Food and Drug Administration (FDA) had approved seven health claims backed by current research.

The FDA allows food labels to point to calcium's value in preventing osteoporosis, a condition in which bones become thin and brittle. Food labels may say that fiber-containing grains, fruits, and vegetables may lower the risk of coronary heart disease and some cancers. And they may claim that a diet rich in fruits and vegetables (good sources of vitamins A and C) may lower the risk of some cancers. In addition, labels may note the link between sodium and high blood pressure, between a low-fat diet and a reduced risk of some cancers, and between a diet low in saturated fat and cholesterol and a decreased risk of coronary heart disease.

The centerpiece of the new label is the Nutrition Facts panel, an easy-to-read chart on the the package. The chart starts with a definition of a "real life" serving size, such as three cookies. A chart shows how many servings are in the food package, as well as the total number of calories and calories from fat in each serving.

A new nutrition reference called Percent Daily Value lets you see at a glance, without complicated calculations, whether a food is high, medium, or low in fat, cholesterol, sodium, carbohydrates, dietary fiber, sugars, protein, vitamin A, vitamin C, calcium, and iron. A Daily Value is a guide to help adults eat a healthful amount of nutrients every day. The goal is for adults to choose foods that provide no more than 100 percent of the Daily Value of fat, sodium, and cholesterol, along with 100 percent of such nutrients as vitamins.

The Percent Daily Values are based on a 2,000-calorie-a-day regimen, the diet recommended for teen-age girls, sedentary men, and most moderately active women (pregnant and lactating women need more). The percentages are somewhat high for the 1,800-calorie diet recommended for sedentary women and older people, and somewhat low for the 2,500-calorie diet recommended for most men, active women, and teen-age boys.

A healthful 2,000-calorie diet allows for no more than 65 grams of fat, including 20 grams of saturated fat; a maximum of 300 milligrams of cholesterol; 300 grams of carbohydrates; at least 25 grams

Going by the numbers

- Serving sizes reflect the amount people are likely to eat and are uniform from one product to another.

- The label shows the total number of calories per serving and calories from fat, helping consumers follow dietary guidelines that no more than 30 percent of calories come from fat.

- The label shows Daily Values for diets of 2,000 calories, the amount recommended for many adults. Some labels also show Daily Values for diets of 2,500 calories a day, recommended for more active adults.

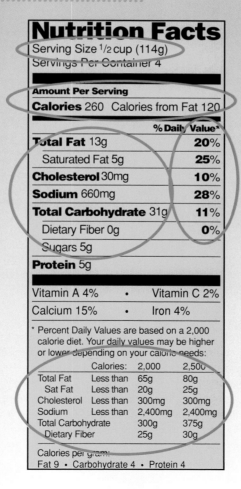

- The label includes information about the content of nutrients that affect health, such as cholesterol, sodium, fiber, calcium, and iron. This information helps consumers get the proper amount of these nutrients in their diet.

- Percent Daily Value shows how a food fits into a daily diet plan. People hoping to consume more iron, for example, can compare the Percent Daily Value for iron on several products to determine the best choice.

- The label lists ingredients in descending order of weight, helping consumers who seek to avoid certain nutrients because of allergies or other health problems.

High and low

You no longer need to guess what the words *high* and *low* mean. Now you can rely on the FDA's new, standardized definitions. For example:

- *High* means that one serving of the food contains 20 percent or more of the daily value for a particular nutrient. For example, a tomato juice that supplies 30 percent of the Daily Value for Vitamin C may describe itself as "high in Vitamin C." Such foods also may be described as *rich in* a particular nutrient, or an *excellent source* of the nutrient.

- *Good source* means one serving supplies 10 to 19 percent of a Daily Value for a particular nutrient. For example, a whole-grain bread that provides 16 percent of the Daily Value for fiber can be called "a good source of fiber."

- *Light* can mean one of two things. First, that a nutritionally altered product contains one-third fewer calories or half the fat of the "regular" product. If a serving of Brand X's regular potato chips provides 150 calories, for example, a serving of Brand X's light chips must provide no more than 100 calories. Second, *light* may mean that the sodium content of a low-calorie, low-fat food has been reduced by 50 percent.

  Light sometimes describes the color or texture of a product, provided that the label makes the meaning clear. Names that have a long history of use, such as *light brown sugar*, still may be used without additional explanation.

- *Reduced* means that one serving has 25 percent less of a particular nutrient, such as fat, sugar, or sodium, than one serving of the "regular" product. For example, if Brand X's mayonnaise usually has 12 grams of fat per serving, it can put *reduced fat* on a version of the mayonnaise that has 9 grams of fat or less per serving. If they prefer, manufacturers may use the term *less* rather than *reduced.*

- *Low-fat* means 3 grams or less of fat per serving, or, if the serving size is very small, per 50 grams of the food.

- *Free* means the product contains only a trace or none of a particular nutrient. For example, a product containing 5 calories or less per serving may be described as *calorie free* and one containing less than 0.5 gram of fat, as *fat free.*

- *More* means the food contains at least 10 percent more of the Daily Value for a particular nutrient (such as dietary fiber, potassium, protein, or an essential vitamin or mineral) than the "regular" version of the product. In this case, manufacturers also may use the terms *fortified, enriched,* or *added.*

- *Lean* is used for meat, fish, poultry, seafood, or game with less than 10 grams of fat, less than 4 grams of saturated fat, and less than 95 milligrams of cholesterol per serving. Lean foods include Spanish mackerel and bluefish tuna.

- *Extra-lean* is used for meat, fish, poultry, or game with less than 5 grams of fat, less than 2 grams of saturated fat, and less than 95 milligrams of cholesterol per serving. Extra-lean foods include haddock and swordfish.

of fiber; and no more than 2,400 milligrams of sodium. Because this diet's Daily Value for fat is 65 grams, the label of a food that has 13 grams of fat per serving would show a 20% Daily Value for fat.

Once you have the label in hand, it's a cinch to use. Key numbers to look for include fat content, amount of saturated fat and cholesterol, amount of carbohydrates and dietary fiber, and minerals such as calcium. If you opt for the 2,000-calorie-a-day regimen, the label makes clear that your diet should not include more than 20 grams of saturated fat. So, one serving of ice cream with 10 grams of saturated fat consumes half of your allowance. The rest of the food you eat that day should provide no more than 10 grams of saturated fat.

It takes practice to use a food label wisely. Once you get in the habit of doing so, however, you're likely to find that it's never been so easy to eat a healthful diet. •••

life consists of about one tablespoon of food per year of age. Older children should be allowed to decide the helping size of each food they eat, as long as a healthful variety is offered. (See FOLLOWING A HEALTHFUL DIET for information about the Food Guide Pyramid.)

Parents can do much to encourage good eating habits in youngsters. By eating healthful foods themselves, parents show the importance of nutrition. By establishing regular mealtimes and snack times, they foster the habit of eating regularly. And by offering a hungry child a starchy snack, such as a bagel, rather than a high-fat snack, such as cake, they build healthy habits.

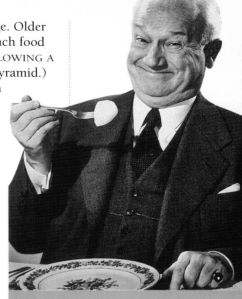

Sustaining teens through rapid growth

After infancy, the most rapid growth spurt occurs in girls from ages 10 through 13 and in boys from ages 12 through 15. During the growth spurt, most teens have large appetites and need more calories than they did previously: for males, about 2,500 calories a day between the ages of 11 and 14, about 3,000 calories between 15 and 18 years, and about 2,900 calories between 19 and 24. Females need about 2,200 calories a day between the ages of 11 and 24. Again, appropriate gains in height and weight indicate the adequacy of calorie intake.

To develop healthful eating habits, teens need not give up favorite foods. Small portions of low-nutrient foods can complement large portions of wholesome foods. A meal of a hamburger on a bun with lettuce and tomato, garden salad, small order of french fries, and low-fat milk is both tasty and healthful.

Adolescents also have some special nutrient needs. Because their bones are growing rapidly, they require about 1,200 to 1,500 milligrams (mg) of calcium daily, supplied in three or more daily servings of such calcium-rich foods as milk, yogurt, and cheese.

Because the teens are a time of rapid growth, adolescents need extra iron to build new cells: about 12 mg daily for males between the ages of 11 and 18, and 10 mg between the ages of 19 and 24. Girls and women need even more of this mineral, about 15 mg daily from the age of 11 to 50. Iron-rich foods include red meat, whole grains, enriched grains, and legumes. Teen-agers can boost absorption of iron by consuming a helping of vitamin C, such as a glass of orange juice, with a meal.

Encouraging good eating habits among teen-age girls is particularly important because adolescent girls concerned about their changing bodies are vulnerable to eating disorders as they try to lose weight. Usually, the most effective strategy when talking with teens about

Making nutrition easier for older people

Many older people consume fewer calories than they need, perhaps because they live alone and find cooking a chore or are struggling to live within a fixed income. Nutritionists say that eating right can be a matter of making a few simple changes.

- Eat regularly, perhaps small but frequent meals.

- Cook large amounts of food, divide the food into individual servings, and freeze.

- Ask grocers to open wrapped, family-sized packages of meat or fresh vegetables and separate into smaller packages.

- Add dried milk to baked goods to boost their nutritional value.

- Keep some easy-to-prepare food on hand for occasional use but avoid relying on processed food.

- Buy fruit that is in various stages of ripeness, so that it can be eaten over several days.

food choices is to focus on immediate, rather than future, benefits of healthful eating. Depending on the teen-ager's interests, adults might emphasize nutrition's role in maintaining health, fitness, and appropriate weight; developing muscles; or boosting energy.

Food for adults

People's bodies stop growing when they are in their late 20's and early 30's, and so they need fewer calories than before. Inactive men aged 25 to 50 need about 2,200 calories a day, and inactive women need about 1,600 calories daily. Active men require about 2,800 calories; active women, about 2,200. Maintaining appropriate weight is a good guide for assessing the adequacy of calorie intake.

Pregnant women have special nutrition needs. A woman of appropriate weight should gain approximately 25 to 35 pounds during pregnancy for her baby to develop properly. During the last six months of pregnancy, women need about 300 additional calories a day, as well as increased calcium. Eating one or two extra servings of dairy products contributes to both goals. In addition, an adequate intake of the B vitamin folic acid—0.4 mg daily—before and during pregnancy helps prevent birth defects. Good sources of folic acid include oranges, liver, leafy greens, legumes, and whole grains. After childbirth, mothers who are breast-feeding require about 500 more calories a day than they needed during pregnancy.

Mothers also must take care to get sufficient iron and calcium. Women who are not pregnant need about 15 mg of iron a day, but this doubles to 30 mg during pregnancy. In the case of calcium, middle-aged women who are not pregnant require 800 to 1,000 mg daily. Pregnant and breast-feeding women require 1,200 to 1,500 mg.

Like all adults, people older than 50 should strive for variety, balance, and moderation in the food they eat. They should also make sure they get enough vitamin D, calcium, vitamin B-12, dietary fiber, and fluids. At least 5 micrograms (mcg) of vitamin D and 800 to 1,000 mg of calcium are recommended to help keep bones strong, though some experts recommend as much as 1,500 mg of calcium for women over 50 who are not on hormone replacement therapy and for all adults over age 65. Fortified milk contains vitamin D, and foods rich in calcium include dairy products and fortified orange juice. Animal products are good sources of the recommended 2 mcg of vitamin B-12, a nutrient needed to produce red blood cells and maintain nerve tissue. As the body ages, it is less able to absorb vitamin B-12, so older people are more likely than others to be deficient in this vitamin. Dietary fiber promotes intestinal health, and is plentiful in fruits, vegetables, beans, and whole grains.

Good nutrition sets the stage for healthful living, from infancy to retirement, and the Food Guide Pyramid provides a useful tool for improving eating habits. Good eating habits developed in childhood can provide benefits throughout life, and parents can do much to foster good habits in their children.　●●●

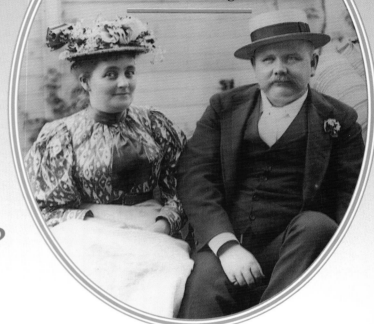

How have guidelines on recommended weights changed, and how much science stands behind the changes?

Ideal
Weight:

Science or Fashion?

By Jeanine Barone

WE TAKE IT FOR GRANTED THAT BEING FAT is associated with health problems. It hasn't always been that way. At one time, people viewed the full figure as a sign of health and prosperity. A large appetite was considered a healthy one, and chubby babies represented the very picture of health. Until the early 1900's, plump women were generally considered to have the ideal body shape. Thinness was believed to increase the risk of pneumonia and tuberculosis—diseases that once took many lives. Doctors told skinny people to gain weight because those extra pounds could help should they get sick. And they advised individuals suffering from a vague malady termed "nervous exhaustion" to eat more fat.

During the 20th century, the study of nutrition became more scientific. From insurance company statistics on death rates, researchers had concluded by the 1930's that excess weight often was linked to an early death. They began to suspect that obesity damaged health. (Obesity is defined today as a body weight that is 20 percent or more over the recommended weight for a person's age, build, sex, and height.) Since the 1930's, health professionals have continued to warn that excess weight poses a serious health threat.

At about the same time that medical professionals changed their views on body fat, so did the fashion industry. Clothing became less

The author:

....

Jeanine Barone is a nutritionist and a contributing editor to the *University of California at Berkeley Wellness Letter.*

restrictive as women emerged from the home, engaged in more sports, and went to work. Those excess pounds, once hidden under voluminous skirts, came into view as skirts became shorter and clothing more fitted. During much of this century, the fashionable female shape has veered between two extremes: the boyish look of the 1920's flapper and the curvaceous hourglass figure exemplified in the 1950's by the actress Marilyn Monroe.

Fashion hit a new low, weightwise that is, in the 1960's when the skinny British model Twiggy came on the scene and suddenly became the fashion ideal. Since then, for most people lean has been in with only one variation: the toned, athletic build introduced during the exercise craze of the mid-1980's.

Even as the thin woman became the 1960's ideal and dieting articles in women's magazines proliferated, the average American's weight climbed. This upward creep in weight has been documented in surveys conducted by the National Center for Health Statistics since 1960. During the 1980's, the center said, Americans gained 8 pounds on average. The center estimates that one-third of American adults today weigh at least 20 percent more than their desirable or healthy weight.

Figuring out the best weight

Figures for recommended body weights typically come from insurance company tables. Today, the most widely used weight tables are those of the Metropolitan Life Insurance Company. To calculate these weights, statisticians use death rates among policy holders of various shapes and sizes.

The tables have seen several revisions. "Ideal weight" tables introduced in 1942 became "desirable weight" tables in a 1959 revision. The more recent versions have been called "healthy weight" tables.

When the tables changed in 1983 and in 1990, the upper limit on recommended weights climbed to reflect more accurately the actual weights of Americans. In the 1959 tables, the maximum desirable weight for a man 5 feet 8 inches tall was 149 pounds. In the 1983 tables, it was 155 pounds. The 1990 tables permit a person to gain 10 to 15 pounds after age 35 and still remain within the acceptable weight range. The same man who should have weighed 149 pounds at most in 1959 could, if he was 40 years old, weigh up to 178 pounds in 1990.

Height and weight tables have their critics. Some suspect that they are inaccurate because they rely on heights and weights reported by policy holders but never actually measured. In addition, policy hold-

Healthy weights

Tables of recommended weights, by height and age, are based on mortality statistics collected by insurance companies. They were last revised by the federal government in 1990. The lower end of the weight range generally applies to women; the higher end, to men. The table defines height without shoes and weight without clothes.

| Height | Weight in pounds | |
	19 to 34 years	35 years and over
5'0"	97–128	108–138
5'1"	101–132	111–143
5'2"	104–137	115–148
5'3"	107–141	119–152
5'4"	111–146	122–157
5'5"	114–150	126–162
5'6"	118–155	130–167
5'7"	121–160	134–172
5'8"	125–164	138–178
5'9"	129–169	142–183
5'10"	132–174	146–188
5'11"	136–179	151–194
6'0"	140–184	155–199
6'1"	144–189	159–205
6'2"	148–195	164–210
6'3"	152–200	168–216
6'4"	156–205	173–222
6'5"	160–211	177–228
6'6"	164–216	182–234

Source: Department of Agriculture; Department of Health and Human Services.

ers usually are younger, better educated, and more affluent than the general population and thus, critics claim, unrepresentative of the population at large.

Furthermore, not all forms of excess weight constitute a health problem. A person can weigh more than the recommended weight as a result of extra muscle or extra fat. The first situation poses no health risk, but the second does. The distribution of fat also can make a difference. Excess weight carried on and above the waist—the so-called apple shape—is considered a greater health risk than weight carried on the hips—the pear shape. Studies have found that the apple shape raises the risk of adult-onset diabetes, high blood pressure, breast cancer, and heart disease.

Excess weight: How much of a risk?

Some health professionals favor a return to the 1959 tables, with their lower weight recommendations. The 1990 tables suggest—erroneously, according to researchers at the Harvard School of Public Health—that a gain of 10 to 15 pounds after age 35 is fine. These researchers say that this weight gain can increase the risk of heart disease.

On the basis of a 14-year study of 115,818 nurses who provided periodic information on their weight and health, the Harvard researchers found that women who gained 12 to 15 pounds after the age of 18 increased their risk of heart disease by 25 percent, compared with women who gained fewer than 11 pounds. And a gain of 17 to 24 pounds raised a woman's risk by 64 percent. A woman 5 feet 6 inches tall and weighing more than 170 pounds has 3 ½ times the risk of a heart attack as a woman weighing less than 124 pounds.

Other researchers, such as Reubin Andres of the National Institute on Aging, believe that people are better off gaining weight as they age. In analyzing 13 studies that looked at changes in body weight and mortality, Andres found that people who gained moderate amounts of weight lived the longest. People who lost weight or put on excessive weight had the highest death rates. Andres uses a "safe" weight table and considers an 8-to-10-pound weight gain every 10 years healthy, provided the person has no history of high blood pressure, elevated cholesterol, or diabetes—conditions that weight gain can worsen. According to this line of reasoning, people who are heavier may be better nourished and their bodies may be better able to fight illness.

Most researchers, however, agree that excess weight is associated with an increased risk of disease and earlier death. Excess weight makes the heart work harder and can lead to heart disease or worsen an existing heart problem. Excess weight puts more stress on the

Health risks associated with obesity
(20 percent above recommended weight)

- High blood pressure
- Adult-onset diabetes
- Heart disease
- Respiratory ailments
- Stroke
- In women, increased risk for cancer of the breast, ovaries, and uterus; in men, increased risk for cancer of the prostate, colon, and rectum

Source: National Institutes of Health.

joints, which can result in arthritis. It also increases the risk of certain cancers, according to the National Institutes of Health. In women, obesity increases the risk for cancer of the breast, ovary and uterus; in men, the risk of prostate, colon, and rectal cancer.

In a study of 19,297 men, Harvard researchers in 1993 reported finding the lowest mortality rate among men weighing 20 percent below the U.S. average (less than 157 pounds for a 5-foot-10-inch tall man). Mortality increased progressively with weight.

But the link between obesity and disease doesn't mean that being underweight is ideal either. Pregnant women who are underweight are more likely to give birth to babies with low birth weights. Very lean women may be getting insufficient calories and protein, particularly if they're active. As a result, their menstrual cycles may stop, increasing their risk for *osteoporosis* (a thinning of bone mass). It's hard to get sufficient nutrients in a calorie-poor diet, so poor eating habits can deprive the body of needed vitamins and minerals.

Why is Lenny lean but Polly plump?

No one knows exactly why some people put on weight more easily than others. The difference may be genetic. Researchers have found that someone with two lean parents has a 7 to 10 percent chance of becoming obese. One obese parent raises the risk to 40 percent; two obese parents, to 80 percent.

Late in 1994, researchers at Rockefeller University in New York City reported on a gene that controls fat storage in animals. They speculate that this gene controls the mechanism by which the brain signals a sensation of fullness. If the gene malfunctions, a person might not feel full and go on eating.

Some researchers believe that the body tries to maintain a certain weight, called a set point, much as a thermostat maintains a constant temperature. According to this theory, an overweight person may simply have a higher set point than a thin person. Backing up the set-point theory is a study reported in March 1995 by Rockefeller University researchers. The study included 18 obese people and 23 who had never been obese. The researchers found that *metabolism*—the rate at which the body burns calories—sped up in study participants when they gained weight and slowed when they lost it. Their bodies adjusted to weight loss by burning fewer calories and storing more fat, bringing their weight back to the set point. Weight-control specialists say that the way to lower the body's set point is with exercise, which increases metabolism so that the body stores less fat.

Overall, health professionals counsel, it's lifelong habits that make the biggest difference. In other words, it's wise to maintain a stable weight over time and take a look at your lifestyle if you gain more than 5 pounds. In most cases, getting back on track means exercising for at least 30 minutes every other day and eating less fat. ●●●

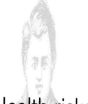

Health risks associated with severe underweight

(20 percent below recommended weight)

- Increased complications after surgery and slow recovery from illness

- Higher death rates, especially among smokers

- In women, menstruation may cease, increasing the risk of osteoporosis

- In pregnant women, increased risk of giving birth to a baby with low weight

Source: Wardlaw and others, *Contemporary Nutrition*.

Restoring Family Mealtime

By Jeanine Barone

Overflowing schedules threaten the family meal, a ritual that serves psychological and nutritional needs.

TELEVISION COMEDIES OF THE 1950's—"Ozzie and Harriet" or "Father Knows Best" —portrayed an idyllic dinner hour: parents and children gathered around the table and engaged in lively conversation as everyone partook of the meal mom had just cooked. How well does this vision reflect reality in the 1990's? Probably not too accurately.

First of all, the nuclear family is less common. Only about one-quarter of American households consist of a father, a mother, and children, according to the 1990 census, and one child in four now lives in a single-parent household. Far more women work outside the home, leaving less time for the activities known as homemaking.

Nor are working women the only ones pressed for time. Eating together has become a challenge as family members are drawn from

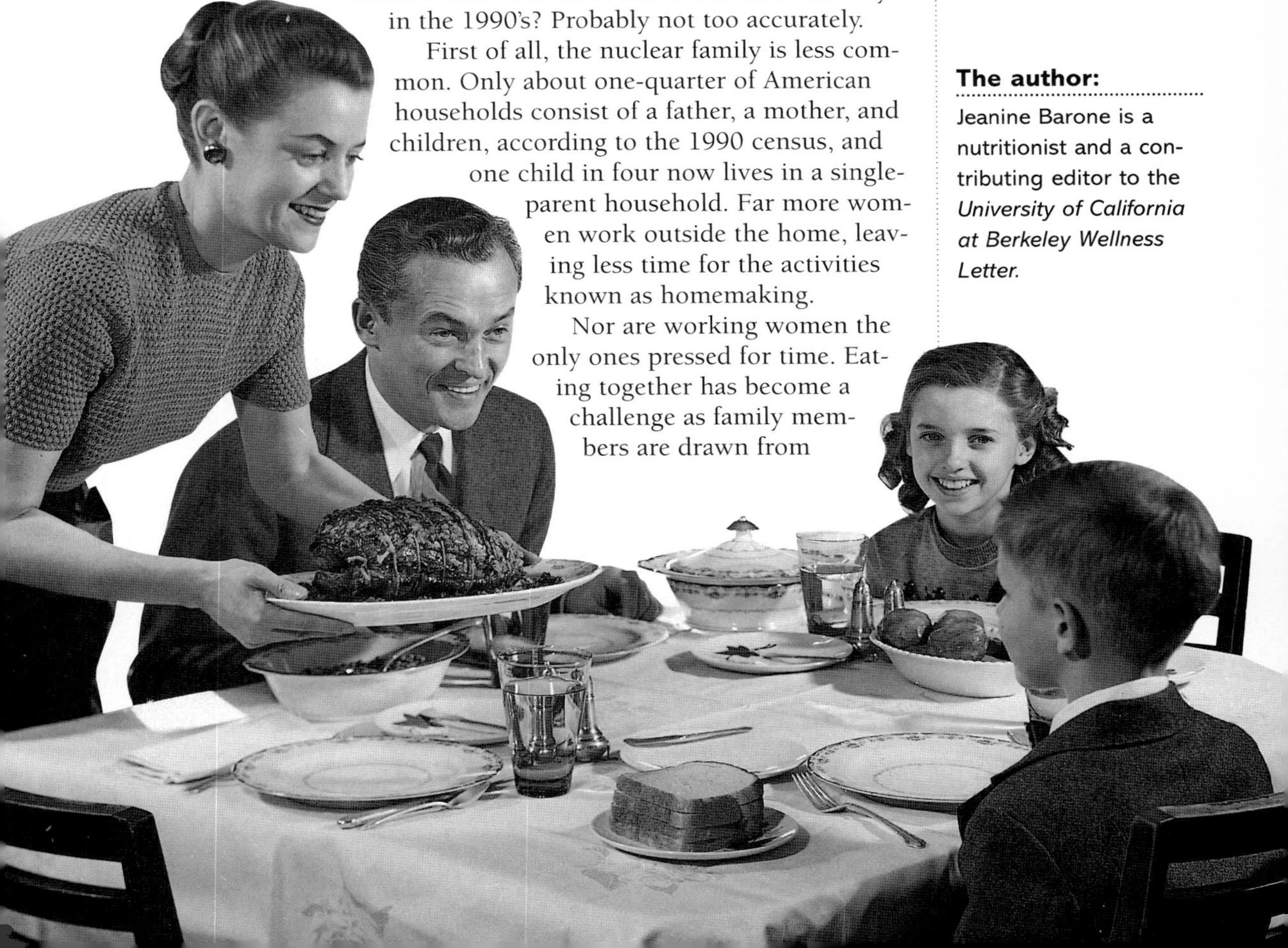

The author:

Jeanine Barone is a nutritionist and a contributing editor to the *University of California at Berkeley Wellness Letter.*

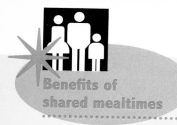

Long work hours, outside activities, and conflicting schedules may make it difficult for families to sit down to dinner together every night. Yet some social scientists say the family meal serves important psychological needs as well as nutritional needs.

- Children may learn social skills by following their parents' example at the dinner table. These skills include table manners, polite conversation, and cooperation.

- The family dinner provides an opportunity for family members to discuss the day's events and make plans for the following day. This exchange can increase the family's sense of togetherness and give children a feeling of security.

- A meal prepared at home and eaten at the dinner table is likely to be more nutritious than one eaten out. Children who develop healthful eating habits early in life are more likely to be healthful eaters throughout their lives.

- Children have an opportunity to participate in adult conversations when the family gathers at the table. This interaction can act as an informal classroom, stimulating children to think about new topics.

home by after-school activities and jobs; adult education classes; church, community, and professional meetings; and long working hours. Getting home late for dinner easily becomes the norm rather than the exception if parents work two jobs, work on different shifts, or have long commutes.

Even if families do manage to sit down and dine together, new made-for-TV movies, popular TV series, or telecasts of favorite sports exert a constant pull. Some may find it easier and more entertaining to stay glued to the TV screen than to converse with other family members.

A tendency to eat alone, rather than as a group, also threatens family mealtime. If mom's eating low-fat to lose weight, dad's still a meat-and-potatoes guy, sister is a vegetarian, and brother is allergic to wheat, it's hard to plan a meal that all can agree upon. "Food has become a form of self-definition, where families have four different menus for the four family members," says Lionel Tiger, professor of anthropology at Rutgers University in New Jersey. By producing single-serving portions, food companies make it easy for family members to eat what they like. With the microwave, even children can prepare their own dinners. "We have 2-year-olds who are miniconsumers and it gives them a false sense of independence," says Tiger.

Dinner: Food for the psyche?

Tiger believes that an organized family mealtime would relieve children of making decisions and give them a sense of routine in what can be an otherwise chaotic day. Others agree that the dinner table satisfies psychological as well as physical needs, especially because it gives family members a chance to gather with people who care about their lives. "Family dinnertime is a harbor you come to after being in the world all day," says Andrew Schwebel, professor of psychology at Ohio State University. It's a check-in time when family members can find out about everyone's day or plans for the week.

That's not the only reason why the family dinner is special, according to those who study human behavior. They point out that children learn manners necessary later in life. If given a task, such as setting or clearing the table, children learn to cooperate and take on responsibility. And they learn to share as food is portioned out. Children also have a chance to learn about adult concerns at the dinner table. "It's a classroom; kids get exposed to issues in adult conversations they would not otherwise be exposed to," says Schwebel.

For couples, dining together is a way to extend their intimacy. Otherwise, says Tiger, "in a two-person family, you may not see each other except to take out the garbage or go to the mall." Besides, dining together can be fun. "If we ate just for the nutrients, we would take pills," says Tiger.

Nutrients do matter, however, and both children and adults are more likely to eat nutritious food and a balanced meal when dining with the family. When eating alone, it's too tempting to eat whatever requires the least effort. In addition, parents can set an example of healthful eating at meals. When children see adults eating vegetables, they may be more inclined to follow suit.

Just what state the family dinner is in remains a topic of debate. In a 1989 survey by the Food Marketing Institute (FMI), a trade association, and the magazine *Better Homes and Gardens,* 56 percent of those polled claimed they eat together as a family every day. Many in the nutrition profession are skeptical about the number of Americans who truly eat together as families. Meals during which people watch TV, they say, do not count. Nor do meals where everyone sits together for the shortest possible time before dashing off to individual activities. (The FMI survey found that even what it counted as a true family dinner was fairly rushed, usually lasting only half an hour.)

Reviving family mealtime

How can Americans return to the family dinner table? One way to start, nutrition professionals say, is by setting a dinner time that everyone can make at least several times a week. It's a good idea to build in some flexibility, especially when negotiating around conflicting schedules. And at the same time, establish some rules about what constitutes a reasonable excuse for missing the meal. Going out with friends might be an unacceptable reason to skip a family dinner, whereas a business trip would be acceptable. If it is too hard to get together at dinner, families can try for breakfast. Or, family members can munch on healthful snacks to stave off hunger pangs until everybody arrives home and dinner can be served.

Another recommendation is to make sure the television set is turned off during mealtimes. To make the occasion enjoyable, meals should consist mostly of foods that everyone eats—perhaps with a few new items as well—and individuals shouldn't be forced to eat foods they dislike. Nor is dinner a time to air grievances.

To prevent dining from being an eat-and-run activity, the meal should take at least half an hour. (In the FMI study, nearly half of respondents said someone left the table before the others.) Families should share responsibility for the meal, with some members planning the menu and purchasing the food, and others cooking, serving, and cleaning up. Putting some of these tips into practice may make dining together a focal point of family life once again. • • •

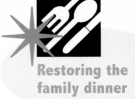

Restoring the family dinner

It may be a challenge, but families can restore the family dinner. The secret lies in making the meal a routine and protecting it from disruption.

- Try to set a fixed time for dinner. Compare schedules to decide on a time that everyone can observe most of the time.

- Try to keep interruptions at a minimum. Turning the television off and ignoring the telephone can help.

- Try to make the meal enjoyable. One way is to serve a variety of foods that everyone likes.

- To reinforce the sense of a shared occasion, try giving all family members some responsibility for the meal. If some members plan the meals and buy the food, others might help with the cooking and cleanup.

Source: Jeanine Barone.

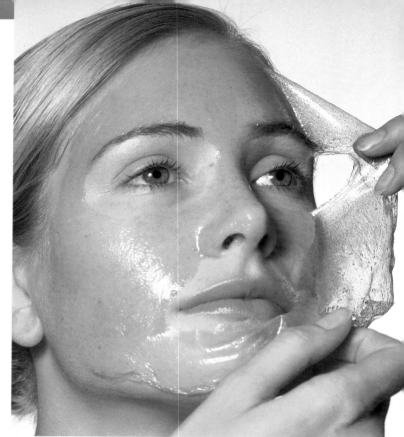

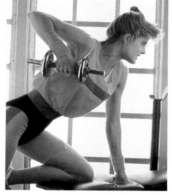

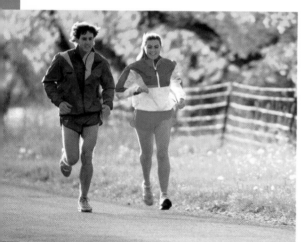

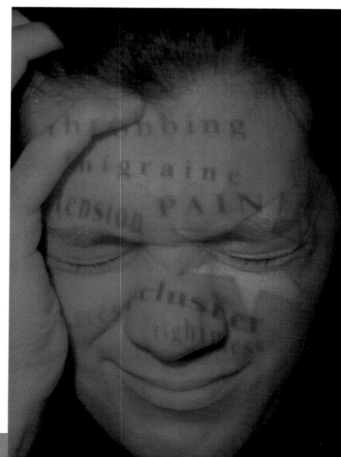

Some people who suffer from cluster headaches compare the pain to being stabbed in the eye with a hot poker. The pain bores into one side of the head, typically the eye socket or the temple, according to descriptions, and it may be accompanied by a drooping eyelid on the affected side. The eye also may become red and teary, and the nose may become stuffed or runny.

Fortunately, cluster headaches are much rarer than migraines or tension-type headaches, affecting from 1 to 3 Americans in 1,000, according to estimates. They are most prevalent among men aged 20 to 40. Smoking heavily and drinking alcohol can trigger cluster headaches in susceptible people.

Headache causes: Standard theories

Physicians also classify headaches as primary or secondary. Primary headaches are themselves the cause of the pain and related symptoms, whereas secondary headaches have other underlying causes, such as an allergic response or sinus infection.

Clinicians have identified more than 300 conditions that can bring on a secondary headache, including sinus inflammation, allergies, vision problems, and overuse of certain medications. Other medical conditions responsible for secondary headaches can be far more serious. These include ruptured blood vessels in the brain that signify stroke; meningitis, an inflammation of the brain's covering; and glaucoma, an eye disease that results from elevated pressure in the eyeball. Physicians advise people to seek medical attention if a sudden headache is accompanied by vision problems, weakness, or difficulty walking, especially if the patient is 55 or older, because the headache could warn of an impending stroke. A headache that is the worst one ever experienced also warrants swift medical attention.

Prior to the 1960's, researchers shared some standard theories about the causes of tension-type and migraine headache pain. But the mechanism behind cluster headaches was as much of a mystery as it is today. Researchers believed that tension-type headaches were caused by excessive tightening of the muscles of the neck and scalp, possibly triggered by stress. Migraine was believed to result from the *constriction* (narrowing) and subsequent *dilation* (widening) of blood vessels in the head. According to the theory, the constriction of blood vessels reduced blood flow in the brain, bringing on the visual and sensory disturbances of the aura and prodromal phase. The subsequent throbbing was attributed to a rush of blood through the vessels, as the body reacted to the drop in blood flow by suddenly dilating the blood vessels.

During the 1960's and 1970's, studies of headache sufferers, coupled with a better understanding of brain function, prompted researchers to challenge the standard theories. Some studies showed that even though muscle contraction occurs during tension-type headaches, many people experience the same muscle contractions without any accompanying headache pain. Nor does stress, which

OTHER COMMON CAUSES OF
head pain
. . . .

Some headaches have a specific underlying cause, unlike the
three main categories of headache. Many of these headaches
can be alleviated with pain relievers.

Type	Symptoms	Causes	Treatments
Arthritis	Pain at back of the neck or head that intensifies with movement.	Inflammation.	Anti-inflammatory drugs, muscle relaxants.
Caffeine withdrawal	Throbbing head pain.	Consuming large amounts of caffeine.	Gradually decreasing caffeine consumption.
Exertion	Generalized head pain during or following exercise or after sneezing or coughing.	Usually related to migraine or cluster headaches in progress.	Aspirin, indomethacin, or beta-blocker.
Eyestrain	Pain, usually on both sides of the head.	Uncorrected vision, astigmatism, eye muscle imbalance.	Eye examination followed by steps to correct vision problem.
Fever	Generalized head pain that develops with fever.	Inflammation of the blood vessels of the head.	Aspirin or acetaminophen.
Hangover	Throbbing pain and nausea.	Dilation of blood vessels surrounding the brain due to alcohol.	Consuming liquids, especially fruit juices.
Hunger	Generalized head pain.	Muscle tension, low blood sugar, and dilation of the blood vessels just before mealtime.	Eating regular meals containing adequate protein and complex carbohydrates.
Menstrual	Migraine-type pain around the time of menstruation or ovulation.	Changes in estrogen levels.	Small doses of vasoconstrictors; anti-inflammatory drugs.
Sinus	Gnawing pain over the nasal area, often increasing in severity as the day progresses.	Acute infection of the sinuses.	Antibiotics and decongestants; surgical drainage of the sinuses in severe cases.
Temporomandibular joint (TMJ)	Pain at the side of the head, where the jaw opens and closes; sometimes accompanied by a clicking sound on opening the jaw.	Poor bite; clenching of the jaw as a reaction to stress.	Relaxation techniques; biofeedback; use at night of a bite plate fitting over the teeth.

Critically reviewed by Richard B. Lipton, M.D., of the Montefiore Headache Unit of the Albert Einstein College of Medicine.

nearly all people encounter, trigger headaches in everyone. Similarly, changes in blood vessels and blood flow in the brain, resembling those associated with migraine, also can occur during exercise or while taking a hot bath, without causing headache pain.

New theories of headache pain

The shortcomings of the standard theories prompted researchers to look for new explanations for headache pain. Even though the pain mechanisms responsible for headaches are still not clearly defined, most experts now believe that the changes in muscles and blood vessels that occur during headaches are orchestrated by complex interactions, malfunctions, and miscommunications within the brain.

Some studies have implicated the trigeminal nerve in the brain stem, which controls blood vessels in the head and also transmits sensory information from the face and scalp to the brain. When this nerve becomes irritated, researchers suspect, it releases chemicals that cause the inflammation and dilation of blood vessels, leading to the throbbing pain of migraine.

How or why the trigeminal nerve becomes irritated isn't well understood, but some researchers believe that a chemical called serotonin is involved. Serotonin is a *neurotransmitter* (chemical messenger that transmits nerve signals in the brain). It is involved in regulating mood, sleep patterns, pain, and a variety of other bodily functions, including blood flow in the brain. Disturbances in the brain's serotonin regulation system, researchers suggest, may be the trigger that sets off the events that culminate in migraine pain.

Serotonin and the neurotransmitter norepinephrine—as well as the natural painkiller endorphin—are involved in regulating a region of the brain stem called the descending pain modulating zone. Researchers describe it as an "antipain" region, because it can halt the transmission of nerve signals from the scalp, neck, and face— signals that are experienced as pain if they reach the brain's outer layer. Malfunctions of these neurotransmitters could allow pain signals to travel through the brain unchecked.

Another phenomenon that may play a role in migraine is called spreading depression. The term refers to depressed or reduced activity of nerve cells in the brain, which gradually spreads. Some researchers believe this phenomenon may account for vision disturbances during the aura phase of a migraine. In animal studies, spreading depression has been linked with inflammation of blood vessels in the brain.

The new theory claims that the constriction and dilation of blood vessels in the head is not the cause of headaches but instead is the consequence of changes in brain activity. As a result of this research into the physiological underpinnings of headaches, new therapies to relieve and prevent headaches concentrate on treating changes in serotonin activity and the consequent inflammation of blood vessels in the head.

WHEN A HEADACHE CALLS FOR

quick action
• • • • • • • • • • • • • •

Most headaches are not medical emergencies. But some can indicate a serious underlying medical condition, such as a tumor or an impending stroke. Doctors recommend that you see your physician as soon as possible if:

- Your headache will not go away.
- It is the worst headache you've ever had.
- You are age 50 or older and it's your first severe headache.
- Your headache is accompanied by weakness, numbness, paralysis, or a tingling sensation in your hands or feet.
- Your headache changes your thought patterns or affects your memory.
- Your headache is accompanied by a stiff neck.
- Your headache was brought on by exertion, such as bending over, coughing, or sneezing.
- Your headache intensifies.
- Your headache is severe and comes on suddenly.

Critically reviewed by Richard B. Lipton, M.D., of the Montefiore Headache Unit of the Albert Einstein College of Medicine.

The road to relief

The road to headache relief begins with a proper diagnosis. Physicians generally begin by taking a headache history to learn about the characteristics of the pain, headache patterns, and suspected triggers. They also conduct a physical examination and may order blood tests to determine overall health and rule out any underlying illness. If the examination suggests an underlying problem, then the physician may order diagnostic imaging procedures, such as a CT (computerized tomography) scan, a cervical spine X ray, or an MRI (magnetic resonance imaging) scan. These scans provide cross-sectional views of brain tissue and help physicians rule out the possibility of a tumor or other abnormality in the brain. They are typically ordered if the onset of the headache is sudden and severe. If headaches are chronic and long-standing, physicians are unlikely to gain useful information from such tests.

If no underlying cause for a patient's headache is found, physicians suggest a treatment aimed at controlling symptoms or preventing attacks. Medications to control symptoms obviously should relieve head pain. If the headache is accompanied by nausea and vomiting, the physician may prescribe antiemetics, drugs that quell stomach distress while enhancing the effects of pain relievers.

Tension-type headaches generally respond to over-the-counter pain relievers such as aspirin, acetaminophen, and ibuprofen. Some of these same drugs are effective for migraine headache as well.

Severe migraine, however, usually requires prescription medication. Some commonly used medications for migraine pain are derived from ergot, a fungus that attacks grain. Researchers believe that ergot compounds, such as dihydroergotamine (DHE), act on serotonin levels and also help reduce inflammation of blood vessels. DHE may relieve migraine pain in as little as 30 minutes. It is especially effective in treating migraines associated with the menstrual cycle. The action of another ergot derivative, ergotamine tartrate, is stronger than DHE, but it can cause nausea. Ergot derivatives also relieve cluster headaches in some people.

Sumatriptan, introduced in 1992, is the newest drug in the headache arsenal. Sumatriptan appears to act on serotonin receptors—sites in the brain that serotonin must bind to in order to affect various physiological functions. By acting on serotonin receptors on the trigeminal nerve endings, sumatriptan prevents them from producing the inflammation that triggers headache pain. The drug also helps quell the nausea and vomiting that can accompany migraine. Sumatriptan has been called the first "designer drug" for headaches because it targets specific receptors involved in head pain.

A study reported in 1994 by researchers at the New England Center for Headache in Stamford, Connecticut, found that sumatriptan reduced the severity of headache pain in 84 of the 100 study participants who received it. However, about half of the participants experienced a recurrence after several hours. Some physicians anticipate that the high price of sumatriptan (about $40 per injection), its short-lived effectiveness, and the need to administer it by injection may limit the drug's use in treating headaches. However, drug companies are working to develop longer-lasting drugs related to sumatriptan that can be taken orally.

When such medications fail to relieve headache pain, physicians may prescribe narcotics such as codeine or drugs called corticosteroids that reduce inflammation. Both have serious side effects. Prolonged use of narcotics can lead to addiction, and prolonged use of corticosteroids can elevate blood pressure, cause swelling, and impair the body's ability to fight infections.

Prevention strategies

Other treatment strategies focus on preventing headaches, especially migraines, or on reducing their duration and frequency. Identifying triggers is one starting point. This procedure can be lengthy, however, because of the number of known triggers. Some physicians recommend that patients narrow the list of possible triggers by keeping a headache diary in which they note the foods they have eaten, changes in weather conditions, hormonal fluctuations, variations in sleep or eating patterns, or other factors that precede an attack. If a trigger is identified, treatment can then center on avoiding it.

In some cases, lifestyle changes can help prevent headaches. For

TREATING—AND PREVENTING—
headaches
· ·

Ideally, people find out what stimuli trigger their headaches and then learn to avoid those triggers. Once a headache begins, an over-the-counter pain reliever may help. If that proves ineffective, a physician may prescribe another treatment. Reducing muscle tension can ease tension-type headaches. Many treatments for cluster and migraine headaches *constrict* (narrow) blood vessels or reduce the inflammation that accompanies dilated vessels.

Tension-type headache

Treatment
- For occasional headaches, over-the-counter pain relievers, such as acetaminophen, aspirin, or ibuprofen.
- For chronic headaches, a prescription antidepressant, which interferes with pain signals.

Prevention
- Relaxation techniques.
- Avoidance of stress.
- Antidepressant medication.

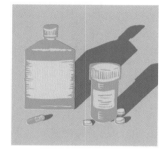

Cluster headache

Treatment
- Prescription drugs such as ergotamine that constrict and reduce inflammation of blood vessels in the head.
- Oxygen inhalation.
- A local anesthetic, such as lidocaine, taken through the nose.

Prevention
- For episodic headaches, an ergot derivative along with corticosteroids that reduce inflammation.
- For chronic headaches, small doses of lithium carbonate, which appears to act on chemicals in the brain.

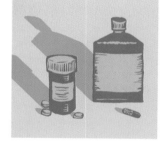

Migraine headache

Treatment
- Ice packs to constrict blood vessels.
- Over-the-counter or prescription pain relievers containing acetaminophen, aspirin, or ibuprofen in combination with caffeine, barbiturates, or narcotics.
- Prescription drugs such as sumatriptan that constrict blood vessels in the head.

Prevention
- Avoidance of known triggers.
- Eating regularly scheduled meals and getting adequate sleep.
- Biofeedback to control muscle tightening and the swelling of blood vessels.
- Beta-blockers and calcium-channel blockers, prescription drugs that appear to act on chemicals in the brain.
- Prescription drugs that reduce inflammation of blood vessels in the head.

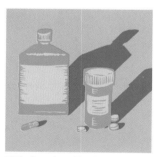

Critically reviewed by Richard B. Lipton, M.D., of the Montefiore Headache Unit of the Albert Einstein College of Medicine.

example, a person might quit smoking, regularize sleeping and eating patterns, or learn relaxation techniques to alleviate stress. For other people, however, medication may be necessary.

Physicians usually prescribe preventive medication only when headaches are disabling or especially frequent, and when other medications have failed to control the pain. The reluctance to prescribe such drugs stems from the side effects that these medications, like all drugs, can produce. Preventive medication is taken daily, regardless of whether a headache is in progress.

Among the drugs most commonly used to prevent migraines are beta-blockers, which were originally developed to treat high blood pressure and certain heart ailments. Although researchers are not sure exactly why beta-blockers prevent headaches, they believe the drugs interact with the neurotransmitters serotonin and norepinephrine. Side effects associated with beta-blockers include fatigue, depression, sleep disturbances, lightheadedness, and weight gain.

Calcium-channel blockers also were developed for treating high blood pressure and heart ailments, and they appear to prevent cluster headaches as well as migraines. The drugs seem to block the release of serotonin, and scientists believe they also prevent inflammation. Calcium-channel blockers have fewer side effects than beta-blockers. The most pronounced side effect is constipation, which occurs in 10 to 20 percent of patients. Some physicians are awaiting additional data before prescribing these drugs.

Antidepressants that interact with serotonin also can be effective in preventing migraines, regardless of whether the sufferer is experiencing depression. The most commonly used are tricyclics; MAO (monoamine oxidase) inhibitors; and serotonin-reuptake inhibitors, such as Prozac. These drugs interact with serotonin and other brain chemicals thought to play a role in migraine. The tricyclics also may be effective in preventing chronic tension-type headaches. Side effects of antidepressants include drowsiness, weight gain, tremor, sleep problems, and dry mouth and eyes.

Medications derived from ergot can be helpful in averting a full-blown migraine attack if taken at the first sign of symptoms. They also are used in the prevention of cluster headaches. However, these drugs must be monitored carefully because they can aggravate stomach distress and may actually cause headaches if they are overused.

Treatment without drugs

Some patients, including women who plan to become pregnant, prefer nondrug alternatives for treating tension-type headaches. Because stress can be a trigger, many patients choose to learn relaxation techniques.

One of the most widely accepted relaxation techniques is biofeedback, in which patients learn to control physiological responses to stress involving blood pressure, pulse rate, skin temperature, and muscle tension. Some people suffering from headaches use biofeedback techniques daily to help reduce pain or to avert a major attack when they experience an early warning.

A technique known as progressive muscle relaxation brings relief to some headache patients by helping them release excess tension. Other patients have found a measure of relief in meditation and the gentle, stretching exercises of yoga.

Another alternative to medication is acupuncture, the Chinese practice of relieving pain by placing long, thin needles at specific sites in the body. Some scientists suggest that acupuncture is effective because it releases endorphins, the body's natural painkillers. However, headache sufferers have reported only limited and temporary success in relieving headache pain through acupuncture.

Some people suffering from cluster headaches find relief by inhaling pure oxygen administered through a face mask. Oxygen con-

A headache diary

The National Headache Foundation recommends keeping a diary in preparation for seeing a doctor about recurring headaches. A headache diary helps you answer specific questions that your physician may ask in determining the type of headache you have and the best treatment for it.

When did you first develop headaches?

How often do you have headaches?

Where is the pain exactly?

How long do the headaches last?

What time of day do the headaches occur?

Do you eat any foods beforehand that may trigger the headaches?

Do you engage in any activities beforehand that may contribute to the headaches?

If you are a woman of child-bearing age, do you get headaches before, during, or after your menstrual period?

What physical or environmental factors might trigger the headaches?

bright lights	changing altitudes
intense odors	loud noises
smoke	stress
sleeping late	weather changes

What symptoms, if any, do you experience prior to the headaches?

nausea	dizziness
vomiting	sound sensitivity
light sensitivity	numbness

Which words would you use to describe your pain?

throbbing	pounding
splitting	piercing
blinding	stabbing
aching	wrenching

Source: National Headache Foundation.

stricts blood vessels, but because experts do not understand the causes of cluster headaches, they also are unsure why oxygen works on some people.

The list of nonmedication therapies is long, and it includes massage, self-hypnosis, and exercise—low-impact aerobics or a brisk walk. Sometimes headache patients are referred for psychotherapy, not because their pain is considered psychological in origin, but as a means to express the anger they feel about the pain.

A word of caution—and hope

In the past few years, alternatives to traditional medicine have grown increasingly popular for a variety of health problems. But experts caution that many practitioners of these therapies are not licensed and may not be thoroughly trained. Patients are advised to tell their physicians if they are using a nontraditional therapy so that it can be taken into consideration in developing any treatment regimen. In fact, patients who seek treatment at specialized headache treatment centers sometimes can receive traditional therapies and nondrug alternatives under one roof.

How and where to seek medical care is an individual choice. But recent research and clinical advances have considerably brightened the therapeutic prospects for people who suffer from chronic headaches. Specialists emphasize that headaches are neither a personal failing nor an emotional weakness, but a treatable illness that need not be endured in silence.   ●●●

For further reading:

The American Council on Headache Education. *Migraine: The Complete Guide.* Dell, 1994.

Lipton, Richard B., and others. *Migraine: Beating the Odds.* Addison-Wesley, 1992.

Saper, Joel R., and others. *Handbook of Headache Management.* Williams & Wilkins, 1993.

For more information:

The National Headache Foundation
5252 N. Western Avenue
Chicago, IL 60625
Within Illinois: 800-523-8858
All other states: 800-843-2256

American Council for Headache Education
875 Kings Highway
West Deptford, NJ 08096
800-255-ACHE

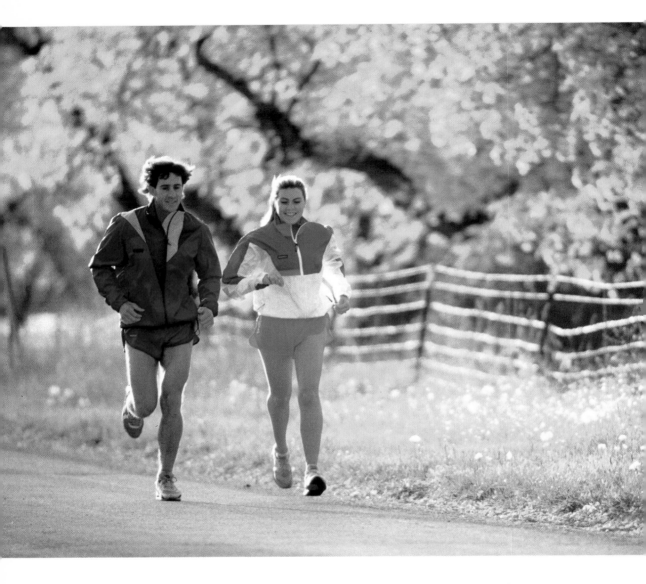

How Much Exercise Is Enough?

Exercise doesn't have to wear you out to yield health benefits, but it should be fairly vigorous.

By Priscilla M. Clarkson

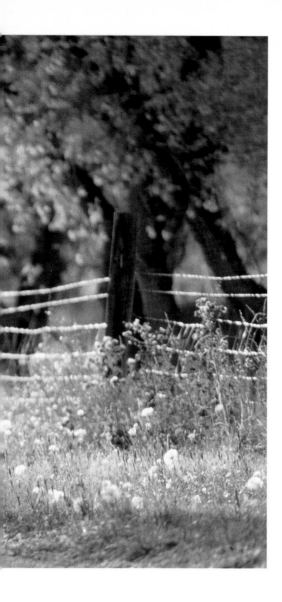

H OW MUCH EXERCISE does a person need to have a good chance of living a long, healthy life? In 1995, two widely publicized reports gave what might seem to be conflicting answers to that question.

"Everyone is confused" about how intense exercise must be to promote good health, admitted physician Ralph S. Paffenbarger, Jr., of Stanford University in California, coauthor of one of those papers. "Even the scientists are confused."

The study Paffenbarger participated in, reported in April 1995, was an analysis of the exercise habits and health of 17,300 male alumni of Harvard University in Cambridge, Massachusetts. Paffenbarger and his colleagues at the Harvard Medical School, Brigham and Women's Hospital, and the Harvard School of Public Health, all in Boston, made a surprising finding. Only men who exercised hard enough to work up a sweat were rewarded with longer lives.

Men in the Harvard alumni group who expended an average of 1,500 calories a week in vigorous physical activities such as fast walking, jogging, and swimming had a 13 to 25 percent lower death rate than alumni who did not take part in such forms of exercise. Nonvigorous activities, such as leisurely walking, were found to have no beneficial effect on mortality.

The Harvard report came close on the heels of a "Special Communication" on exercise issued jointly in February 1995 by the Centers for Disease Control and Prevention (CDC) in Atlanta, Georgia, and the American College of Sports Medicine in Indianapolis. That report—based on a review of research papers and other evidence— concluded that exercise of only moderate intensity, such as gardening or walking, for at least 30 minutes every day produces many health benefits.

The investigators said that health gains can also be derived from intermittent short periods of exercise throughout the day that add up to 30 minutes. Examples of such exercise could include walking up and down a flight of stairs several times, pedaling a stationery bicycle for 15 minutes while watching TV, and performing 10 minutes of housecleaning activities.

The Special Communication was examining general health benefits, while the Harvard study concerned itself only with death rates. But there is obviously some connection between the two, and that is where the confusion arose. To soften the impact of their findings, Paffenbarger and his colleagues pointed out that low-key exercise has been shown in many studies to produce some measurable benefits, such as reducing blood *lipids* (fats), even if it may not greatly prolong life. They concluded, "We strongly believe that even nonvigorous exercise is preferable to sedentariness."

Nonetheless, there is little doubt that vigorous exercise is best and the more such exercise you get, the better off you're likely to be. Summing up the extent of current knowledge, a newsletter from the University of California at Berkeley School of Public Health said, "Any exercise is better than none. But more exercise—enough to give your heart and lungs a real workout—is better." So if you want to increase your chances of living a long time and staying healthy, find an exercise or activity you enjoy that gets the blood pumping and engage in it on a regular basis.

The three kinds of exercise and their benefits

The vigorous exercise the physicians were advocating is known as aerobic exercise because it increases the body's oxygen intake. (The word *aerobic* is derived from the Greek words for *air* and *life*.) Aerobic exercises include such activities as jogging, swimming, bicycling, rowing, and fast walking. These exercises elevate the heart rate to get blood pumping faster, so that the blood delivers more oxygen to the muscles for energy production.

Research has shown that aerobic exercise benefits the body in a number of ways, particularly by improving *cardiovascular* (heart and blood vessel) fitness and helping keep body weight under control. Aerobic exercise also builds stronger bones and reduces mental stress. For greatest benefit, researchers have found, aerobic exercises should be performed continuously for 20 to 60 minutes and get the heart pumping at 50 to 85 percent of its maximum rate. (To calculate your maximum heart rate, subtract your age from 220.)

Aerobic exercise is one of three kinds of exercise that are necessary to achieve the greatest health benefits and all-around fitness. The other two are resistance exercise, which increases muscle strength, and flexibility exercise, which keeps joints limber.

Resistance exercises, such as weight-lifting or pushups, can be used to build muscles or prevent the loss of muscle mass that results from inactivity. These exercises, in which muscles work to overcome weight or other forms of resistance, can also be helpful in correcting certain problems that arise from weak muscles. For example, strengthening the abdominal muscles can help keep the spine in proper alignment, thereby reducing lower-back pain. For a minimum workout to maintain strength, the American College of Sports Medicine recommends that resistance exercise be done at least twice a week for at least 30 minutes at each session.

Flexibility exercises, by stretching muscles, allow for a greater

The author:
....

Priscilla M. Clarkson is associate dean and professor of exercise science at the University of Massachusetts at Amherst's School of Public Health and Health Sciences.

60

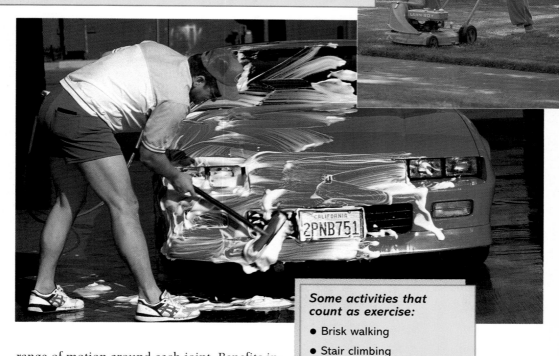

"Exercise lite"—what counts and what doesn't

Doctors have found that many everyday activities can provide people with the exercise they need to live a longer, healthier life. A total of 30 minutes a day of such exercise is the recommended minimum. To qualify as exercise, an activity must be fairly vigorous, causing the body to burn extra calories. Some activities are not strenuous enough to produce beneficial health effects.

Some activities that count as exercise:

- Brisk walking
- Stair climbing
- Moving the furniture
- Gardening and yardwork
- Scrubbing floors
- Shoveling snow
- Washing the car
- House painting
- Square dancing

A few that don't:

- Dusting the furniture
- Ironing clothes
- Watering the lawn
- Making beds
- Vacuuming
- Strolling

range of motion around each joint. Benefits include greater ease of movement, fewer *musculoskeletal* (muscle and skeleton) problems, such as back pain, and a reduced risk of straining or pulling a muscle. The American College of Sports Medicine recommends that stretching exercises be done for about 20 minutes or more, at least three days a week. But take it easy—muscles should never be stretched to the point of pain.

Resistance and flexibility exercise can make us stronger and more limber, but it is aerobic exercise that holds the greatest promise of reducing the risk of disease and early death by strengthening the cardiovascular system. Achieving cardiovascular fitness can help ward off the two forms of cardiovascular disease that kill the most Americans each year: coronary heart disease and strokes. In 1995, the American Heart Association predicted, some

Working toward maximum fitness

Those who wish to get into top physical shape should combine an array of aerobic exercises—activities, such as cycling, that significantly increase the body's oxygen uptake—with resistance, or muscle-strengthening, exercises, such as weight-lifting. Flexibility exercises, which stretch muscles to increase the range of motion around joints, are also part of a well-rounded exercise program.

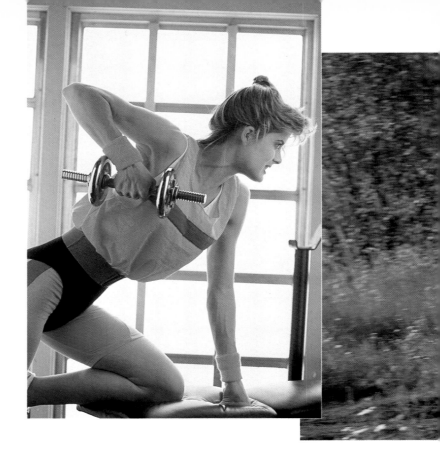

500,000 Americans would die of heart attacks and as many as 150,000 would succumb to strokes. Although the incidence of cardiovascular disease has been dropping since the mid-1960's as more and more people have adopted healthier lifestyles, it is still the number-one cause of death in the United States.

A 1993 CDC report on deaths from heart disease in the United States in 1986 attributed 205,254 of the more than 500,000 deaths to lack of adequate exercise. Exercise can help prevent such deaths by improving a person's blood-cholesterol levels and by lowering moderately elevated blood pressure.

Exercise can also help prevent unwanted weight gain. Being overweight increases the risk not only of cardiovascular disease but also of several other health problems, including diabetes and arthritis of the knees, hips, and ankles.

There are two ways to lose weight: by eating less or exercising more. Physicians caution, however, that decreasing calorie intake too much can result in inadequate nutrition. On top of that, quick weight loss is often followed by the "rebound syndrome," in which the individual regains the lost weight as well as a few extra pounds.

Because of these problems with dieting, weight-control experts are virtually unanimous in advocating a combination of sensible eating and regular aerobic exercise for controlling weight. Resistance exercises can be added for extra benefit. What the individual should

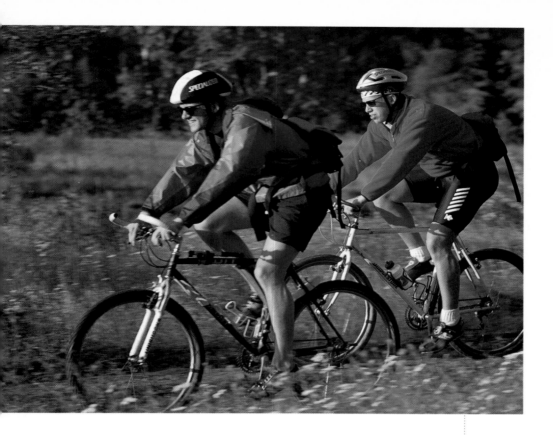

strive for is a whole new way of living, not just a short-term plan that will be discarded as soon as the desired weight goal is achieved.

Aerobic exercise not only helps the body by reducing the amount of weight it must carry, it also strengthens bones. The stooped posture of many older people is primarily due to decreased levels of minerals, notably calcium, in the bones. The process of bone loss, called *osteoporosis,* increases the risk of bone fractures in older adults. Inadequate calcium intake over a period of years is a major contributing factor to this disorder, but so is physical inactivity. Exercises such as walking and jogging, which put weight on bones, can prevent bone loss and may even increase bone mass. Studies have found that thin people are at greater risk than others for osteoporosis, probably because their bones carry less weight.

Finally, regular aerobic exercise seems to help many people control psychological stress. Studies of physically active individuals have found that they usually report feeling a greater level of emotional well-being than sedentary people.

Embarking on a healthy new life

Most healthy adults will not need a physician's approval to begin a program of moderately intense exercise. However, anyone with a chronic disease, or who has risk factors for cardiovascular disease or

Tailoring your exercise to your health goals

It is possible to obtain health benefits, including a lower risk of heart disease and various other illnesses, with as little as 30 minutes a day of moderately vigorous exercise, such as brisk walking or gardening. More ambitious goals, including losing weight or achieving optimal physical fitness, require more strenuous exertions, such as jogging and rowing, usually done for a more prolonged period. Exercise can be put into three main categories:

Aerobic exercises—exercises that significantly increase one's pulse rate and oxygen uptake for a prolonged period, thereby improving *cardiovascular* (heart and blood vessel) fitness. These can include everyday activities such as yardwork and climbing stairs or more sporting activities such as fast walking, running, bicycle riding, swimming, and skiing.

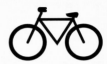

Resistance exercises—exercises designed to increase muscle strength. These include weight training and various floor exercises, such as push-ups and sit-ups, in which the muscles contract while overcoming resistance.

Flexibility exercises—stretching exercises aimed at improving the range of motion around joints.

Health goal	Type of exercise	Recommended frequency
A healthier life	Moderately vigorous activities and exercise	30 minutes daily
More immediate physical benefits, such as increased energy and endurance	Aerobic exercise	20 to 60 minutes, 3 or more times a week
A high level of physical fitness	Vigorous aerobic exercise	20 to 60 minutes daily
	Resistance exercises	30 minutes, twice a week
	Flexibility exercises	20 minutes, 3 times a week
Weight loss	Aerobic exercise	60 minutes, 5 times a week
	Resistance exercises	30 minutes, 3 times a week

Sources: American College of Sports Medicine; Centers for Disease Control and Prevention; Harvard Alumni Health Study.

other illnesses, should consult a physician before starting an exercise program.

Healthy individuals whose goal is just to stay healthy and feel good could start by adopting the guidelines of the CDC and American College of Sports Medicine and aim at getting a total of at least 30 minutes of aerobic activities daily. This can be accomplished to a large extent through changes in one's daily routine—walking rather than driving, taking the stairs instead of the elevator, and working around the house and yard. People who have not been exercising should start slowly and gradually build up to 30 minutes.

The CDC and American College of Sports Medicine said people should aim at burning at least 200 extra calories a day during that 30 minutes of exercise. Moderate activities such as brisk walking and recreational cycling burn 4 to 7 calories a minute. More strenuous exercises, such as fast walking, rowing, and running, expend 7 to 12 calories a minute. A few of the most intensive exercises, including running up stairs and shoveling wet snow, burn 15 calories or more a minute. The heavier a person is, the more calories are expended in a given activity, because it takes more energy to move a greater amount of weight.

People who want to significantly increase their cardiovascular fitness can tailor their own aerobic-exercise program. And for those who are really motivated, combining intense aerobic activities with flexibility and resistance exercises will lead to maximum fitness. But whatever one's goal, the most important thing is to get started.

It's never too late to change sedentary ways, though it gets progressively harder. Beyond a certain age, many inactive individuals may simply find exercise too physically taxing, or they may conclude that it would be fruitless. And at that point, their ability to fully enjoy life could decline. A lack of physical activity in one's later years can hasten the aging process, thereby diminishing the prospect of leading an independent life.

The best time to start exercising is early in life. Children should be encouraged to acquire healthy exercise habits when they are young so that they will continue to exercise regularly when they reach adulthood.

Regular exercise can energize one's life, and it is one of the best investments people can make for their future health. If people give exercise a try, they may even find it habit-forming.   •••

For further reading:
Nieman, David C. *Fitness and Sports Medicine. A Health-Related Approach.* Bull Publishing Company, 1995.
University of California at Berkeley Wellness Letter Editors. *The Wellness Guide to Lifelong Fitness.* Rebus Incorporated, 1993.

Drawing From Your Own

Blood Bank

The public blood supply has never been safer, but donating your own blood before surgery can eliminate the slight chance of disease transmission.

By Judy Reiss Berlfein

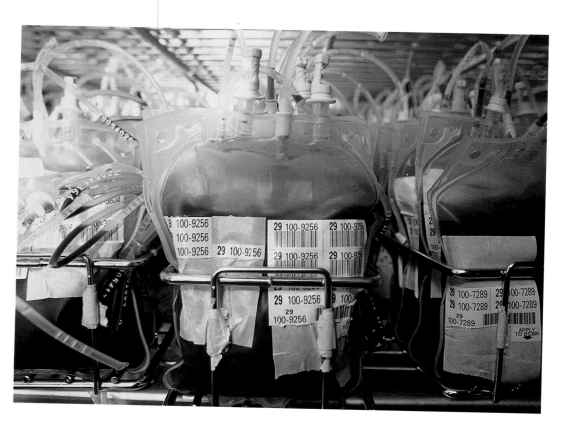

WHEN TIM SCHEDULED HIS BACK SURGERY, he wanted to be certain all would go in his favor. From his perspective, the outcome seemed to rest solely in the surgeon's hands, yet Tim himself was able to contribute to the operation's success. At his physician's suggestion, Tim donated two units (approximately two pints) of his blood in the weeks prior to surgery. If a transfusion became necessary, the surgeon would infuse Tim's own blood back into his veins. When the surgery finally took place, Tim was grateful. He needed a transfusion, and the surgical team filled his depleted vessels with his own blood.

Why did Tim bother putting his blood in the bank? Most people who donate blood to themselves—a procedure known as *autologous* (self-derived) donation—do so before surgery. In the event of significant blood loss during surgery, these donors avoid the small possibility of infection from viruses that might contaminate a transfusion of blood from another donor.

Health officials insist, however, that the chances of contracting an infectious disease through donated blood are extremely slight. They have determined that only a handful of diseases pose enough of a risk that blood banks need to test for them. All blood banks in the United States test donated blood for HIV, the virus that causes AIDS; syphilis; the liver diseases hepatitis B and C; and a virus that can cause a form of the blood cancer leukemia.

Despite these precautions, a slight risk of infection from donated blood still exists. Hepatitis C poses the biggest risk—about 1 in 3,300 transfusions carries the hepatitis C virus, according to the Food and Drug Administration (FDA), a federal government agency that oversees blood donation in the United States.

For HIV and hepatitis B, the risks are smaller still—about 1 in 250,000 carries the hepatitis B virus, and about 1 in 420,000 units of blood carries HIV, according to the Red Cross. The screening for HIV tests for the presence of disease-fighting cells called antibodies, and antibodies to HIV do not appear until about 25 days after infection. Most HIV-contaminated blood comes from infected donors in whom antibodies have not yet appeared.

Aside from eliminating the risk of infection, autologous donation can limit other potential complications from transfused blood. If the body's immune system identifies the donated blood as "foreign" and potentially harmful, it may react adversely. Immune system responses are usually mild, causing fevers, headache, wheezing, or skin rash. In a severe response, however, the patient's immune system destroys the donated red blood cells, which can lead to abnormal bleeding, fever and chills, kidney failure, and even death.

To prevent such immune system reactions, samples of the donated blood and the patient's blood are usually mixed together before the transfusion to see if they are compatible, a procedure called a cross-match. In the event of sudden and unexpected blood loss, however, there might not be time for a compatibility check before a transfusion. In such an emergency, doctors often give blood type O, which

The author:

Judy Reiss Berlfein is a free-lance medical writer.

67

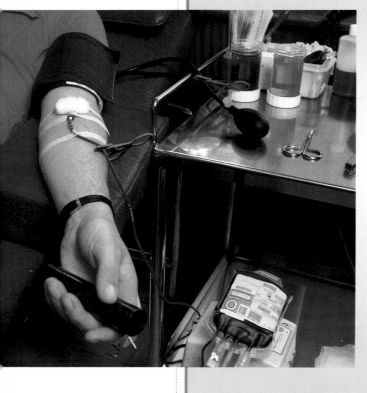

Preparing to donate to yourself

Donating blood to yourself is more complicated than donating to the general public. These tips should make it easier.

- Discuss the donation schedule with your physician to make sure there is time to donate sufficient blood before the operation. Most donations begin six weeks before the operation.

- Make sure you give the appropriate amount of blood for the scheduled surgery. Transfusions from the general blood supply will be required if you donate too little of your own blood.

- Tell the blood bank if the date or location of the surgery changes, or if the surgery is cancelled. Failure to do so may result in delivery of your blood at the wrong time or to the wrong location.

- Give correct personal information. If hospital records and blood bank records do not match in all aspects, you may have trouble convincing hospital staff that the blood you donated is really your own.

is known as the universal donor type because almost all patients can use it without a reaction. Autologous donation eliminates the possibility of incompatibility, but it doesn't ensure the availability of the blood in an emergency. In very rare instances, medical workers give patients the wrong blood type, a mistake that can have deadly consequences.

Most physicians recommend autologous blood donation only for patients who are likely to require a limited amount of blood during planned surgery. Physicians discourage people from donating their blood simply to have it available in case of an emergency. One reason is that blood must be frozen if it is kept more than a few weeks, and storage costs for frozen blood are high. In addition, donors may be hundreds of miles from their blood supply when it is needed. If a scheduled surgery must be postponed, however, freezing the patient's donated blood becomes a workable option.

Some operations carry more risk of blood loss than others. Minor surgeries such as removing a *cataract* (clouding of the lens of the eye) or appendix usually require no extra blood. But in other operations when a transfusion is required, the average amount of blood used is 3.4 units, according to the American Association of Blood Banks in Bethesda, Md., an agency that inspects and accredits blood banks in the United States. A unit of blood contains 450 milliliters (15 ounces) of blood plus 63 milliliters (2 ounces) of a preservative solution. Common elective operations for which people donate autologous blood include hip replacement and certain types of heart surgery. Autologous donation is not an option before organ transplants, and certain other major operations because of the high volume of blood—as many as 30 units—required.

People who donate blood to themselves do so a few weeks before their surgery. Patients can donate autologous units as often as every fourth day, but they should allow three days before the operation to permit their blood volume to return to normal.

Medical problems may prevent some people from becoming autologous donors. Patients with unstable heart conditions, for example, may be poor candidates for autologous donation, because blood removal might disrupt their blood pressure and cause a heart attack. A bone infection called osteomyelitis also rules out autologous donation because of the presence of bacteria in the blood. Bacteria can easily multiply in stored blood, releasing *toxins* (poisons) that can cause severe shock if reinfused into the patient.

The process of autologous donation

Donating blood to oneself is fairly easy. The American Association of Blood Banks requires all blood centers to offer such a service. Autologous donors give blood alongside other donors, whom blood banks call community donors, and everybody follows the same basic procedures. To draw the blood, a medical attendant inserts a needle at-

---

Who should not give blood

Physicians recommend that people with certain medical conditions not give blood. Those generally prohibited from giving blood include:

- People with a serious heart condition, such as angina or congestive heart failure. The loss of blood from blood donation, though small, could trigger a heart attack.

- People with the bone infection osteomyelitis, which can enter the blood. Reinfusing tainted blood could cause reinfection or worsen an existing infection. Bacteria could also reproduce while the blood is in storage.

- Cancer patients whose disease has spread to the bloodstream. There would be little point in removing a cancerous tumor if cancer cells were infused back into the bloodstream during the operation.

- People whose surgery requires many transfusions. Time constraints prevent people from donating more than six units of blood before an operation. Most people donate one unit a week before surgery, and blood cannot be stored for more than six weeks without freezing.

- People with severe anemia—a disorder that results in a reduced red blood cell count.

Source: The American Red Cross.

Salvaging blood

Donating blood before surgery is not the only way of avoiding a transfusion of someone else's blood. Blood salvage involves suctioning blood from the surgical cavity and reinfusing it into the patient. This technique is most often used in heart surgery and surgery involving the bones—procedures that typically require large amounts of blood.

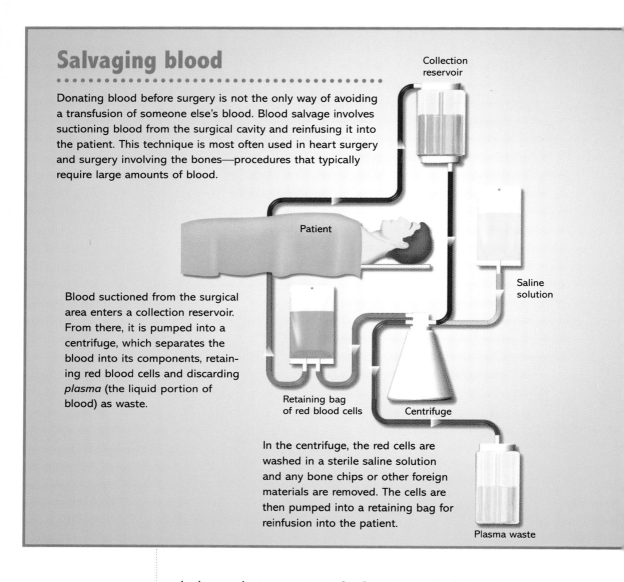

Collection reservoir

Patient

Saline solution

Blood suctioned from the surgical area enters a collection reservoir. From there, it is pumped into a centrifuge, which separates the blood into its components, retaining red blood cells and discarding *plasma* (the liquid portion of blood) as waste.

Retaining bag of red blood cells

Centrifuge

In the centrifuge, the red cells are washed in a sterile saline solution and any bone chips or other foreign materials are removed. The cells are then pumped into a retaining bag for reinfusion into the patient.

Plasma waste

tached to a tube into a vein in the donor's arm. Each donation takes about an hour, and, contrary to fears that some people have, donating carries no risk of contracting infection.

All donors answer questions concerning their general health beforehand. Blood banks screen donors to protect both the donor and the recipient. On one hand, donors must be healthy enough to give up a pint of blood, and on the other hand, their blood must be sufficiently safe to pass on to someone else.

Because their blood does not enter the public supply, autologous donors are able to bypass many restrictions placed on other donors. The usual minimum donor weight of 110 pounds (50 kilograms) is often waived for autologous donors, for instance. If a patient falls at the low end of the scale, the blood bank will simply draw smaller

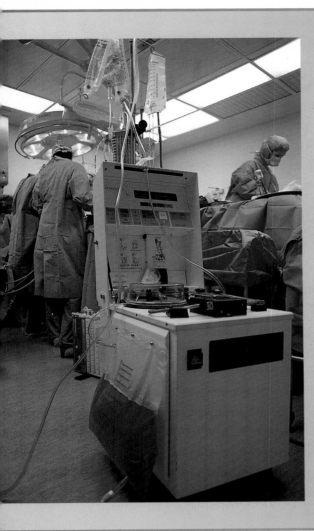

A blood salvaging machine collects blood from a heart surgery patient during an operation. The machine filters the blood for reinfusion into the patient and helps reduce the need for donated blood.

quantities of blood. Children as young as 10 years of age, who generally do not meet the weight requirement, can donate to themselves, as can older people who fall below the weight limit. Together, the patient's personal physician and the blood bank personnel make the final decision about autologous donation.

The FDA also allows people infected with HIV or hepatitis B to donate and receive their own blood, if their physician requests it in writing and blood bank personnel are informed of the patient's infection before the donation. Viruses, unlike bacteria, do not multiply rapidly in stored blood and do not produce toxins, according to Richard Davey, chief medical officer for the American Red Cross.

Autologous blood can cost two times as much per unit as blood from community donors. Much of the added cost stems from an at-

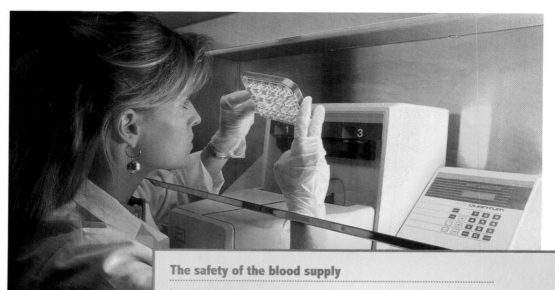

A laboratory technician at a blood bank tests donated blood for infection with hepatitis.

The safety of the blood supply

Improved monitoring and testing have made the blood supply safer than ever. But a slight risk still remains of contracting HIV or the liver diseases hepatitis B and hepatitis C through a blood transfusion. The risks of contracting HIV and hepatitis B are far smaller than the risk of death from other common activities:

- Contracting HIV through blood transfusion: 1 in 420,000 transfusions.

- Contracting hepatitis B through blood transfusion: 1 in 250,000 transfusions.

- Contracting hepatitis C through blood transfusion: 1 in 3,300 transfusions.

- Dying in a car accident: 1 in 11,000 motorists in any given year.

- Dying in a home accident: 1 in 65,000 people in any given year.

Source: The American Red Cross.

tempt by blood banks to make up for the lost money they would normally receive from the sale of each unit of blood from community donors, according to Roslyn Yomtovian, chairperson of the autologous transfusion committee for the American Association of Blood Banks. Blood banks usually separate units of whole blood from community donors into three components: red cells, *plasma* (the liquid portion of blood), and *platelets* (disklike structures that help stop bleeding). Blood banks sell each component separately. But because autologous blood is not broken into components, blood centers make up the difference in revenue by charging more for whole autologous units. The special care that goes into accommodating autologous donors also makes the costs high. According to blood bank personnel, much of the extra expense comes from processing blood that is never used. In addition, autologous blood must be treated specially, stored in a separate location, and transported to a specific hospital and patient.

Reducing the need for a transfusion

Patients can reduce the risks associated with donated blood in other ways than autologous donation. During operations such as open-heart surgery, in which a patient loses large quantities of blood, the surgical team can salvage the blood by suctioning it from the area of the body being operated on and returning it to the patient. In some operations, such as abdominal or bone surgery, fecal matter, fat, or bone chips can contaminate the blood, and it may be unsuitable for reinfusion into the patient. In other surgeries, doctors can reinfuse the blood directly into the patient.

Surgeons do not recommend blood salvage for all operations, however. Surgeons may decline to perform blood salvage during cancer surgery, for example, if there is a possibility that cancerous cells have contaminated blood around the surgical area. Blood also cannot be salvaged if the patient has osteomyelitis.

Another technique for protecting against blood loss is hemodilution, which involves thinning the blood. Immediately before surgery, the patient donates blood and receives in exchange a solution containing essential body fluids and salts but no red blood cells. This substitution reduces the concentration of red blood cells so that fewer of these crucial oxygen-carrying cells are lost during surgery. When the operation is completed, the surgical team reinfuses the initial donation, enriching the body once again.

Some people ask friends and relatives with the same blood type to donate blood, but blood bank personnel caution that this well-intentioned approach may not work as anticipated. Acquaintances who have never given blood before may experience more difficulty than regular donors. If friends or family members feel pressure to donate, they may withhold vital information about their health status that could disqualify them as donors. If their blood later fails to pass the screening tests, health workers destroy it, and the blood bank has wasted time and resources collecting unusable blood.

There is little doubt that autologous blood donation protects donors against the slight, but serious, risks of receiving blood from the community blood supply. Since the chances of infection from blood donation are so small, the biggest benefit that autologous donation provides may be psychological. But that may be the only incentive many people need. ●●●

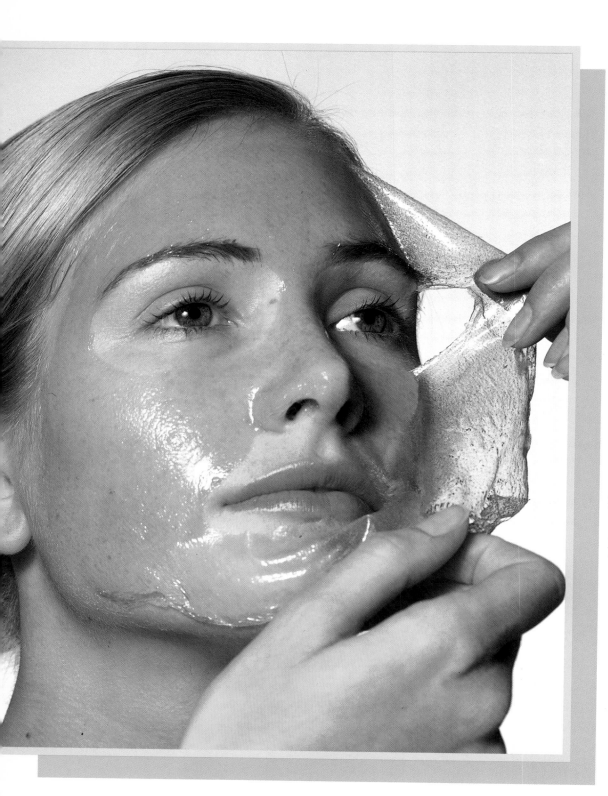

Wrinkle Removal:

An Antidote to Aging Skin?

By Richard G. Glogau

AS BABY BOOMERS ENTER THEIR 40's AND 50's, the problem of aging skin has moved to the forefront of consumer consciousness. In response, the cosmetics industry has flooded the market with products that claim to remove wrinkles and reverse aging. The line-up of skin-care products, once limited primarily to substances for hiding blemishes or moisturizing and toning skin, has expanded with the help of the medical profession. Today, it includes Retin-A, alpha-hydroxy acids, chemical peels, collagen injections, and sunscreens. Confronted with so many choices, consumers may well wonder which products, if any, live up to their claims.

Worries over aging skin have become so prevalent largely because of social and economic changes that took place after World War II (1939-1945) and turned Americans into sun lovers. A booming economy gave people more leisure time and more money to spend on recreation, often outdoors. They soon came to view a tan as glamorous and a sign of wealth and leisure, rather than a mark of laboring in the fields.

Promoting this change in attitude was the growth of the motion-picture industry in southern California, which linked stardom and sunny locale. Moreover, soldiers who served in the Pacific theater during the war returned with an expanded view of sunny climates. And a postwar real estate boom sparked migration to the Sun Belt. At about the same time, American fashion began to copy such trend-setters as England's Duke of Windsor and his friends, who introduced more revealing bathing suits. Never before had people appeared at the beach or pool in such a state of undress.

This massive change in exposure to the sun has doubled as an experiment on the long-term effect of exposure to the damaging ultraviolet (UV) radiation in sunlight, an effect called photoaging. The

> Various products and procedures promise to remove wrinkles, but it's important to find out about the cost, time, and risks involved beforehand.

75

most damaging consequence of photoaging is skin cancer, which has grown astronomically in prevalence, to an estimated 800,000 new U.S. cases in 1995. Earlier signs of photoaging are even more widespread. One sign is a shift in skin color, from the rosy blush of youth to the yellow-grey sallowness of age. Another is the wrinkle.

Skin develops wrinkles in response to several factors. First and foremost is chronic exposure to the UV radiation in sunlight and in artificial sources such as sun-lamps and tanning booths. Repeated exposure causes changes in the skin's structure that are visible under a microscope. Two fibers in the skin, collagen and elastin, become fragmented and disordered. As a result, skin gradually loses its natural resiliency and elasticity. Like an overstretched rubber band, the skin can no longer snap back. It begins to hang in folds and show small, fine wrinkles. Some of this change in elastin and collagen fibers results from the aging process, but most dermatologists agree that chronic sun exposure is the main cause of wrinkles.

Heredity also plays a role, affecting photoaging in two ways. First, people who inherit dark skin appear to photoage at a slower rate than those born with fair skin, possibly because the additional pigment in dark skin acts as a shield against UV radiation. Second, people of the same age and skin tone may photoage at different rates, depending on their skin's inherited ability to heal after a sunburn. People whose skin heals poorly after sun damage tend to photoage more rapidly. You can assess your genetic risk of photoaging by looking at the condition of your parents' skin.

Sun exposure damages all skin types, whether dry or oily. Oily skin confers no protection, nor do moisturizers unless they contain a sun block. There is no such thing as a healthy tan.

Gravity and facial movements accentuate the lines and wrinkles caused by photoaging. Gravity, for example, accelerates the development of folds along the side of the mouth. Repeated squinting—a reflex action to protect the eyes from UV radiation—produces lines near the eyes known as crow's feet. Scowling and frowning lead to vertical lines between the eyebrows and horizontal lines across the forehead. Smoking fosters wrinkles, especially around the mouth, because it requires repeated pursing and sucking. It also adds to wrinkling by exposing smokers to carbon monoxide, which lowers the blood's oxygen content—oxygen that the skin needs for healing.

The author:

Richard G. Glogau is clinical professor of dermatology at the University of California at San Francisco.

You can take several steps to help prevent wrinkles. First and most important, use a sunscreen with a Sun Protection Factor (SPF) rating of 15 or higher. Apply the sunscreen daily, whether the sky is cloudy or clear. The UV radiation that causes wrinkles and skin cancer travels right through the thickest clouds. Second, avoid going outdoors between 10 a.m. and 2 p.m., when the sun's rays are strongest. Third, don't smoke. Fourth, weigh your genetic risk. If you have the pale skin typical of people of northern European descent, you are at particular risk. If you have dark skin, however, do not assume it protects you completely from wrinkles. It does not do so.

When you look in the mirror and see wrinkles you would rather not see, you have a number of options. They include medicated lotions, chemical peels and other techniques that resurface damaged skin, and injections. These therapies vary in cost, risk, and results.

To understand how wrinkle-removal therapies work, it's necessary to know something about the skin's three layers. The skin that we see is part of the epidermis, the outer layer, which also contains cells that produce pigment and give skin its color. Underneath lies the dermis, which is made up of blood vessels and connective tissue that nourish the skin. The skin's innermost layer, the subcutaneous tissue, consists mainly of connective tissue, blood vessels, and fat cells.

Chemical peels strip away part or all of the epidermis and sometimes part of the dermis as well. Peels consist of

Wrinkles: A sign of sun and age

Wrinkles develop as the skin loses its natural elasticity, but we don't all develop creases and folds at the same rate. Heredity and the effects of gravity play a role, but most dermatologists agree that chronic sun exposure is the main cause of wrinkling.

- Over time, ultraviolet radiation from the sun, sunlamps, or tanning booths breaks up fibers of collagen and elastin in the skin. As a result, the skin loses its resilience and begins to hang in folds and show fine wrinkles.

- Fair skin wrinkles more rapidly than dark skin, possibly because the additional pigment that gives dark skin its color also acts as a shield against ultraviolet radiation.

- Skin that heals quickly after sunburn appears to wrinkle more slowly than skin that heals slowly. The rate at which a person's skin heals appears to be hereditary.

- The pull of gravity accentuates wrinkles and speeds the development of folds, such as those that come down from the mouth.

- Frequently repeated facial movements can produce wrinkles. Repeated squinting, for example, produces crow's-feet, the tiny lines that fan out from the eyes.

- Smoking promotes wrinkles, especially around the mouth, because of the repeated pursing of the lips and sucking it requires. Smoking also reduces the blood's oxygen content, which may slow healing after sunburn and so increase the rate of wrinkling.

Source:
Richard G. Glogau. M.D.

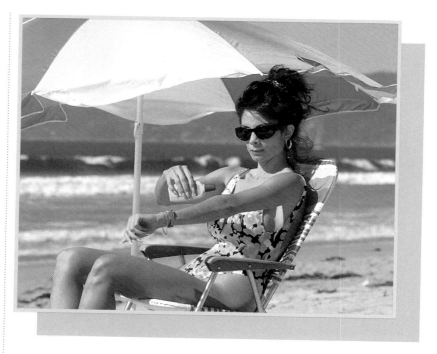

Prolonged exposure to sunlight is the main cause of wrinkles, according to most dermatologists. Sunlight's ultraviolet rays fragment fibers in the skin, so that it loses elasticity and begins to sag and develop fine lines.

various acids, including the newly popular alpha-hydroxy acids, which produce a mild to heavy burn when applied to the skin. Peels can be superficial or deep depending on the application technique and on the type, strength, and amount of the acid used.

Superficial peels, which remove only cells in the epidermis, can improve skin color and give skin a smoother feel, but they have little, if any, effect on wrinkles. Photoaged skin often appears mottled and muddy because of uneven deposits of the pigment melanin. As the skin heals from a superficial peel, new deposits of melanin appear, evening out skin color. A deep chemical peel removes all the epidermis and part of the dermis. As the body repairs this damage, it produces new collagen and elastin, which make the skin appear smoother and firmer

Chemical peels containing alpha-hydroxy acids (AHA's) are available in a range of formulations and concentrations. Those available at salons or physicians' offices contain higher concentrations of AHA's than those sold for home use. AHA's also appear in weak concentrations in lotions and creams sold over the counter.

AHA's occur naturally in such substances as milk (lactic acid), fruit (citric, malic, and tartaric acids), tea (tannic acid), and sugar cane (glycolic acid). The most widely used is glycolic acid. Low-strength AHA peels, which typically contain from 20 to 30 percent glycolic acid, lead to slight peeling of skin over a few days and generally cause no significant reddening. They also produce little permanent change in skin and none of the changes seen with deeper peels. High-strength AHA peels consist of 40 percent to 70 percent acid and can safely be left on the skin only a short time. Improperly applied, strong AHA peels can cause chemical burns, brown or white spots, and permanent scarring.

Deep chemical peels, whether based on AHA's or other acids—such as trichloroacetic acid (TCA)—produce the most dramatic results and pose the highest risks, including changes in skin color and scarring. Skin tone can lighten with the removal of melanin-producing cells. Olive skin, for example, may turn several shades lighter, but pale skin usually shows no change because such skin has little melanin to begin with.

Healing typically takes several weeks after a deep peel but only a few days after a superficial peel. Yet even superficial peels pose some risk of delayed healing and changes in skin color. For this reason, all peels are best done under the supervision of a physician who is well versed in peeling techniques. Charges for peels range from less than $100 to several thousand dollars, depending on the depth of the peel and the areas being treated.

AHA's also are used in cosmetic lotions in concentrations that vary from 6 percent to 20 percent. Most over-the-counter products have concentrations of about 14 to 16 percent. According to cosmetics firms, AHA lotions accelerate the rate at which the skin sheds its top layer of dead cells. As fresh cells replace the discarded cells, the skin appears tighter and smoother, and skin color may become more even. When used repeatedly, AHA's also may increase the skin's ground substance, the "glue" that holds together the dermis. Increases in the ground substance generally are associated with younger, healthier skin. No studies have looked at the long-term consequences of using AHA's, however.

Not all skin reacts the same way to AHA's, so it's important to pay attention to the concentration in any product you buy. If your skin is sensitive, even a low-dose AHA may irritate it. Prices vary greatly, with some creams costing less than $10. Competing claims by cosmetics firms for the effectiveness of their formulations are not backed up by any published evidence, and an expensive product may provide no more benefits than a drug store brand. The best way to select a cream is through trial and error, until you find one that makes your skin look and feel good.

While peels use chemicals to thin the epidermis, skin sanding does the same thing mechanically. Dermatologists have used skin sanding, also known as dermabrasion, for many years to resurface sun-damaged skin, particularly around the mouth but often over the whole face. Healing takes two weeks, and skin color returns to normal after several more weeks. The cost of skin sanding ranges from hundreds of dollars to thousands of dollars. Dermabrasion, like medium to deep peels, carries some risks of scarring and permanent change in skin color.

Laser technology, specifically the development of short-pulse car-

Wrinkle removal: Results

Dermatologists attack wrinkles, such as folds along the nose and mouth, in several ways. They may inject substances under the fold to plump it out, *right,* or treat the skin with chemicals to make it smoother or even out color, *far right.*

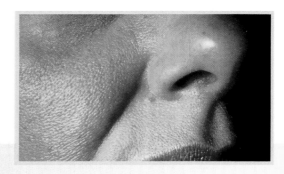

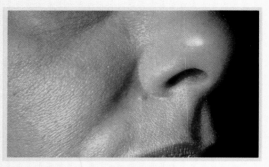

To remove the fold from this patient's face, a dermatologist injected it with collagen extracted from cowhide. Collagen—a substance that occurs naturally in human skin—normally firms the skin. But when collagen fibers are damaged by sun exposure or aging, the skin begins to hang in folds and show small wrinkles. Although the collagen injection smoothed the fold, *bottom,* the line will return in a month or two.

bon-dioxide lasers, has created a new technique for skin resurfacing. Proponents say these lasers emit such short bursts of energy that they can vaporize outer layers of skin without damaging its deeper layers. If so, this would give physicians a dependable method of treating the fine wrinkles of sun-damaged skin, particularly around the mouth and eyes. Controlled clinical studies comparing this method with chemical peels and skin sanding were already underway in 1995.

Retinoic acid, sold under the trade name Retin-A, is an acne cream that has been studied for its antiaging effect. Like AHA's, Retin-A increases the ground substance in the skin's dermis and tightens the epidermal layer. Retin-A also increases blood flow into the skin, which helps keep the skin moist.

Retin-A is classified as a drug, and so its use is regulated by the U.S. Food and Drug Administration (FDA). Although the FDA has approved Retin-A for treating acne, it has not yet granted the manufacturer permission to market Retin-A as a wrinkle cream. Retin-A comes in cream, gel, and liquid form at various strengths, but it is available by prescription only.

Retin-A can irritate the skin, which makes it difficult to find the right balance between the medication's strength and the frequency of its application. Newer retinoid drugs are likely to evolve, and these may provide less irritation and more benefits to skin than Retin-A.

In the 1950's and 1960's, estrogen was an ingredient of many com-

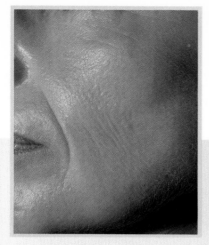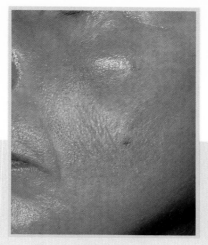

A dermatologist minimized fine lines on this patient's face with three glycolic acid peels, one consisting of 20 percent acid and two consisting of 35 percent acid. The acids loosened and removed layers of dead skin cells that accumulate on the surface of the skin. The slight reddening of the skin, which often occurs immediately after the procedure, *right,* disappears in a few days.

plexion creams. Estrogen can help clear acne, though no evidence suggests that it reverses photoaging when applied to the skin. Moreover, the body absorbs almost all of the estrogen, and so estrogen creams lead to the same range of side effects as estrogen taken by mouth, including breast tenderness and bleeding between menstrual periods. Because of these side effects, estrogen creams fell from favor in the United States, but estrogen remains an essential part of European antiaging creams.

Materials that are injected into the skin or just beneath it can treat individual lines and wrinkles. The injectable material most widely used is Zyderm collagen, which is extracted from cow hides. Dermatologists use it to plump up folds along the mouth, soften crow's feet and wrinkles of the upper lip, and enlarge the lips. The injections are expensive ($300 and up for a single injection) and their effect is temporary, typically lasting only a month or two. These injections are popular, however, because they can be done during an office visit and require little recovery time. About 2 percent of patients are allergic to the material, however.

Fibrel is an injectable substance made from the patient's own serum, a liquid that is part of the blood. Although similar in price to Zyderm, Fibrel has failed to gain widespread use, probably because the patient's blood must be collected to prepare the material, making the procedure time consuming.

Dermatologists also use a potent natural poison to temporarily remove deep vertical frown lines between the eyebrows. The toxin, *Clostridium botulinum,* causes the food poisoning known as botulism

How wrinkle treatments compare

A number of treatments are available for minimizing wrinkles. In general, the more effective the treatment, the greater are the risks it involves. A physician should perform, or at least supervise, any procedure entailing risk, including peels, skin sanding, and injections.

Treatment	How it works	What it claims to do	Limitations and risks	Cost
Alpha-hydroxy lotion or peel	Applied to the face, it peels the skin's outer layer and may add to the "glue" binding the skin's underlying layer.	Smooths the skin's outer layer and plumps up the underlying layer, making wrinkles less visible.	Lotions and low-strength peels have no permanent effect and may irritate sensitive skin. Strong peels can cause burns, spots, or scarring.	Peels: $100 to more than $1,000 Lotions: Under $10 and up
Chemical peel	Applied to the face, it burns part of the skin's outer layer. Healing gives the skin new collagen fibers, which firm it.	Low-strength peels may even out skin color; deeper peels may make the skin appear smoother and firmer.	Superficial peels may alter skin color. Deep peels require weeks of healing time and can cause scarring and permanent change in skin color.	From $100 to more than $3,000
Collagen injection	Injected into the skin, it can treat individual wrinkles.	Plumps up folds and softens wrinkles.	Temporary effect lasting only a month or so. Some patients are allergic to the collagen used.	$300 per injection
Retin-A®	Applied to the face, it may add to the "glue" binding the skin's underlying layer. It also increases blood flow to the skin.	Smooths the skin's outer layer, plumps up its underlying layer, and adds to its moisture.	May irritate the skin.	From $25 to $45
Botulinum toxin injection	Injected into the forehead, the toxin weakens or paralyzes muscles that produce deep frown lines.	Removes deep frown lines in the forehead.	Spontaneously reversible effect lasting several months.	Less than $500
Skin sanding	Mechanical abrasion strips part of the skin's outer layer.	Removes facial wrinkles, particularly around the mouth.	Two-week healing time; some risk of scarring or permanent change in skin color.	From $100 to more than $3,000

Source: Richard G. Glogau. M.D.

when consumed. When small amounts are injected into the forehead, the toxin weakens or paralyzes the muscles that cause frown lines. Inactivating these muscles allows the wrinkled skin to become smooth. This effect lasts for several months. The procedure costs less than $500, requires no incisions, and is performed during an office visit. It can be repeated months later if the lines reappear after the paralyzed muscle awakens.

Remedies for sun damage do not address the effects of gravity and age: drooping muscle, skin, and jowls. Facelifts do so, but they are expensive, starting at several thousand dollars. Facelifts are surgical procedures that carry the risks of all surgeries, including scarring, infection, bleeding, prolonged healing, bruising, and discomfort.

Choosing a treatment for wrinkled and photodamaged skin boils down to balancing the risks and benefits. When considering a certain treatment, ask yourself what benefit you desire and what degree of risk you will assume to achieve it. Can you take three weeks off from work, the minimum required for a deep peel? Or is your only option a therapy that doesn't require a noticeable break in your daily routine? Finally, how much money are you willing to spend?

A physician should perform, or at least supervise, all procedures that entail some risk, including peels, skin sanding, injections, and, of course, surgery. It's a good idea to get the opinion of more than one physician before deciding on a procedure. Ask about risks, and get a detailed explanation so that you can intelligently weigh them. In particular, ask what is the longest possible healing time. It is highly improbable that any procedure claiming to magically erase wrinkles is free of risk.

As a general rule, if an over-the-counter product sounds too good to be true, it probably is. So far, the FDA has been having difficulty monitoring claims made by the cosmetics industry, because cosmetics, as defined by the FDA, are products whose sole purpose is to improve appearance. If a product affects a body structure or function, it is classified as a drug, and the manufacturer must demonstrate that it is safe and effective. With the use of ingredients such as AHA's, however, the line between cosmetics and pharmaceuticals has become blurred. The FDA was considering the regulation of these new "cosmeceuticals" in 1995, but whether it had sufficient resources for the task was unclear. • • •

For more information:

To obtain more information about various procedures or about physician services in your area, telephone the American Academy of Dermatology at 708-330-0050 or the American Society of Dermatologic Surgery at 800-441-2737.

Treating Hemorrhoids

By James L. Franklin

Hemorrhoids are among the most common ailments of Americans, but there's no need to suffer from them.

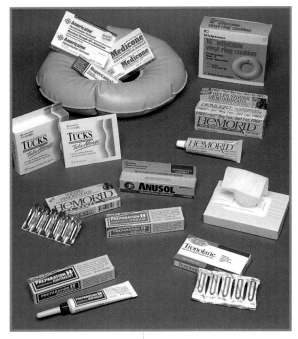

The variety of over-the-counter products to ease the discomfort of hemorrhoids testifies to the high incidence of this ailment.

HEMORRHOIDS ARE AMONG THE MOST COMMON DISORDERS in the United States, affecting an estimated 10 million people at any one time. The likelihood of the condition increases with age: As many as half of Americans over age 50 have a hemorrhoid.

A hemorrhoid is a swollen vein in the lining of the *rectum* (the lower end of the large intestine) or the *anus* (the opening at the end of the rectum). Depending on location, hemorrhoids are classified as internal or external. Internal hemorrhoids develop above the point where the rectum and anus meet; external hemorrhoids, below this point. As an internal hemorrhoid enlarges, it may *prolapse* (slip down) and protrude through the anus.

Although many hemorrhoids produce no discomfort, others cause pain or itching. Hemorrhoids that prolapse typically cause the greatest discomfort. The pain and itching that accompanies many prolapsed hemorrhoids results from inflammation of the mucous membrane around the swollen vein.

Several symptoms can indicate a hemorrhoid, though these symptoms are not confined to hemorrhoids alone. Probably the most common sign is the appearance of blood in the toilet bowl or on toilet tissue, or blood that drips from the rectum at the end of a bowel

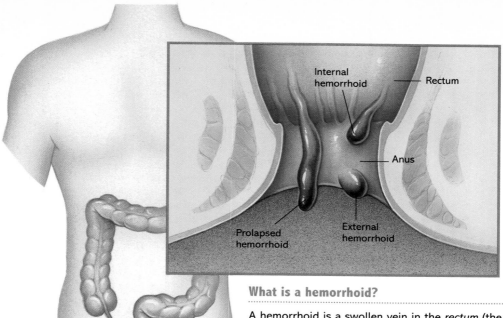

The author:

James L. Franklin is associate professor of medicine at Rush-Presbyterian-St. Luke's Medical Center in Chicago.

What is a hemorrhoid?

A hemorrhoid is a swollen vein in the *rectum* (the lowest part of the large intestine) or the *anus* (the extension and opening at the end of the rectum. Internal hemorrhoids occur above the site where the rectum and anus meet; external hemorrhoids, below this point. In some cases, internal hemorrhoids *prolapse* (slip down) and protrude through the anal opening.

movement. Bleeding occurs as a result of tiny tears in hemorrhoidal tissue—the swollen vein and the mucous membrane covering it.

Another sign is the sensation of a mass in the rectum, which results when hemorrhoidal tissue prolapses. Prolapsing may occur all the time or only during a bowel movement. A prolapsed hemorrhoid can soil underclothes with fecal matter, blood, or mucus, and the soiling can contribute to irritation or itching.

A hemorrhoid can become extremely painful if blood clots form in the swollen vein and obstruct circulation. This condition is known as thrombosis, and it usually prevents the prolapsed hemorrhoid from moving back into the anus or rectum.

What causes hemorrhoids?

Physicians do not know the precise cause of hemorrhoids. The condition appears to develop as a result of pressure on the many veins in the lining of the anus and rectum. The act of defecation normally causes these veins to *distend* (expand from pressure). Prolonged straining—from constipation, for example—may exaggerate this distention and lead to hemorrhoids. An extended bout of diarrhea also can distend the veins in the lining of the anus and rectum.

A study by a British researcher found that hemorrhoids are exceedingly rare in rural Africa and other developing regions, in sharp

Removing hemorrhoids

Mild cases of hemorrhoids can generally be treated with an ointment or suppository to relieve symptoms. But when a hemorrhoid becomes painful or bleeds, the physician may decide to remove it. The method chosen depends on the hemorrhoid's severity. Sclerotherapy and rubber band ligation can be performed in a physician's office, but the surgical removal of a hemorrhoid usually requires a hospital stay.

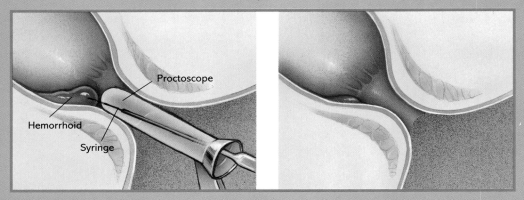

Sclerotherapy
In sclerotherapy, a physician injects a chemical solution into the hemorrhoid, using a syringe inserted through a tube called a proctoscope, *left*. The solution causes the hemorrhoid to harden and shrink, *right*. Physicians typically chose sclerotherapy for removing hemorrhoids that do not prolapse.

contrast to their high prevalence in developed Western nations. One explanation for the discrepancy is the low amount of fiber in most Western diets. People who eat little fiber have fewer bowel movements, pass harder stools with less bulk and lower water content, and are more likely to become constipated than are people whose diet is rich in fiber. All of these factors contribute to straining during a bowel movement.

Heredity also may play a role in the development of hemorrhoids. Just as varicose veins (swollen and twisted veins) occur more frequently in some families than in others, so may certain families be predisposed to hemorrhoids.

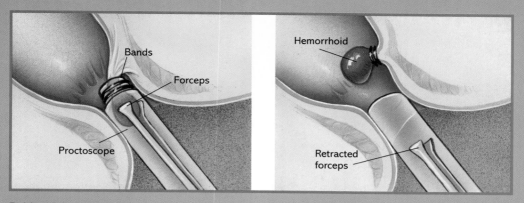

Rubber band ligation

In rubber band ligation, a physician uses a forceps to gently pull the hemorrhoid into a proctoscope, where a rubber band is placed around the hemorrhoid, *left*. The rubber band cuts off blood flow to the hemorrhoid, causing it to wither, *right*. Physicians generally choose rubber band ligation for removing hemorrhoids that prolapse during bowel movements only.

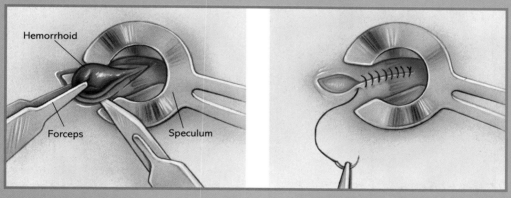

Hemorrhoidectomy

In a hemorrhoidectomy, a physician grasps the hemorrhoid with a speculum and forceps and cuts away the tissue with a knife, *left*. The wound is then closed up, *right*. Physicians generally choose surgery for constantly prolapsing hemorrhoids.

Certain medical conditions also increase the likelihood of hemorrhoids. Pregnancy, for example, often brings on hemorrhoids, presumably because pressure from the woman's enlarged uterus impedes the normal flow of blood through the veins of the anal canal. Large pelvic tumors can have the same effect. A type of liver damage known as cirrhosis can elevate blood pressure in the veins of the abdomen, including those veins that continue to the rectum. This condition can lead to markedly enlarged hemorrhoids and severe rectal bleeding.

It's important to see a doctor at the first sign of rectal bleeding, especially if you're over 40, because such bleeding can also be a sign of

Preventing hemorrhoids

Hemorrhoids are caused primarily by pressure on veins in the rectum or anal area. Straining during bowel movements puts pressure on these veins, and the best means of preventing hemorrhoids is to avoid straining. Physicians recommend the following steps:

- Keep the stool soft so that it passes easily. This can be accomplished by eating a diet high in fiber and drinking lots of liquids. High-fiber foods include fruits; vegetables, especially leafy kinds; and whole grains, especially bran.

- Exercise. Even moderate exercise, such as walking, helps prevent constipation and subsequent straining.

- Respond quickly to the urge to move your bowels, thereby avoiding possible difficulty later on.

- Avoid sitting too long on the toilet because it increases pressure on veins in the rectum.

Source: National Institute of Diabetes and Digestive and Kidney Diseases.

a much more serious condition, such as colon cancer. To diagnose a hemorrhoid, the physician examines the anal canal and rectum. As an aid to diagnosis, the physician may use an anoscope—a short, lighted tube that often is equipped with a slot into which the hemorrhoidal tissue slips.

To rule out any other causes of a patient's rectal bleeding, the physician is likely to examine larger areas of the rectum and colon. A variety of viewing instruments enable the physician to detect growths such as polyps or tumors that may lurk just above the anal canal and that could be responsible for the bleeding. Other possible causes of rectal bleeding that the physician may look for include inflammatory bowel disease and ulcerative colitis.

Treatment options

The treatment for hemorrhoids depends upon their severity, and the classification system physicians use for hemorrhoids reflects severity. First-degree hemorrhoids, the least advanced of all, remain in position within the anal canal. Second-degree hemorrhoids prolapse during defecation but spontaneously recede afterward. Third-degree hemorrhoids prolapse all the time but can be reduced by hand and pushed back into position. Fourth-degree hemorrhoids are large and prolapsed and do not respond to manipulation. Alleviating symptoms may suffice for treating first-degree hemorrhoids, whereas more advanced hemorrhoids may need to be removed.

Over-the-counter preparations or stronger prescription medications can reduce such hemorrhoidal symptoms as pain and itching. In addition, the physician will probably recommend strategies to reduce straining and relieve pressure on hemorrhoidal tissue. Most physicians advise adding fiber to the diet, either in foods or in supplement form. Foods high in fiber include fruits, vegetables, and whole grains. These foods, like such fiber supplements as psyllium (sold as Metamucil) or unprocessed bran, add bulk to stools and soften them. Laxatives can relieve constipation that may be contributing to straining.

If the symptoms cannot be controlled, physicians can perform a variety of procedures in their office that remove first- and second-degree hemorrhoids by shrinking them. These techniques include sclerotherapy, rubber band ligation, and infrared photocoagulation. They require no anesthesia and produce little discomfort.

In sclerotherapy, the physician injects a chemical solution into the hemorrhoid, which hardens and shrinks it. In rubber band ligation, the physician uses an instrument to grasp the hemorrhoid and place a rubber band around the tuft of swollen tissue. Strangling the hemorrhoid cuts off blood circulation to it, and the ensnared tissue withers away as a result.

Infrared photocoagulation also cuts off blood supply to a hemorrhoid but does so with a short burst of infrared radiation. The physician uses a gun-shaped instrument to deliver from half a second to three seconds of radiation, which scars the hemorrhoidal vein and stops blood flow into it.

Turning to surgery

Surgical removal, known as hemorrhoidectomy, is the standard treatment for third- and fourth-degree hemorrhoids. Techniques used less often, because of the expense of the equipment, are cryodestruction, which halts blood flow to hemorrhoidal tissue by freezing it, and laser removal, which uses a concentrated beam of light to vaporize a hemorrhoid.

Before a hemorrhoidectomy, the patient receives a local anesthetic, and the surgeon then makes a triangular incision that outlines the tissue to be removed. The tissue is grasped and cut, and the edges of the wound are closed with suture. Most patients are able to leave the hospital within 24 hours.

Hemorrhoidectomy, like all surgeries, entails some risks. Among the complications that sometimes occur immediately after surgery are bleeding, retention of urine, and impacted fecal matter. Other complications that may develop later also include bleeding, in about 2 percent of patients, and *stenosis* (narrowing) of the anal canal, in about 1 percent of patients. Pus-filled skin openings, known as abscesses of fistulae, occur in about 1 patient in 10,000.

Avoiding the problem

The best treatment for hemorrhoids is prevention, and the best means of preventing hemorrhoids is to keep the stool soft so that it passes without straining and to empty bowels as soon as possible after feeling the urge to do so. Physicians advise patients to avoid sitting on the toilet for long periods, which puts pressure on the veins. They also advise eating foods high in fiber and drinking six to eight glasses of nonalcoholic liquid daily, which makes it easier to empty the bowels and so reduces straining. Exercise also helps prevent constipation and consequent straining.

Hemorrhoids can be prevented. And when necessary, they can be treated to stop discomfort. ●●●

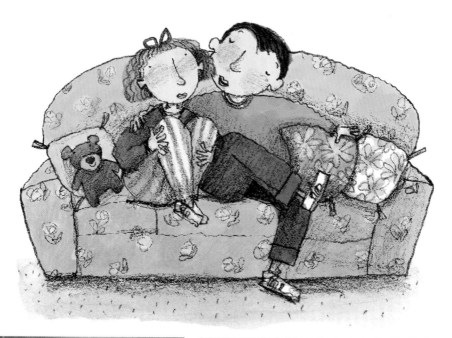

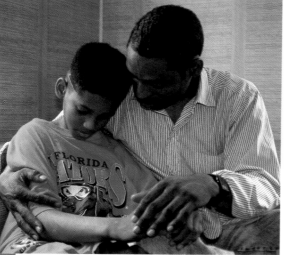

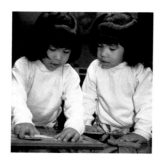

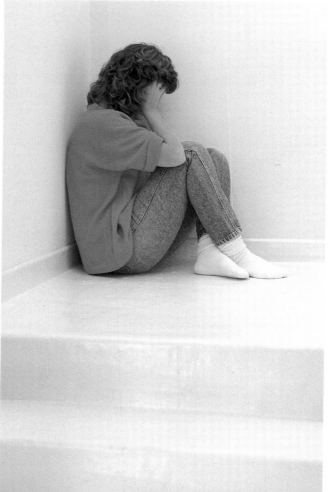

A Healthy Family

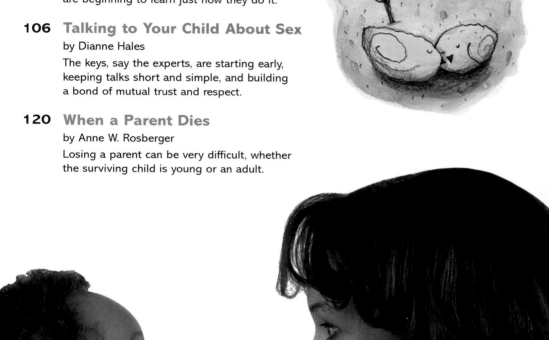

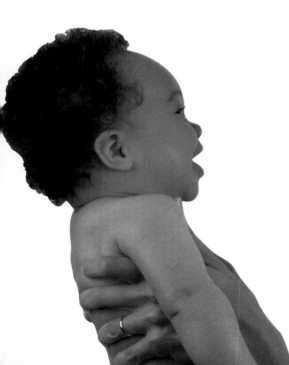

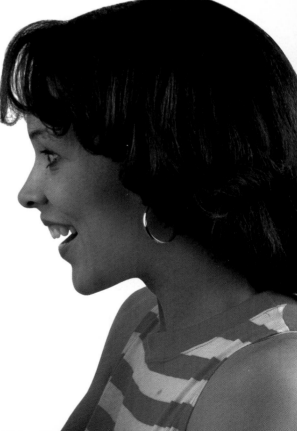

How Children Learn to Talk

By Kathy Hirsh-Pasek and Roberta Michnick Golinkoff

It takes only a few years for children to understand and use language effectively. Researchers are beginning to learn just how they do it.

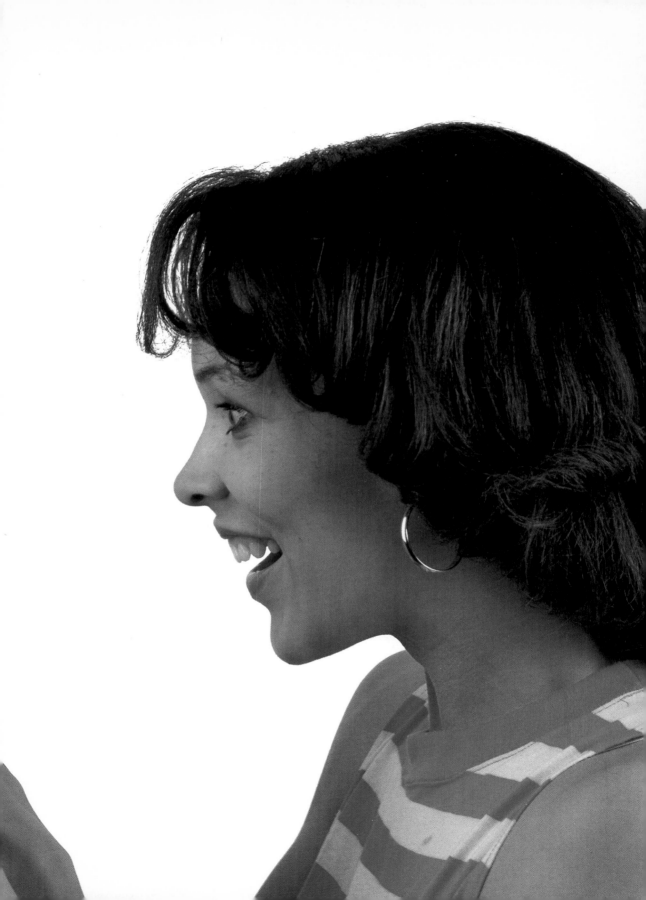

- **Five-year-old Michael:** "Mom, did you know that baseball games need a vampire?"
  Mother: "A vampire?"
  Michael: "Yes, the vampire stands in back of the catcher and catches any of the balls that the catcher misses."

- **Four-year-old Lisa:** "Nobody doesn't like me."
  Father: "You mean, 'Nobody likes me.'"
  Lisa: "OK, nobody doesn't like you."

MICHAEL AND LISA, LIKE YOUNG CHILDREN THE WORLD OVER, are engaged in one of the most difficult tasks they will ever perform: mastering the complex system we call language. To use language, a person must combine sounds into words and words into phrases and sentences—an effort that requires the mind to select from among countless possible arrangements. It is no wonder that scientists regard language as among the most complicated behaviors of the human species.

From a child's point of view, though, language is not complex at all—no more so than flying is to young birds. The errors preschoolers make when they speak mask the fact that children seem to learn language almost effortlessly. By the end of their first year, children can understand many things said to them and may have spoken their first words. By the time they are 2, most children can speak in short sentences and use language to influence the world around them. A 3-year-old can do what the most advanced computer cannot: share thoughts and ideas with others and represent events in the past, present, and future. And a 4-year-old can produce complex sentences and have rich and varied conversations.

Psychologists like ourselves who study how children acquire language are engaged in *psycholinguistics,* a discipline that combines elements of both linguistics and psychology. Psycholinguistics took off in the mid-1950's, sparked by the work of scholars such as the linguist Noam Chomsky. Whereas earlier researchers focused on describing the rules of specific languages and their development over time, Chomsky and others were concerned with how these rules take shape in the mind, and how they get translated into ordinary speech.

In the 1960's and 1970's, psychologists who studied children's language gathered data by observing children at home and school and by asking parents to keep records of their children's speech. Later, lightweight tape recorders, videocameras, and other devices enabled researchers to test their ideas in the laboratory as well as through more traditional methods. As a result, psychologists in the 1980's and 1990's have gained insights that go far toward explaining how children learn to use and understand language.

Although most people think of language as spoken language, language is not the same as speech. People with medical conditions that keep them from speaking still have language. Similarly,

The authors:

Kathy Hirsh-Pasek is associate professor of psychology at Temple University in Philadelphia. Roberta Michnick Golinkoff is professor of psychology, linguistics, and educational studies at the University of Delaware in Newark.

What is language?

Linguists describe language as having four distinct components: sound (or its sign language equivalent); meaning; grammar; and *pragmatics*, or language use.

The first component, sound, includes stresses that characterize words and sentences, such as the way English uses rising pitch to signal a question. It also includes rules governing individual sounds. In English, the last letter of the word *hats* is pronounced s, but the last letter of *heads* is pronounced *z*. This is because English speakers pronounce the final s in a word according to whether the consonant preceding it is spoken with the voice, as is *d*, or simply by moving the lips and tongue and releasing air, as is *t*.

The second component, meaning, has to do with the content of words and word groups, such as phrases and sentences. Meaning is complicated by the fact that words can mean different things in different contexts. A street sign reading "Slow Children," for example, means that drivers should progress with caution, not that children in the area dawdle. Another problem is that the relationship between most words and their meanings is arbitrary: that is, there is no obvious connection between the word and what it stands for—unlike, say, *hiccup*, which sounds like what it means. Many theorists believe that children link words to their meanings in part by forming categories, recognizing, for example, that though dogs can be large or small, they all share features that distinguish them from cats or elephants.

Grammar refers to the way people put sentences together, combining nouns, verbs, and other parts of speech in acceptable ways. Grammar allows us to combine a finite store of words into an infinite number of sentences. Grammar is also an important part of expressing meaning. The English sentences "The cat ate the mouse" and "The mouse ate the cat" use the same words, but they have opposite meanings, only one of which is likely to be true.

Pragmatics, the fourth component, governs how we use language to accomplish goals and to interact with others. It includes the use of words and phrases for social purposes, such as *please* and *thank you*. It also includes rules for carrying on conversations, such as taking turns and sticking to the subject. And it includes the use of language to joke, hint, persuade, and fill any other purpose of communication. A 4-year-old violates a rule of pragmatics when she responds "Yes" to the telephone caller's query, "Is your mother home?" The 4-year-old does not understand that the caller is making an indirect request, not asking for information.   [K. H.-P. and R. M. G.]

---

the sign languages used by deaf people are genuine languages that rely on hand movements and facial expressions instead of speech.

Scientists regard language as having four components: sound (or its sign language equivalent); meaning; grammar; and *pragmatics*, or language use. Each component has a set of rules that children must master. For more information on the components of language, see WHAT IS LANGUAGE? above.

The normal course of language development

Newborn infants hear only long, meaningless strings of sound. Before they can understand and use language, children must learn to break apart those strings into words, phrases, and other units. They must puzzle out the relationship between words and what they represent, and they must learn how sounds and words can be combined to express meanings. Finally, they must discover all the ways people use language to influence and interact with others.

The journey toward language begins before birth. That fetuses

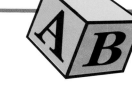

Milestones in children's language

Children acquire language at different rates. But most children reach the major milestones in language learning at roughly the following ages:

● 2 months	Coos and smiles.
● 6 to 10 months	Babbles repeated syllables, usually with one or more of the consonants *m, n, b, p, d,* and *t* (for example, *ninini* or *dadada*).
● 9 to 18 months	Produces speechlike gibberish.
● 10 to 12 months	Understands some words and simple phrases. Begins to point to people and things as a prelude to naming them.
● 12 to 18 months	Speaks first words.
● 18 to 24 months	Can say about 50 words. Makes two-word combinations.
● 2 years	Can take turns talking. Uses language to influence and relate to others.
● 2 to 2½ years	Begins to make three-word combinations.
● 2½ to 3 years	Begins to relate experiences.
● 3 to 4 years	Understands and uses basic rules of grammar, including past tense and questions. Vocabulary includes some prepositions and common adjectives.

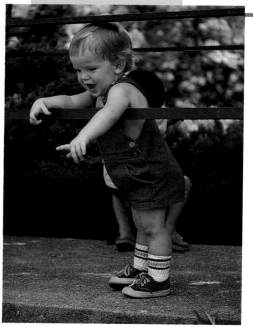

can hear sounds was discovered through experiments using a specially designed pacifier connected to an audiotape player. In one 1988 experiment, psychologists working in Paris found that French newborns sucked faster when they heard a recorded voice speaking French than when the same voice was speaking Russian, whereas newborns from non-French and non-Russian households did not alter their sucking for either language. The French infants even increased their sucking upon hearing their native tongue when the sound was electronically filtered, muffling the consonants and vowels. This suggests that the babies were responding to the melody of the language, which they had become accustomed to while in the womb, rather than to its specific sounds.

At first, babies produce few sounds other than grunts and cries. But at about 2 months, they begin to coo, making vowel sounds such as *ahhh* and *oooh*. Young infants have trouble producing consonants other than g or k. This is partly because an infant's relatively large tongue fills much of the mouth, making it awkward and inflexible. Also, a newborn's larynx—the voice box, where the vocal cords reside—sits high in the throat. This keeps the nasal passages open so the infant can breathe through the nose while swallowing, but it also hampers the movement of the tongue.

During the first year, the larynx descends deeper in the throat and the child begins to babble syllables. The first sounds to appear, usually by 7 or 8 months, are *b, p, d, t, m,* or *n,* which are made at the front of the mouth and so are fairly easy to pronounce. Linguists believe this is why in most languages, children's words for *mother* contain the letters *m* or *n* and their words for *father* contain *b, p,* or *d*—for instance, *mommy* and *daddy* in English, *imah* and *abah* in Hebrew, and *anuka* and *apuka* in Hungarian.

A month or two after babbling begins, most children start emitting strings of repeated syllables, like *babababa* and *dididi.* Just why babies do this is unknown, but researchers note that it is just one of many repetitive activities—like banging the arms and scissoring the legs—that babies enjoy around this time. Soon, however, babies begin to vary the sounds they babble, and they start producing speechlike gibberish. This kind of babbling can continue until the baby is about 18 months old.

Beyond coos and babbles

Around the time that babies start to babble, they also begin to recognize individual words. Researchers have evidence that babies can pick words out of the speech stream by about 9 months. In a study reported in 1994, psychologist Peter Jusczyk of the State University of New York at Buffalo repeatedly played a recorded story to 8½-month-old infants. Afterward, Jusczyk played various words through a loudspeaker for up to 20 seconds each and measured how long the babies looked toward the source of the sound. The children looked longer at the speaker when it played words that had appeared many times in the story than when it played other words, indicating that they recognized the sounds of those words they had heard more often.

Probably the first word that actually has meaning for a baby is his or her own name. By 6 or 7 months, a baby will turn if called by name. Gradually, children begin to associate more and more words with the objects and ideas they represent. In a 1994 study, psychologists at San Diego State University distributed a list of some 400 common words to parents and asked them to mark off those they believed their children understood. The psychologists concluded that most babies enter their second year comprehending about 100 words, though they speak only a few at most.

Another leap forward occurs during the second half of the first year, as babies learn to use sounds and gestures to communicate. By catching her mother's eye, reaching toward the mantelpiece,

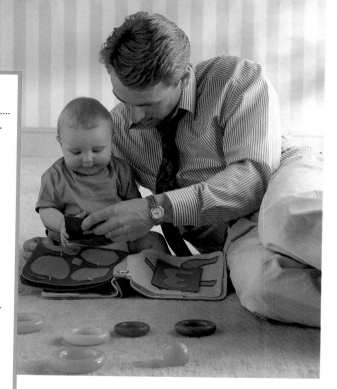

Encouraging language development in your child

Most experts agree that parents cannot "teach" language to a child. But parents can help strengthen and enrich a child's language.

From the beginning

- Talk to the baby about objects and events that the baby is involved with. Talking about the here and now helps babies link words with the meanings they represent.

- Ask the baby questions and answer them. ("Are you hungry now? You are? Let's get your cereal.")

- Describe to the baby your daily activities . . . but pause often to let the baby "talk" too.

- Imitate the baby's sounds.

- Play language-related games such as peek-a-boo and pat-a-cake.

- Read and sing poems, songs, and nursery rhymes. Children thrive on rhythm, rhyme, and repetition.

- Read aloud to the child often.

As the child learns to talk

- Rephrase and expand the child's talk. (Child: "Kitty go 'way." Parent: "Yes, the kitty went away. The kitty ran behind the couch, didn't it?")

- Ask questions often, especially those requiring more than a yes-or-no answer.

- Talk about what you read and see in picture books. For instance, ask what the child thinks about events described in a story or shown in its illustrations.

and emitting an insistent "Uh," a 9-month-old can indicate that she is interested in the shiny vase standing there and would like to examine it close up. Communication becomes even more effective when the baby learns to point, usually at 10 to 12 months. Through the extended forefinger, the child can now refer directly to things in the world—an important step on the road to language.

Shortly after pointing begins, children say their first words. Now, for the first time, toddlers can refer to things even when they are not visible, a major milestone in language development.

Babies the world over start talking with the same types of words. Most early words stand for things the baby handles, such as *bottle* and *sock*, or things that move, such as *dog, car,* and *mama.* Other words, such as *up* and *more,* have to do with the baby's daily routine. A baby's words may not mean what adults mean by them. The word *go,* for instance, might stand for cars, trains, or buses. The baby might use *all gone* to mean "I ate my lunch" or "The bird flew away" and *more* to mean "Give me more" or "Do it again."

At first, the child's spoken vocabulary grows slowly. By 18 to 24 months, most children can say about 50 words, though these are not always pronounced in easily recognizable ways. For reasons that are not well understood, this 50-word threshold marks the start of a period of rapid word growth. By some estimates, babies 18 to 24 months old learn an average of 9 new words each day. Psychologists often refer to this period as the naming explosion.

The 50-word watershed is also important for another reason: It heralds the beginning of grammar, when children combine words for the first time in truly creative ways. Before this point, some children learn whole phrases or sentences, such as "What's that?" or "I love you." But from the child's perspective, researchers believe, such productions represent one long word, *whatsthat* and *iloveyou*. The child is unable to separate out individual words and replace them with others to produce, for instance, "I love kitty."

From words to sentences

The beginning of grammar dramatically expands the ideas a child can express with a limited store of words. In their grammatically incomplete way, children can now talk about people doing things ("Daddy throw"), people and their possessions ("Mommy sock"), and interesting events ("Plane fly"). Children's early word combinations are often called telegraphic because they leave out all nonessential elements, including words like *the, to, my,* and *is,* and word endings like *s, ing,* and *ed.*

Just as children comprehend many words well before they can produce them, they seem to understand more grammar than they can produce. In experiments beginning in the 1980's, we showed toddlers pairs of videotapes featuring characters from the television program "Sesame Street." On one screen, the children—who were 17 months old on average—saw Big Bird tickling Cookie Monster, while on the other they saw Cookie Monster tickling Big Bird. A recorded voice then instructed the children to "Find Big Bird tickling Cookie Monster" or the reverse. The children consistently showed they understood the instructions by looking longer at the correct screen.

As children approach and then pass their second birthdays, their sentences grow longer and their grasp of grammar becomes more refined. Gradually, children add the grammatical forms that were missing from their two-word utterances. For instance, a 20-month-old who doesn't want her sandwich might say "No eat" or "No lunch." By 27 months, the child might produce a three-word sentence, "No eat lunch." A few months later, the sentence might include a subject: "I no want lunch." Finally, by 3 years or so, *no* gives way to the grammatically correct *don't*: "I don't want lunch."

Children add grammatical structures to their speech in a predictable order, beginning with the most common ones and concluding with those that are less often used or more complex. In English, one of the last structures children master is the passive voice. Many children have difficulty with such sentences as "The

Varying rates of language development

Some children reach language milestones a year or more after others their age without its being a cause for worry. Factors that can affect the rate of language development include:

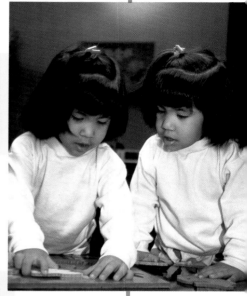

- The child is a boy.

- Some experts believe boys tend to reach language milestones slightly behind girls, perhaps because parents tend to spend more time talking with their daughters than their sons.

- The child is a younger sibling.

- The pressures of caring for a larger family may leave parents less time to talk with a younger baby. Older brothers and sisters also may interpret for the baby, leaving him little need to speak for himself.

- The child is a twin.

- Twins, like younger siblings, spend less time talking alone with parents than single children do.

- The child is learning more than one language.

- Children being raised in bilingual households need time to sort out one language from another.

boy was kicked by the horse" until their elementary school years.

By age 4 or 5, though, children's use of grammar is approaching that of adults—as is their grasp of the pragmatics of language. A 2½-year-old, for instance, told to "watch your head," would probably interpret the command literally—causing the child much puzzlement. A 4-year-old would correctly interpret the command as an indirect warning to be careful.

How parents can help

Although children pass through the stages of language learning in the same order, they don't do so at the same time. Some children who are developing normally speak their first words, start combining words, or reach other milestones as much as a year after others in their age group. In general, observers have noted, first-born children seem to talk earlier than younger siblings, perhaps because the demands of a larger family leave parents less time to talk with their younger children. Also, children being raised to speak two or more languages may take some time to sort out one language from another, a feat they typically accomplish by age 3.

To keep a child's language on course, experts advise, parents should talk with the child as much as possible, even before the baby can respond. Talking about the here now and helps babies link words to the events and objects they represent. Experts suggest that as parents play with their babies or perform various tasks, they should describe what they are doing, saying, for example, "Daddy's changing your diaper now." Parents also can encourage babies to express themselves by imitating the baby's own sounds and by giving the child a chance to "talk"—for instance, asking questions and waiting for the baby to coo in response.

With toddlers and preschoolers, parents can employ a technique sometimes called scaffolding to help strengthen and enrich the child's speech. In scaffolding, parents expand a child's utterance into grammatically correct speech, then prompt the child to venture additional talk. If a child says "Puppy wet," for instance, the parent might say "Yes, the puppy wet the bed. What should Mommy do?"—prompting a response such as "Mommy dry bed." In general, parents can encourage children to talk by favoring questions that require more than a yes-or-no answer, asking, for example, "What is the cat doing?" rather than "Do you see the cat?"

When language development lags

When children are given many opportunities to hear and use language, what appear to be problems in most cases correct themselves. Sometimes, though, children fail to reach language milestones along with others their age because something is hindering their language development. Parents should trust their instincts if they think something is wrong and consult a doctor or specialist in language disorders.

Specialists who deal with disorders of speech and language are called speech-language pathologists. These professionals can evaluate a child's ability to understand and produce language. They can then design a program tailored to the aspects of language the child needs to work on.

If a child seems not to be reaching language milestones, especially if the child does not react to others' speech, the problem could be a hearing impairment. Using computerized hearing tests, audiologists—specialists who diagnose and treat hearing defects—can screen even newborns for hearing problems. Testing for such problems early is crucial, doctors say, because failure to treat or compensate for hearing loss can lead to long-term language delay.

Most cases of hearing impairment in young children are temporary and easily treatable. A common cause is *otitis media*—an infection of the middle ear that results in a build-up of pus and mucus behind the eardrum. Sometimes, the fluid drains out naturally. But more often, it remains in the ear, muffling hearing. If untreated, the fluid build-up and impaired hearing can last for months or

Potential warning signs

The following signs suggest a child may have a speech or language problem. Parents also should trust their instincts, experts say, and consult a doctor or speech-language pathologist if they are concerned about their child's language.

- The child does not coo or babble during the first 6 months.
- The child does not understand simple phrases without visual cues by 12 to 18 months.
- The child has not said a few words by 18 months or put two words together by 24 months.
- The child has trouble chewing, sucking, or swallowing.
- The child repeats words or phrases without understanding them and without ever venturing meaningful speech.
- Stuttering is severe or persists after age 3.
- The child relies primarily on gestures to communicate after age 3.
- By age 4, the child does not use basic grammar, including question forms.

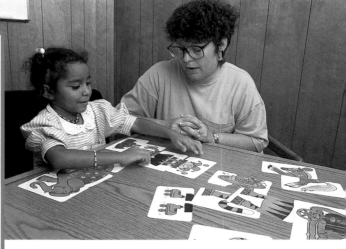

Specialists in speech and language can evaluate a child's language abilities and design a program tailored to the child's needs. A speech-language pathologist evaluates a preschooler's skills, *above*.

even years, often without producing obvious symptoms.

According to the American Speech-Language-Hearing Association (ASHA), based in Rockville, Md., about a third of American children suffer three or more bouts of otitis media by age 3. Studies have found that some of these children start to talk later than their peers, though they seem to catch up in most areas by age 4.

A doctor can diagnose otitis media by looking in the ears through an instrument called an otoscope. Usually, the condition can be treated at home with antibiotics. If a child has frequent ear infections, the doctor may recommend a procedure in which surgeons implant a tiny tube in the ear to allow fluid to drain out. The tube is removed when there is no longer a risk of infection.

About 1 in 1,000 American children have permanent hearing loss severe enough to affect language, according to ASHA. In many cases, a doctor can fit the child with a hearing aid or other device to enhance any remaining hearing. Some children can regain some hearing through a cochlear implant, a device that is surgically implanted in the ear. (In the section On the Medical Frontier, see COCHLEAR IMPLANTS: DELIVERING SOUND TO THE DEAF.)

Many experts recommend that children whose hearing cannot be helped by a hearing aid or other device be exposed to people fluent in a sign language as early as possible. Deaf children who learn to sign develop language the same way hearing children do, researchers believe, whereas those not exposed to either speech or sign language may always have poor language skills.

Unexplained language delay

In addition to hearing loss, rare conditions such as severe mental retardation interfere with language development. In children with the form of retardation known as Down syndrome, for instance, studies suggest that language development is commensurate with the child's mental age rather than chronological age.

But for some children whose language development is not progressing on course, doctors can find no obvious explanation. Specialists refer to these children as language-delayed. Some experts estimate that delayed language affects between 1 and 3 percent of American preschoolers.

Delayed language does not necessarily represent a serious problem. Some children have no difficulty understanding speech but, for unknown reasons, do not begin to speak until they are 4 years old or even older. Some medical problems, such as poor muscle development in the jaw, can keep a child from trying to produce speech. If a doctor does not diagnose such a problem, many specialists say, parents need not worry as long as the child's understanding is developing on course.

For other children, delayed language is more critical. As they grow into adolescence and beyond, these children may have trouble learning and recalling new words. They may find it hard to produce or understand long or complex sentences. They also may have difficulty with pragmatic aspects of language, such as understanding indirect requests.

Researchers do not understand why some children become language-delayed. A likely explanation in many cases, specialists say, is that children with this problem have some underlying disorder affecting areas of the brain important for language learning. Researchers are exploring new techniques, including scanning devices that produce images of the brain, which, they say, may begin yielding answers to this puzzle by the year 2000 or 2005. In the meantime, early diagnosis and treatment offer the best hope for language-delayed children. Researchers have found that by using specific strategies—such as teaching children to imitate particular

When parents need not worry

Many parents mistakenly fear their child's language is not developing on course. The following situations are common in children with normally developing language abilities.

- **Stuttering.** Many children stutter for a time around age 2, when their need to express themselves far outpaces their ability to shape thoughts into words. Parents should consult a speech pathologist if a child continues to stutter after age 3.

- **Irregular verbs.** At 2½ or 3, many children say *goed* for *went, breaked* for *broke*, and the like. Children learn general rules, such as the rule for forming the past tense by adding "-ed" to a verb, before they memorize exceptions.

- **Pronunciation.** It can take until age 8 for a child to become adept at *articulating* (pronouncing) certain sounds, such as *th, y, l,* and *r.* Unless the child's articulation embarrasses the child or hampers communication, experts advise letting the child's speech mature on its own.

- **Late talking.** It's all right for a child not to talk, even as late as 18 months, experts say, as long as the child understands as much as others at the same age. Some children simply start to talk late.

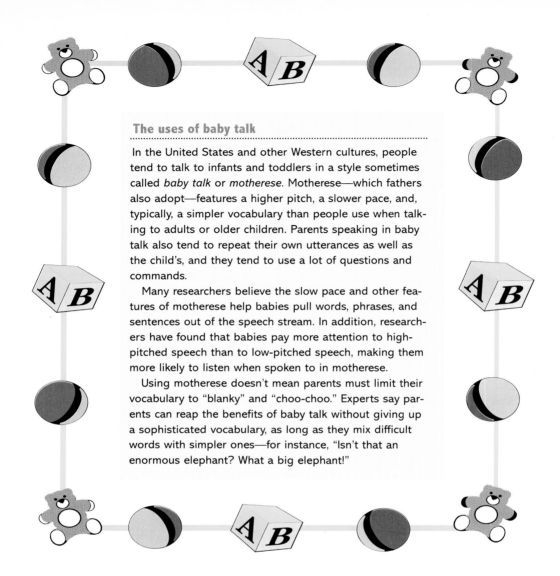

The uses of baby talk

In the United States and other Western cultures, people tend to talk to infants and toddlers in a style sometimes called *baby talk* or *motherese*. Motherese—which fathers also adopt—features a higher pitch, a slower pace, and, typically, a simpler vocabulary than people use when talking to adults or older children. Parents speaking in baby talk also tend to repeat their own utterances as well as the child's, and they tend to use a lot of questions and commands.

Many researchers believe the slow pace and other features of motherese help babies pull words, phrases, and sentences out of the speech stream. In addition, researchers have found that babies pay more attention to high-pitched speech than to low-pitched speech, making them more likely to listen when spoken to in motherese.

Using motherese doesn't mean parents must limit their vocabulary to "blanky" and "choo-choo." Experts say parents can reap the benefits of baby talk without giving up a sophisticated vocabulary, as long as they mix difficult words with simpler ones—for instance, "Isn't that an enormous elephant? What a big elephant!"

utterances—speech-language pathologists can help these children overcome at least some language deficits.

How do they do it?

Researchers have come a long way toward understanding the normal course of language development and the circumstances that can interrupt it. A more difficult question is *how* children acquire language. How are children transformed from gurgling newborns into linguistically creative preschoolers?

One camp in the debate over this issue consists of psycholinguists who believe that the human brain is genetically programmed to learn language. These researchers argue that exposure to speech triggers the emergence of language, much as water and sunlight trigger the germination of a seed. A second camp holds that the driving force behind language is the desire to communicate. These

Although schools may incorporate some discussion of sexuality in the early elementary grades, most such classes focus on correct anatomical terms and reproduction in animals. Even when they offer more comprehensive discussions, classes should be viewed as a complement to, rather than a substitute for, conversation. "You could leave the job of sex education to the schools," Kelly notes, "but parents are the ones who can emphasize values most effectively."

First steps toward sex education

Even before they speak, children absorb their first lessons in sexuality. The way parents clean a baby's genitals, their responses to toilet training, their looks of approval or disapproval in response to a youngster's words and actions contribute to a child's self-image and sense of sexuality.

Being prepared for questions

To a child, questions about body parts or where babies come from are the same as questions about anything else. If a question comes up in an inappropriate location, such as a supermarket line or a crowded restaurant, tell the child you'll answer it later and make sure you do. If you don't, children will draw the conclusion that they shouldn't ask questions about sex.

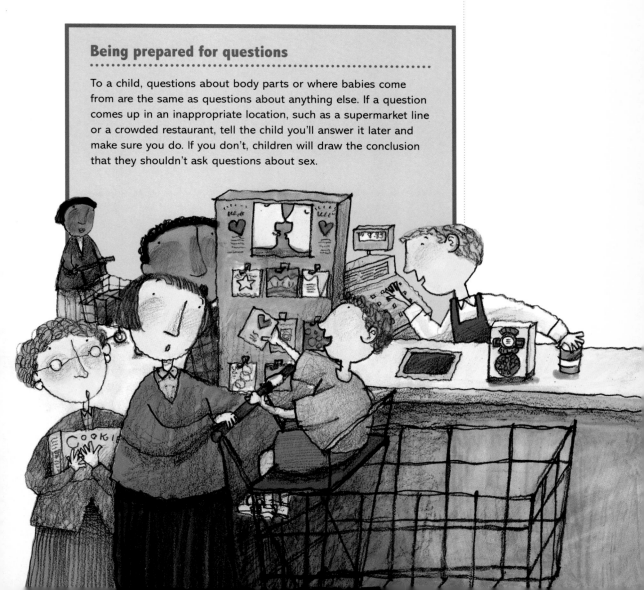

"Much of what children learn about their own sexuality and the sexuality of others comes from the ways their parents behave, not from what their parents say," observes psychologist Larry Kutler, author of *Parent and Child*. "The sexual values and beliefs that express themselves forcefully in adolescence and adulthood are rooted, in part, in children's early concepts of themselves."

A child's very first lessons in sex education may not have anything directly to do with sex. "The mechanics of sex are probably the least important aspects of sexuality that children learn," says Kutler, who points out that the bad outcomes of sexual activity that parents fear most—unwanted pregnancy, rape, sexually transmitted diseases—do not come about solely because of sexual behaviors.

"They all involve issues related to how people feel about and treat others and how they handle issues of responsibility. Far more critical to children than learning the details of intercourse at a young age is understanding that they should think of others as independent and worthwhile human beings. It is especially important that they learn to think of themselves as worthy of others' respect and capable of making their own decisions, for that will inoculate them against many forms of sexual exploitation when they become older."

The most effective way for parents to impart these qualities is by modeling them in their everyday interactions. By taking good care of their own bodies, parents demonstrate the importance of healthy behavior. By encouraging children to express their feelings and opinions, they show that they're interested in their youngster's point of view. By listening without judging, they encourage open communi-

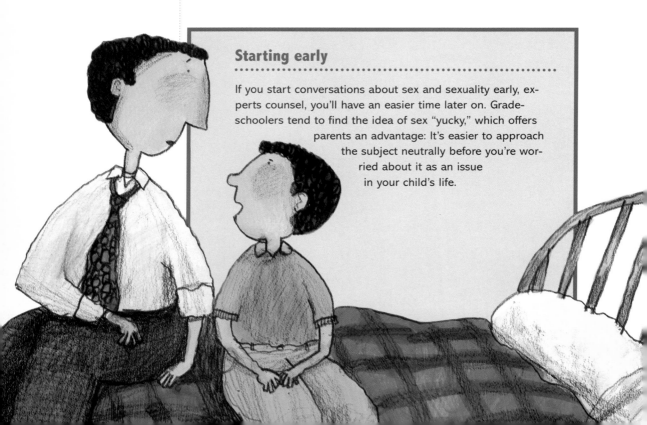

Starting early

If you start conversations about sex and sexuality early, experts counsel, you'll have an easier time later on. Grade-schoolers tend to find the idea of sex "yucky," which offers parents an advantage: It's easier to approach the subject neutrally before you're worried about it as an issue in your child's life.

cation and trust. And by emphasizing sensitivity to the feelings and needs of others, they instill in their youngsters an understanding of responsible, caring relationships.

General guidelines

When a discussion does turn to sex, the tone parents adopt is as important as content. Parents should be respectful, never laughing at a child's questions or comments or dismissing them as silly or trite. Children who learn early that they can bring up sex without fear of ridicule, rebuke, or embarrassment develop a trust that can endure into adolescence.

Because sexual attitudes and values are highly personal and can provoke deep emotion, parents should think through what they most want to communicate to their children. In addition to providing basic birds-and-bees information, they may want their youngsters to grow up with positive feelings about their bodies and about being a boy or a girl. Or, remembering painful or embarrassing experiences of their own, they may want to reassure children that sexual thoughts and feelings are normal or to warn youngsters about the dangers of sexual exploitation or abuse.

For parents who find even the thought of talking about sex with their children intimidating, preparation can help. There are excellent basic books about human sexuality, as well as guides for talking with youngsters, available in libraries and bookstores. Practicing what you'd like to say, either alone or with a partner or friend, often is useful. "It also may help to put an emotional distance between you by pretending for a few minutes that you're talking with someone else's child," suggests Kelly.

If you still feel nervous, admit it to your child. You might say, "I know this feels kind of awkward for both of us. But when I was growing up, I wished I could have talked to my parents about sex. Even though it may be a little embarrassing at first, I want you to know that in our house it's okay to talk about sex, and I'll try to be as open and honest as I can."

One of the best ways of introducing sex into daily conversation is by looking for "teachable" moments. Often family pets offer opportunities for explaining basic sexual biology. When psychologist Selverstone brought home two gerbils—which he believed to be males—his family was surprised by the birth of five babies. "It was a wonderful teachable moment, and we talked about how gerbils make babies, about the penis and the vagina, about the fact that human beings have babies in the same way. And our daughter, who wasn't ten yet, just went, 'Yuck!' and ran away. But she came back in a couple of weeks and said, 'Remember you were talking about the penis and the vagina? Tell me some more about that.'"

Such conversations show children that sex is woven into the fabric of daily life and that they needn't be afraid to ask or talk about it. If children aren't yet ready to absorb what parents have to say, at least they learn that they can turn to you when they do want to know more.

Watching television with children also can provide plenty of chances to converse about sex. If there are comments about virginity, for instance, you might explain that a virgin is a person who has never had sexual intercourse and that many young people remain virgins until they're more mature and involved in a committed relationship. If a man and a woman go into a clinch, you might ask what your kids think (under-tens will find such displays gross). Ask what a girl seems to find attractive about a boy and vice versa, how your child might feel in a similar situation, if it would make a difference if he were a girl or she were a boy.

You also can use characters on a TV show to introduce the concept of sexual decision-making and responsibility. If two teenagers on screen talk about having sex, you might comment that you hope that your youngsters will wait until they're older before taking such a big step and raise questions about birth control and safe sex. Rather than lecturing, try to draw youngsters out so they can start thinking about these issues.

Answering a young child's questions

With young children, conversations about sex should be simple and brief. Each talk adds to your youngster's understanding and helps you become more comfortable discussing sex—something that will help as children get older and ask for more detailed information.

Sex education may begin informally with the naming of various body parts, including sexual ones. Children invariably notice when parents don't mention their genitals or use special names for them. Most sex educators advise teaching the correct anatomical terms in a matter-of-fact way. However, such terms can sound disconcerting coming out of the mouths of babes. To avoid the embarrassment of a curious preschooler asking Great Aunt Martha if she has a vagina, parenting advisor Marguerite Kelly suggests using the correct terminology in conversations at home but allowing more euphemistic language in public places or with people other than immediate family members. However, as children mature, using precise terms to explain sexuality makes the subject less difficult, confusing, and awkward—for parents and youngsters.

When preschoolers ask about sex, they often choose less than perfect places or times. While you don't have to respond in the supermarket line or a crowded restaurant, let your child know that you will answer his question just as soon as you get to the car or arrive home. Once you are in a quiet spot, bring up the subject. If you don't, children may assume you don't want to talk about sex—or that they did something bad by asking.

One of the most common mistakes parents make, say sex educators, is telling very young children more than they can understand or ever wanted to know. "Children understand sex the same way they understand anything—according to the level of their thinking," Kelly notes. At 3 or 4, when children start asking where babies come from, their minds are incapable of grasping the complex process of reproduction. Explaining that a baby grows inside a Mommy usually suffices. Listen carefully and answer only the questions they ask. A 4-year-old who asks where he lived inside Mommy doesn't need a lecture in anatomy but a simple explanation that he grew inside a special place called a uterus. "You need to spread out information in many small talks, repeating what you've already said several times, so children can assimilate what you've said before you give them more," Kelly says.

At 5 or 6, children will ask for more detailed explanations of their origins. This is an ideal time for parents to explain and to talk about taking care of babies, thereby introducing the concept of sexual relationships and responsibility. At 7 or 8, children will want more specifics about sex: How does the sperm get inside the vagina? Is it like going to the bathroom? How does the baby get out? Simple, clear explanations are best. Be brief, and don't be surprised if youngsters find what you say so repulsive that they're sure sex is some-

Looking for teachable moments

One of the best ways of introducing the topic of sex and sexuality, experts advise, is by finding teachable moments. Pregnancy provides an opportunity for a discussion with a young child. Messages about sex and sexuality from television, movies, or advertising present opportunities for discussion with an older child. Rather than lecture, try to draw the child out and see what he or she thinks.

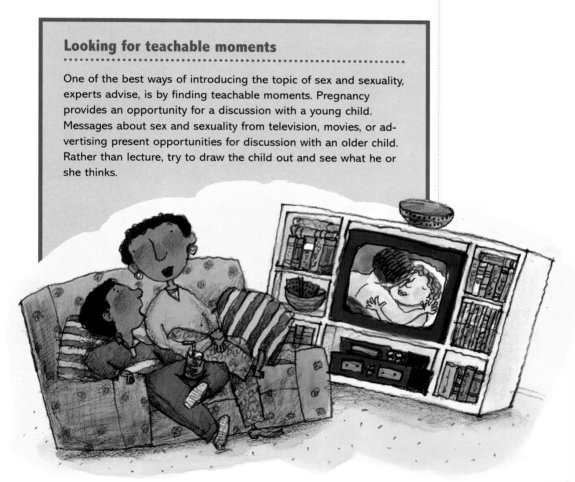

thing they'll never, ever do. "That's a natural reaction," observes noted sex therapist "Dr. Ruth" Westheimer. "Sex only makes sense when it's connected to feelings for another person. Kids don't have these feelings yet and won't really understand them until they do."

But the very fact that grade-school children aren't caught up in the tumult of emotions and hormones is an advantage for parents. "The early grade school years are a gift in terms of laying the groundwork for good communication," says Adler. "Once you're worried about sex as an issue in your child's life, you can't approach it neutrally, and the messages get a lot more complicated."

If a grade-schooler doesn't ask about sex by age seven, take the initiative and bring it up. "The longer you put off The Talk, the more awkward it will be," observes Kelly. You might bring home carefully selected books from the store or library and suggest reading them together, offer them to your youngsters, or leave them where they can read them in private (and they will). Volunteer to answer any questions—or ask questions yourself. Getting a sense of how much your children know can help you decide where to start a discussion and how much information to impart. It can also bring out misconceptions youngsters have picked up from their peers, providing you with an opportunity to correct them

Discussing sex and sexuality with an adolescent

If you haven't been talking about sex casually through the years, your initial conversations with a preteen or teen are bound to be awkward. To prepare yourself, do some homework. "Parents today usually don't have all the knowledge they need to pass on to their children because they weren't necessarily given the information themselves when they were young," observes sex educator Wise. In particular, parents may want to gather up-to-date information on sexually transmitted diseases (STD's), birth control, and safe sex. But don't feel you need to know everything a youngster might possibly ask. If you don't have an answer, simply say so. Then you, or you and your youngster, can do some research and find out.

With 11- to 13-year-olds, one unspoken concern almost always is, "Am I normal?" These self-conscious youngsters need reassurance that their bodies, changing before their eyes, are developing as they should. "Young people constantly check themselves out in comparison with others," says Selverstone. While they can see obvious changes, there are many aspects of sexual development they can't see. Boys may be confused and embarrassed by their unpredictable erections. Girls may fear that their breasts are too big, too small, or never going to develop at all.

Often the best way for parents to approach such sensitive subjects is by disclosing some information about themselves. "If a mother wants to bring up the subject of getting one's period with her daughter, she might tell her daughter how she first felt," says Wise. "That sets up a safe environment for the child and establishes an opportunity for dialogue. There's vulnerability and disclosure on both sides, not just a lecture from a parent and a disclosure from the child. Parents also have to remember not to be judgmental. If a child asks a question, they must give an honest answer and separate fact from opinion. They can give both—but they should identify them as what they are."

Youngsters also need reassurance that their sexual feelings and thoughts are normal—and, despite their surprising force, controllable. Parents might point out that, while sexual desires come from the body, decisions about what to do about them are made in the head. And the best decisions—about sex or any other important aspect of life—are made carefully, slowly, and thoughtfully.

Promoting responsible behavior

Most parents would prefer that their children wait until they are mature before entering sexual relationships. Researchers have found that children armed with information, good self-esteem, and a sense of values tend to delay sexual activity. Letting children know you trust their ability to make decisions and giving them the information with which to make those decisions, sex educators point out, keeps lines of communication open and makes sexual acting out less attractive as a way to rebel.

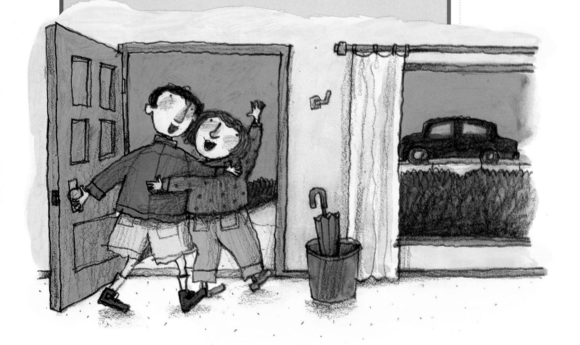

Helping adolescents set limits

Parents might encourage youngsters to think about setting limits on sexual behavior in advance so they don't get into situations where they're forced to make a split-second decision about sexual activity. As they watch television or videotapes with youngsters, parents might point out that each person in a relationship often has different expectations: Some boys think girls should set the limits. Girls may think boys will know when to stop—and will always accept a "no" as a "no." Both have to understand that truly caring, committed partners respect each other's feelings and words. Parents also should point out that alcohol or drugs can make it harder for teens to think clearly or to stick to a decision not to have sex.

Because of what they see in the media and hear from peers, teens may feel that everyone else their age is having sex. To balance this message, parents might note that there are many ways other than intercourse for people to be sexual—holding hands, kissing, hugging—and that just because somebody a youngster is dating wants sex doesn't mean he or she has to want it too.

Parents also should underscore the seriousness of deciding to have intercourse. Among the questions they might suggest that teens consider: Am I ready to have sex? Is someone pressuring me to do it? What might happen after I have sex with this person? What if I get an STD? What if sex results in pregnancy, even if we use birth control? Would I want to raise a child on my own? Would I want to get married? Will I regret having had sex later if I meet someone I truly love? Will I be hurt if I find out my partner is only interested in sex, not me? Will I feel guilty afterward? Will I get a bad name or reputation? Will I feel bad about myself?

Deciding to go all the way, as Dr. Ruth tells teens in *Dr. Ruth Talks to Kids*, is a very serious matter for a number of reasons. First of all, sexual intercourse can result in an unwanted pregnancy. In addition, it carries the risk of contracting of a sexually transmitted disease, including the most dangerous one of all, AIDS. Furthermore, Dr. Ruth points out, sexual intercourse can end in disappointment or unhappiness if it does not occur in the context of a warm, loving, and joyous relationship and is not shared by two people who feel strongly about each other and know exactly what they're doing. "That's why it's sometimes called 'making love.' It's such a powerful experience that no teen-agers I know are ready for it."

Parents might also acknowledge that saying no, especially to someone you care for, is hard. In its guide for teens, "Deciding to Wait," the American Academy of Pediatrics offers specific responses for resisting sexual pressure: "I like you a lot, but I'm not ready to have sex." "You're really fun to be with, but I wouldn't want to ruin our relationship with sex." "You're a great person, but sex isn't something I do to prove I like someone." "I'd like to wait until I'm married to have sex."

Because rebellion is normal in adolescence, communication between parents and teens on any and all subjects, including sex, may

Helping your child handle peer pressure

Peers play an extremely important role in adolescent development, and not conforming to peer group standards can be difficult for a teen. To help adolescents avoid hurting themselves or others, the American Academy of Pediatrics suggests that parents:

- Talk with children about the importance of caring relationships and what they hope the child will gain from and contribute to such relationships.

- Encourage the child to think through feelings about a relationship before it gets serious and to decide what he or she wants from the relationship. This can help the child avoid making a split-second decision on a date.

- Explain to adolescents that it's a good idea to know their limits and not let anyone talk them into going beyond those limits. Remind them that, though saying no isn't always easy, it's better to say no than to be pressured into doing something they don't want to do.

- Acknowledge that an adolescent may be afraid of hurting the other person's feelings by saying no. Some things that an adolescent might say: "I like you a lot, but I'm just not ready to have sex." Or "You're a great person, but sex isn't how I prove I like someone."

- Point out that there are ways of expressing sexuality other than intercourse, such as holding hands, kissing, and hugging.

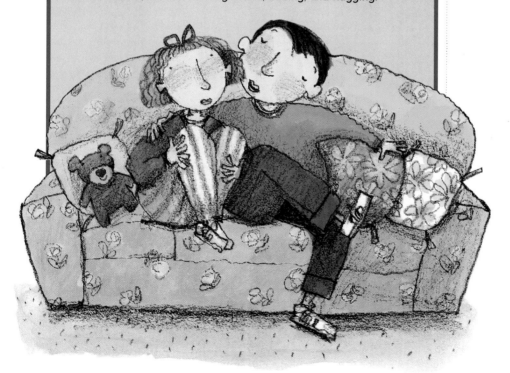

be difficult at times. "Parents have to try extra hard to be there for their teens," says Selverstone. "They have to understand that they frequently will be rejected and encourage children to make up their own minds. This means that though their children may not follow their peers, they also may not follow their parents. Parents need to have been good role models and been accepting of other points of view so the child has the courage to reject the peer group and delay sexual activity."

A nonjudgmental, trusting approach can help. "Let your children know that you respect their ability to make their own decisions about these issues," advises Kutler. "The fear that your child will make the wrong decision often turns into a self-fulfilling prophecy. The idea that you can control your children's sexual activity is an illusion. Demonstrating faith in their ability to make decisions regard-

Having the facts and getting started

For parents who feel uneasy about talking to their children about sex, preparation can help. A number of books and videotapes are available to help parents get started.

Readings:

- Calderone, Mary. *Talking with Your Children About Sex: Questions and Answers for Children from Birth to Puberty.* Ballantine, 1983.
- "Deciding to Wait: Guidelines for Teens." American Academy of Pediatrics, P.O. Box 927, Elk Grove Village, IL 60009.
- Johnson, Eric. *Love and Sex and Growing Up.* Bantam, 1990.
- Mayle, Peter. *Where Did I Come From?* Lyle Stuart, 1973.
- Mayle, Peter. *What's Happening to Me?* Lyle Stuart, 1975.
- Meredith, Susan. *Where Do Babies Come From?* EDC Publishing, 1991.
- Schaefer, Charles, and Teresa DiGeronimo. *How to Talk to Your Kids About Really Important Things.* Jossey-Bass, 1994.
- Westheimer, Ruth. *Dr. Ruth Talks to Kids.* Macmillan, 1993.

Videotapes:

- "Questions Children Ask About Sex." Children's Television Workshop.
- "What Kids Want to Know About Sex and Growing Up." Children's Television Workshop.

ing sex and providing them with the information they need to make those decisions help keep the lines of communication open between you. It also makes sexual acting out less attractive as a way to rebel."

Preventing risky behavior

As with other sexual subjects, it's a good idea to address the risks early in a child's life. According to health experts, most grade-schoolers have heard about HIV and AIDS and are both curious and concerned. Children between 5 and 7 years of age need reassurance that HIV is not like the "bugs" that cause colds and flus and cannot be spread by everyday activities, like using a public water fountain or restroom. Between ages 8 and 10, youngsters should be told that a person with HIV can pass it on through intimate sexual contact and dirty needles used to inject illegal drugs. They also should be told that playing with a child who has AIDS is safe and that young-sters with AIDS deserve understanding and kindness. Let children know that many people are afraid of AIDS and that talking about such concerns can help.

Conversations about sexual risks can serve as an opportunity to discuss healthy behaviors and responsible decision-making. Rather than delivering moralistic lectures, parents might ask youngsters how they think they can protect themselves. Typically, adolescents are convinced that nothing bad—be it an unwanted pregnancy or a sexual infection—could ever happen to them. Even sexually in-formed teens will cling to myths, such as the mistaken notion that a girl can't get pregnant during her period or that you can somehow "tell" whether a potential partner has HIV. Parents might take note of examples—in the newspaper, on television, in the community— of teens who did indeed become pregnant or develop AIDS. They can use these cases in point to ask questions, such as, "What do you think they could have done to protect themselves?" "How would you feel if you were in their place?" Because it bears repeating often, parents should note that the only sure protection against pregnancy and STD's is abstinence.

Raising sexually responsible children

As parents, we teach our youngsters about all sorts of subjects in the hope of preparing them for a happy, healthy, fulfilling life. The goal in talking about sex is the same: to raise responsible children who make decisions carefully and thoughtfully and can resist the pres-sure of peers. We know that, within a loving, mature relationship, sexual intimacy can be one of the most rewarding experiences our children will ever know. We also realize the very real dangers of irre-sponsible sexual behavior. By offering both information and insight, by placing sex in a context of caring, we equip our children to face the future with a true understanding of both the rewards and the risks of sexual behavior.

•••

When a Parent Dies

By Anne W. Rosberger

Losing a parent
can be very
difficult, whether
the surviving child
is young or
an adult.

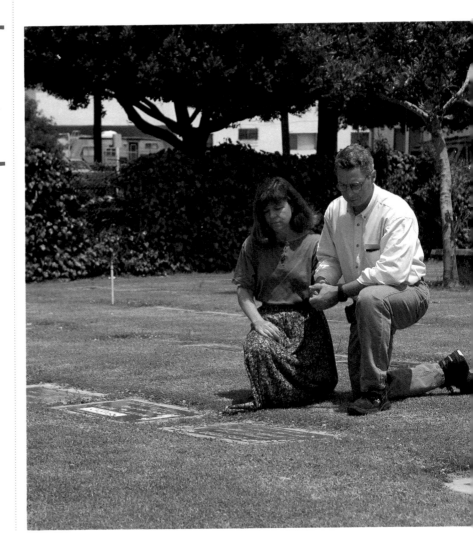

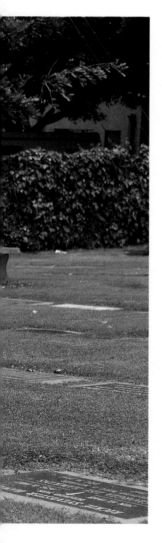

KATHERINE WAS 40 YEARS OLD when her mother died after a long battle with breast cancer. Katherine had watched, feeling helpless, as her mother lost weight, hair, energy, and finally her life. Even though Katherine had done everything she could to support her mother throughout her illness, she could not let go of the sense that she could or should have done more. Could she have chosen better doctors or forced her mother to try another treatment regimen? Their relationship had been good, but there still seemed to be so much left unsaid. Katherine longed to tell her mother one last time how much she loved her and needed her. She yearned for a chance to erase past arguments. Subsequent family milestones in Katherine's life—her own daughter's first birthday, for example—brought tears of loss and loneliness over her mother's absence. Katherine feared she would never feel strong, happy, and whole again.

Katherine's reaction exemplifies the anguish felt by many of the people I counsel as director of the Bereavement and Loss Center of New York. Losing a parent can be one of the most emotionally shattering experiences of a lifetime. Whether the surviving child is young or old, the sense of loss and abandonment and the fear of being left alone in the world can be overwhelming.

The attachment between parent and child is among the most emotionally intense of human bonds and is tied closely to an individual's sense of self-worth, dependence, and vulnerability. As newborns, we depend completely on our parents. As we grow older, the nature of our attachments and needs may change, but the powerful quality of the parent-child connection remains. Even if the relationship with our parents is riddled with problems—and sometimes because of those very problems—the bond is enduring.

Losing a parent can shake a person's very foundations, robbing individuals of the sense that someone is shielding them, if not in a physical sense, then in an emotional way. Although the experience of losing a parent varies dramatically from one person to another, experts recognize certain common themes of grieving. Some reactions to a parent's death are common to children, others are common to adults, and still others span the ages. Although reactions may differ, one thing is common to all human beings: the ability to move past grief and rebuild our lives.

A time to prepare

When family members know that a parent's death is imminent, the result perhaps of an incurable illness, they have time to prepare. Even though the pain of the experience cannot be erased, it is possible to lessen the burden at the most stressful time by preparing emotionally and making practical arrangements in advance.

First, professionals say, it's important for people to recognize their feelings about a parent's approaching death. At this time, they might let themselves mull over, talk about, even write down their emotions. Grief counselors find that acknowledging feelings and facing the reality of the impending death makes it easier to accept the death when it actually occurs.

Being open about feelings can be difficult. In the short term, talking about pain is more difficult than hiding it. But bottling up despair, anger, and fear may prolong grief, interfering with the ability to cope with the pain of the parent's absence and to move on.

Additionally, professionals advise families to use the months or weeks before a parent's death to make decisions about the funeral or memorial service, cremation or burial, and other ways of honoring the deceased. This may be a time to talk with a parent about his or her wishes and for family members to share their thoughts. Making practical arrangements just after the death can be very difficult because emotions are running high and people often are unable to communicate clearly or calmly. Getting as much as possible under control before the death—choosing a funeral home and burial site, for example—will make things easier when the unhappy day arrives. Drawing up a checklist can be helpful, as can a division of tasks so that no one person bears the brunt of the arrangements.

Preparing for a parent's death also offers a chance to bring a sense of closure to the relationship. Many people who lose a parent unexpectedly are plagued by the frustration that they were never able to say good-by. Those who have time to prepare may want to end a long-lasting feud, make promises or apologies, or express love, gratitude, remorse, and other emotions. At the same time, professionals caution, there is no way to say everything to a dying parent. The parent-child bond and the experiences of a lifetime, together or apart, are simply too complex to sum up in several sittings. But, an adult child can express important sentiments in the time remaining.

Sudden death is especially unfortunate for survivors in that it robs them of the opportunity to express these sentiments. At the same time, survivors should remember that a sudden death may be more serene for the parent.

No rules for grieving

There is no step-by-step manual on how to grieve the loss of a parent—or any other death. Grief is a deeply personal experience. Experts note that several factors affect how we respond to the loss of a parent. These factors include our personality, the relationship we

The author:

Anne W. Rosberger is Executive Director of the Bereavement and Loss Center of New York in New York City.

had with the deceased parent, the relationship we have (or do not have) with the surviving parent, and the circumstances of the parent's death. A problem-ridden relationship with the deceased parent, for example, can leave behind regret and guilt.

If the death has been the result of homicide or suicide, survivors are plagued with questions of why and may be left with a great sense of unfairness, powerlessness, and frustration. In the case of suicide, they may suffer from guilt and a sense of shared responsibility as well.

A time to mourn: Four stages of grief

While no two people mourn alike, professionals recognize stages of grieving that are common to many of us. Four stages in the grieving process were named and described in the late 1960's by John Bowlby, a British psychiatrist and the author of a fundamental study of bereavement. People may shift back and forth among the stages, Bowlby wrote, though all four are evident at one time or another after the loss. It's important to remember that these stages vary greatly in intensity from one person to another.

The first stage is often a period of shock, disbelief, and denial, during which the survivor does not or cannot admit that the loss has occurred. The person may feel that "it just can't be" and may walk around as if in a daze. Feelings of numbness may alternate with intense distress during this first stage, which can last from a few hours to a week or more.

The second stage of grieving is one of yearning and searching for the dead parent. During this period, mourners may obsess over the loss and feel that no one understands their grief or is trying to help them "recover" the lost parent. A rush of emotions at this time can include anger and extreme irritability, an urge to blame someone, and a sense of isolation.

This stage may also be marked by a sense that the pain is too hard to manage and the loss too great to survive. Mourners may cry, wail, and hug items that belonged to the parent, or worry about forgetting some aspect, such as the parent's face or voice. The mind may race with anxieties, and the mourner may jump from activity to activity. Or the opposite response can occur: The person may sleep excessively, hiding from the reality and the magnitude of the loss. This second stage can last from a few months to several years after the death.

The third stage of grieving, according to Bowlby, is marked by depression, disorganization, and guilt. When the anger and blaming of the second stage fail to bring the loved one back, only retreat and sadness may seem to remain. At this stage, the mourner may feel overwhelmed, almost beaten by the loss. Concentration and judgment may be poor, and tasks may seem to require too much effort to complete. Grief counselors have found that guilt is one of the most prevalent and painful emotions following any death. The agonizing

Preparing for the death of a parent

When a death is anticipated, family members have time to prepare themselves emotionally and to make practical arrangements. Advance preparations can ease the burden and make the grieving period less difficult when the death occurs.

Preparations for adult children

- Acknowledging feelings about a parent's impending death and discussing these feelings with others, grief experts find, often makes the death easier to accept when it occurs.

- Reaching decisions about the funeral or memorial service and the burial or cremation in the months or weeks before a parent's death can spare family members the burden of making these decisions at the time of death, when emotions run high. This may also be a time to talk with the parent about his or her wishes.

- Finding an occasion to say or do that which they always intended can help adult children bring a sense of closure to the relationship. They may want to end a feud, apologize, make promises, or express love, gratitude, remorse or many other emotions.

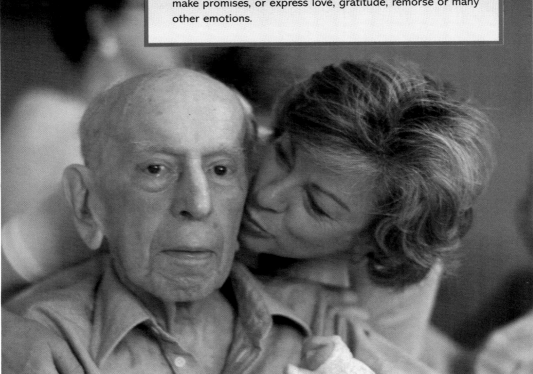

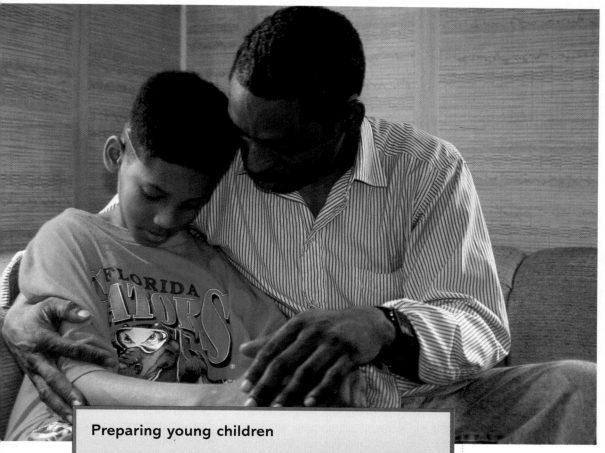

Preparing young children

- Being open and honest, experts advise, helps prepare children for the death of a parent. Adults should answer a child's questions candidly and raise the issue of the impending death if the child does not ask questions.

- Preparing children for the physical signs of illness they will see, such as extreme weight loss or pallor, can make the experience less frightening.

- Apprising children of what life may be like without the parent can prevent them from developing unwarranted fears.

- Including children in funerals or other memorial services, most professionals believe, enables them to benefit from the sense of closure that comes from honoring the deceased. It's a good idea to explain beforehand what the child should expect.

- Assuring children repeatedly that they will always be loved and cared for even in the parent's absence can help ease children's fears.

questions about what one did or did not do or could have done differently or better can plague survivors for many years after the death.

Many of these emotions are intensified when a parent dies as a result of homicide or suicide. In the case of suicide, the survivors' guilt may be overwhelming. Even when a person knows rationally that he or she is not to blame, emotions win out over intellect, and guilt often remains.

Stage four is a period of resolution in which the mourner moves forward into a new life without the deceased and learns to live happily again. In contrast to the disorganization of stage three, bereaved survivors regain control over their lives and emotions in Bowlby's fourth stage.

People often cherish memories of the deceased parent at this stage, though some guilt may linger from a fear that the parent is being forgotten in the survivor's effort to get on with life. Overall, however, a sense of peace replaces guilt in stage four. Life is not as it once was, but it becomes acceptable under new conditions.

Grieving takes a toll

Grief can have physical manifestations as well as emotional consequences. Emotional pain may be expressed in such physical ailments as stomachaches or headaches, by both adults and children. Researchers have found evidence that deep grieving can interfere with the body's ability to fight off disease and that people are more likely to become ill or accident prone during mourning. As scientists become better acquainted with the delicate interactions between the emotions and various systems of the body, we will better understand the connection between grieving, depression, and general health. Because of the powerful link between mind and body, bereavement specialists feel it is especially important to seek help if you are struggling with the process of grieving.

The death of a parent can exact a toll on all family members, sometimes tearing at the fabric that binds brothers, sisters, and other close relatives. The tensions and emotional pain arising from the death can lay bare, or bring about, painful rifts in families. Sibling rivalries may flare, and anger, guilt, blaming, and resentment are common. According to one theory, these sibling conflicts and emotional outbursts serve to block out the actual grief and divert attention from the psychological pain of losing a parent. Group or family therapy can be extremely helpful if these conflicts persist and become unmanageable.

Surviving children may also face the reality of becoming the older generation. Some adult children find it frightening to realize that they are next in line to die. They may also find the prospect of moving forward as fully independent people, in charge of their own lives both practically and emotionally, a difficult and lonely process.

Stages of grieving

Although grieving varies greatly from one individual to another, many grief experts recognize four commonly experienced stages. These stages were identified by British psychiatrist John Bowlby in the 1960's.

Stage 1

A period of shock, disbelief, and denial often follows a death. During this time, mourners may have difficulty admitting that the loss has occurred.

Stage 2

A period of yearning and searching for the dead parent may follow the stage of denial. It may be accompanied by a rush of emotions that can include anger, anxiety, and irritability.

Stage 3

A period of depression, disorganization, and guilt may follow, after the anger of the second stage fails to restore the dead parent. Guilt over what was done or not done may plague the survivor.

Stage 4

A period of resolution finally brings peace, and the survivor learns to move ahead with life under its new terms.

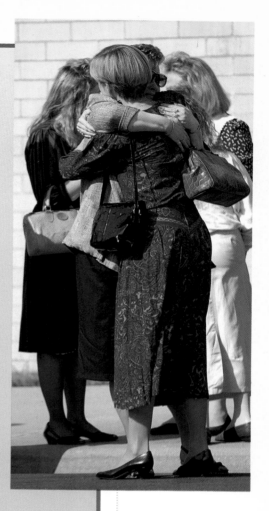

Helping children prepare

Even as they are coping with their own grief, adults may have to prepare their children for a death. This task often falls to the surviving parent, grandparents, or older siblings. Their own suffering makes the job all the more difficult. But experts recognize that children whose needs are overlooked at times of family grief can suffer long-term emotional damage.

Grief counselors generally agree that if there is one rule in preparing children for the loss of a parent, it is to be open and honest. Adults should answer children's questions candidly, and they should raise the issue of the impending death with children who do not ask questions themselves. Silence does not mean the child is unaware of

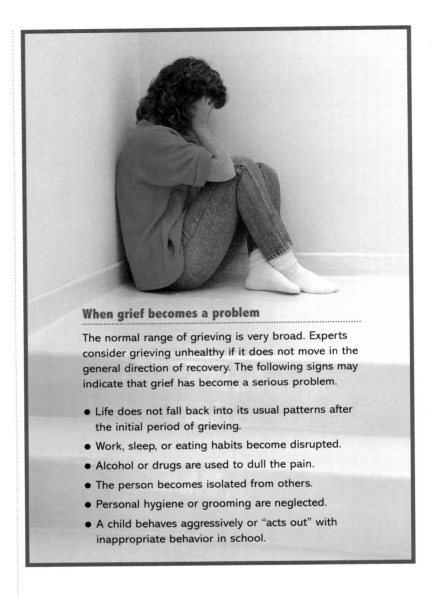

When grief becomes a problem

The normal range of grieving is very broad. Experts consider grieving unhealthy if it does not move in the general direction of recovery. The following signs may indicate that grief has become a serious problem.

- Life does not fall back into its usual patterns after the initial period of grieving.
- Work, sleep, or eating habits become disrupted.
- Alcohol or drugs are used to dull the pain.
- The person becomes isolated from others.
- Personal hygiene or grooming are neglected.
- A child behaves aggressively or "acts out" with inappropriate behavior in school.

the family's distress, but it may indicate that the child is afraid to broach the subject or does not know how. If children are to trust the surviving adults in their lives, they need honest information, even when that information is difficult to give.

How and what to tell a child about a parent's impending death depends on the child's age. Researchers have found that children's comprehension of death varies considerably with age. A very young child may believe that when mommy dies, she continues living as she did before but in a different place—usually heaven—and that she will return someday. Some counselors feel that adults should explain the permanence of death so that the child does not harbor unrealistic expectations. Older children and teen-agers will expect more detailed explanations of death and dying, including information about society's rituals for dealing with death.

To ease possible fears, adults should prepare children for what they will see in a dying parent. Witnessing the physical signs of illness, such as weight loss or paleness, can be startling and painful for an adult, and the experience can be even more unsettling to a child. Emotional changes in the dying parent—from depression or in reaction to pain or medication, for example—can also be upsetting and should be explained.

Children should also be apprised of what life may be like without the parent, to prevent them from developing unwarranted fears and so that they know what to expect. Above all, adults should constantly reassure children that they will always be loved and cared for, even in the parent's absence.

A child may also wonder what is to become of the deceased parent. The nature of this discussion will depend upon the family's beliefs about heaven, the afterlife, disposal of the body, and other related issues.

Most professionals believe that children should not be "spared" the experience of funerals or other memorial services. Like adults, children need the sense of closure that comes with honoring and saying good-by to the deceased. Children also benefit from the support, love, and bonding that are often expressed among mourners. Grief experts sometimes find that children who have been excluded from these group grieving experiences become further isolated and emotionally hurt.

It's a good idea to explain to a child beforehand what to expect— for example, people giving talks, people crying, the body on view, and so on. The more adults tell a child about the process of death, the more comfortable the child will feel about expressing grief and taking solace in the support and love of others.

How children respond to grief

Children may not always express emotional pain openly when a parent dies. Adults are often unaware of the extent of a youngster's distress because children may mask their suffering with other fears and unusual behaviors or express their pain through other physical and emotional complaints. For example, after losing a parent, some children develop fears of leaving the house, going to school, or carrying on other normal activities outside the home.

Professionals find that bereaved children may want to remain at home out of fear that another painful event will occur in their absence. After a parent's death, children often fear for the life of the surviving parent, for other loved ones, and for themselves. Children who lose their parents lose their own childhoods, it is often said, as these children are catapulted into a world of grieving, loneliness, and mortality.

Immediately after a parent's death, young children may engage

The healing process

As difficult as the loss of a parent may be, all human beings share the ability to recover from grief and move on with their lives. During the recovery process, it's important to accept the support of friends, family, and others who want to help—and to let them know how they can help.

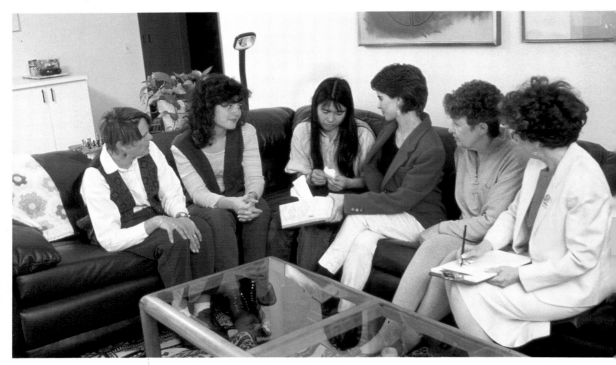

Participating in a therapy group guided by a trained bereavement counselor can help overcome the painful feelings surrounding a death.

in what seems to be inappropriate behavior—such as playing, laughing, or fighting—instead of mourning in ways that are typical of adults. Professionals say that for children to act this way is common and normal, and they suggest that adults not criticize children for such actions. At the same time, adults should continue openly discussing their feelings about the death, even if the child appears to ignore the death. Children often absorb more than is apparent to adults, and they are as watchful of adult behavior in grief as at other times.

After losing a parent, young children may cling unusually hard to the surviving parent. Another common response of children is to become emotionally detached from the surviving parent, teachers, grandparents, and other loved ones. Placing a distance between themselves and others is a way of trying to protect themselves from the pain of future losses. Children may feel that if they do not become close to someone, they cannot be hurt if the person dies or

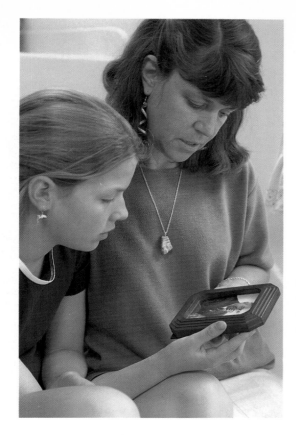

Sharing memories
of a deceased parent
can be a healthy part
of recovery.

goes away. As a bereaved child alternates between clinging and distance, it is extremely important that trusted adults openly express
their commitment to love and care for the child, even if the child repeatedly pushes them away. At this time, more than ever, children
need unconditional love.

In an effort to understand the death, children often question what
they did to contribute to it, and they may feel guilt. They may recall
having disobeyed a parent's instructions, having said something
cruel in an argument, or even having yelled or thought "I wish you
were dead" or "I wish you were not my daddy." It is vital that surviving adults, especially the surviving parent and other close relatives,
alleviate a child's guilt clearly and repeatedly. Children suffering
from the burden of guilt and responsibility must be told as often as
possible that they were not at fault, that the deceased parent loved
them, that surviving adults love them, and that there was nothing
they could have done to prevent the death.

Physical symptoms of grief are common, especially among young
children who may not be able to express their bereavement in
words. Stomachaches, headaches, and similar complaints may be the
physical manifestations of grief. Adults should be alert to this possibility and attend to children's unstated emotional pain as well as to

their physical discomfort. Because the child's pain may originate from the loss, treatment should also include attention to emotional wounds.

A time to heal

The range of normal grieving is enormous. We all mourn in our own ways and on our own schedules. Normal grieving may intensify and subside and then resurface at unexpected times, even many years after the death. However, if the general direction is one of recovery, with a growing sense of peace within, professionals consider the grieving normal.

Experts consider the grieving process abnormal when it does not move in the general direction of healing, even long after the death has occurred. When the ability to function is impaired over the long term—the person cannot work, sleep, or keep up important relationships, for example—grief has become a serious problem. When someone turns to alcohol or drugs to dull the pain, grief has become unhealthy. In some cases, a bereaved person shows no outward signs whatsoever of having experienced a loss. Grief experts believe that this apparent lack of emotion may indicate unhealthy grieving. Professional counseling or therapy can help when an individual's life does not fall back into place after a reasonable period of grieving has passed.

Grief and how to handle grief has become an important area of study among mental health professionals, and support through the grieving process is available in many forms, including individual counseling and group or family bereavement therapy. Specialized bereavement centers have sprung up around the United States. Many hospitals, mental health clinics, and institutes also offer bereavement counseling.

The goal of bereavement therapy is to help survivors overcome the painful emotions, such as guilt, rage, resentment, and alienation, that can obstruct the return to a healthy life. Counselors help survivors express their feelings so they can deal with difficulties directly. Sometimes, therapy begins with a chance to vent painful emotions by crying, wailing, or screaming. After that, talking and healing can begin. By expressing and better understanding their feelings, people reduce the tendency to create emotional moats around themselves that can prevent close relationships from thriving.

For healing, it is important to accept the support of friends, family, and others who want to help during the process of bereavement—and to let them know how they can help. It can be soothing just to have someone listen. Expressing emotional needs helps the grieving person establish the emotional openness that is so vital in overcoming the pain of loss. If talking about the pain is difficult, it may help to find someone who has been through a similar loss and can empathize. The love and support gained by reaching out eases the rough process of putting a life back together.

Although the period of raw emotions shortly after a parent's death is usually the most difficult to endure, certain occasions renew the pain of the loss and seem to reopen the emotional wounds. These occasions include the anniversary of the death, family holidays such as Thanksgiving, the deceased parent's birthday, or one's own birthday. It helps to do something on these days to face the pain and to honor the lost parent in some way, such as writing a heartfelt letter to the deceased, engaging in an activity that the deceased would have appreciated, or talking to other loved ones about your feelings. Over the years, these holiday pangs subside and are replaced by warm memories.

The pain of losing a loved one, especially a parent, can seem unspeakable and unbearable. But it can be overcome. With the help of loved ones and the complex process of grieving, it is possible to move past the pain and go forward, memories intact, to lead a full and meaningful life once again. ● ● ●

For further reading:

Bowlby, John. *Attachment and Loss, Volume III: Loss: Sadness and Depression*. Basic Books, Inc., 1980.

Donnelly, Katherine Fair. *Recovering From the Loss of a Parent*. Berkley Books, 1993.

Gordon, Audrey K., and Klass, Dennis. *They Need to Know: How to Teach Children About Death*. Prentice-Hall, Inc., 1979.

Kubler-Ross, Elisabeth. *On Death & Dying*. Macmillan, 1970.
A groundbreaking book that discusses the five stages of grief that a dying person experiences.

Myers, Edward. *When Parents Die: A Guide for Adults*. Viking Penguin Inc., 1986.

Schaefer, Dan, and Lyons, Christine. *How Do We Tell the Children? A Parent's Guide to Helping Children Understand and Cope When Someone Dies*. Newmarket Press, 1986.

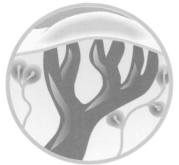

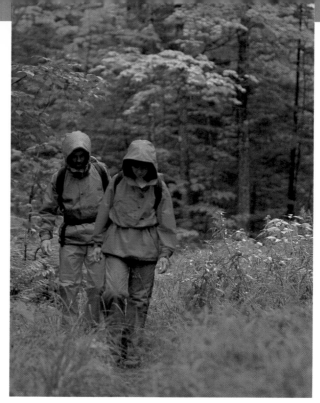

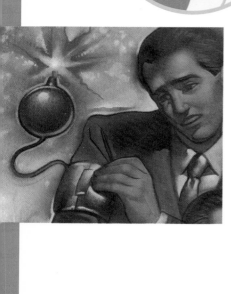

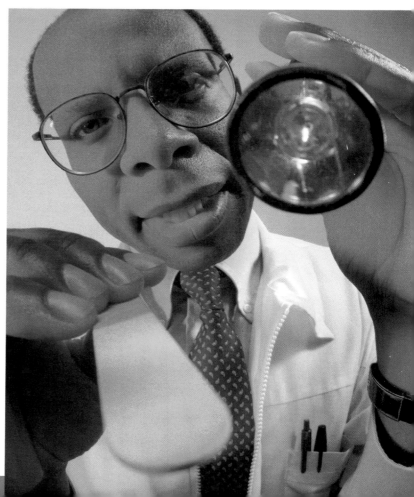

MEDICAL AND SAFETY ALERTS

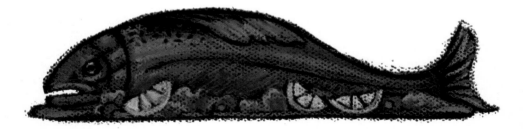

High blood pressure can cause
serious harm while producing few
symptoms. But it can be controlled.

Hypertension: A Ticking Time Bomb

By Richard Trubo

A SINISTER AND SILENT DISEASE IS RAMPANT in the United States. Often unnoticed, it threatens the health of 50 million people, even jeopardizing the lives of many. It plays no favorites among men and women, and once it appears, it can remain for a lifetime.

The disease is high blood pressure, also known as hypertension. Nearly everyone has heard of it, yet many people who have it are unaware that this medical time bomb is ticking inside them. High blood pressure usually causes no symptoms, and thus when doctors diagnose it, patients are often stunned. "I feel great," they typically reply. "How could I possibly be sick?"

Because one in four adult Americans has high blood pressure— and another 2 million people develop it each year—health officials consider hypertension an epidemic demanding attention. In 1994, the National Coalition for Hypertension Education and Control was created, with the goal of improving awareness of high blood pressure and offering screening programs to identify the disease.

Blood pressure is the force exerted on artery walls by blood flowing through them. Each time the heart beats, it squeezes blood into the arteries, creating pressure on vessel walls. If blood vessels become *constricted* (narrowed), a condition that usually accompanies hypertension, the heart has to work harder to propel the blood, and the pressure against vessel walls increases.

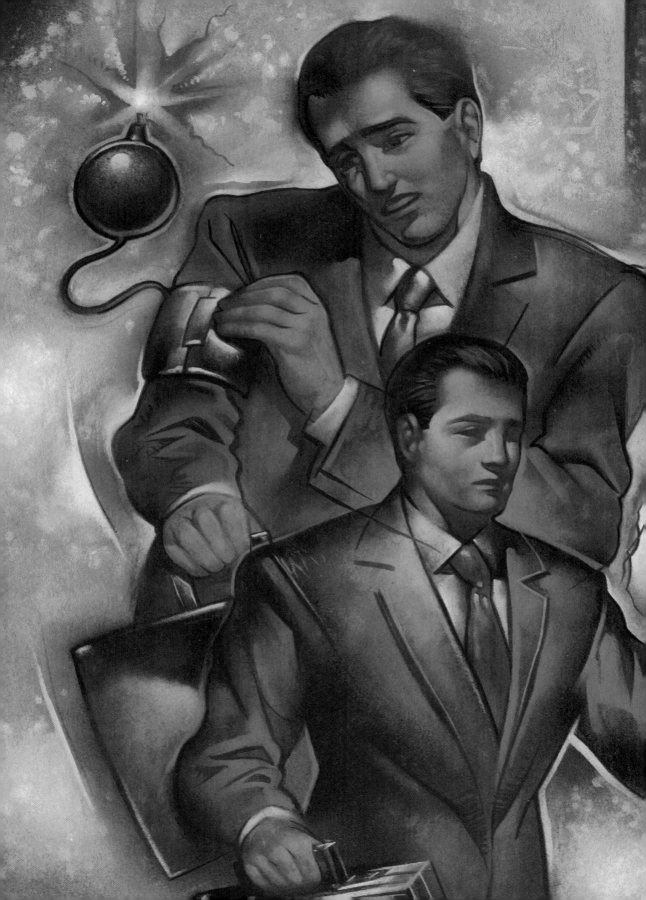

Glossary

Angiotensin: A protein that raises blood pressure by tightening the muscles in the walls of blood vessels.

Arterioles: Smaller blood vessels that narrow to cause hypertension.

Diastolic pressure: The lower portion of a blood pressure reading, which indicates the pressure of blood against blood vessel walls as the heart rests.

Hypertension: Elevated pressure of blood against blood vessel walls that results from a narrowing of blood vessels.

Sphygmomanometer: A blood pressure cuff used to measure blood pressure.

Systolic pressure: The upper portion of a blood pressure reading, which indicates the pressure of blood against blood vessel walls as the heart pumps.

The author:

Richard Trubo is a free-lance medical writer.

When blood flows through arteries and smaller blood vessels at a higher-than-normal pressure, it can create havoc in the human body. The heart may enlarge as it strains to meet the body's need for blood and the oxygen that blood carries. The enlargement can eventually weaken the heart muscle and lead to heart failure, the inability of the heart to pump sufficient blood. Over time, high pressure inside arteries can damage their inner linings, creating rough areas that promote the buildup of fatty deposits. Such deposits can narrow vessels further and leave them less elastic—a condition known as atherosclerosis—further limiting their ability to deliver blood throughout the body.

Hypertension more than any other single factor puts people at risk for stroke—damage to the brain from a disruption in blood flow. Hypertension also is a major risk factor for blockage of the arteries that supply blood to the heart, a condition known as coronary heart disease. Prolonged hypertension can damage the delicate blood vessels in the kidneys, reducing the kidneys' ability to filter wastes from the blood. It can cause blindness by damaging sensitive vessels in the eyes.

I't's no wonder that physicians have declared war on hypertension when the consequences are so severe. What makes the disease even more sinister is that, in most cases, it has no symptoms until it's well advanced. By the time a person experiences such symptoms as *palpitations* (fluttering heartbeats) or shortness of breath, serious damage to the heart may already have occurred.

Although hypertension cannot be cured, a growing number of treatment options—from lifestyle changes to medications—can help bring the disease under control. Signs that this disease can be contained are encouraging. The estimated prevalence of high blood pressure in the United States fell from 58 million people in 1980 to 50 million in 1991. The death rate from high blood pressure fell by 8.6 percent from 1982 to 1992, thanks to increasing knowledge about hypertension and better methods for managing it. At the same time, deaths from strokes and coronary disease fell as well, in part because people had begun to control their hypertension.

Doctors do not know the specific cause of 90 to 95 percent of all cases of high blood pressure. In cases where no underlying cause is identified, the patient is said to have essential hypertension. Factors that may contribute to essential hypertension include atherosclerosis and constriction of arterioles, the vessels that link arteries to smaller capillaries. Researchers suspect that abnormalities in the heart, kidneys, nervous system, or the complex system that maintains normal fluid volume in the body could be at the root of hypertension.

In cases where an underlying disease causes blood pressure to rise, the person is said to have secondary hypertension. Kidney disease or *Cushing's syndrome* (a disorder of the adrenal glands), for example, can elevate blood pressure. When physicians treat the under-

Understanding blood pressure

Blood flowing through blood vessels creates pressure against the vessel walls. Blood pressure is a measure of that pressure taken at two stages. The higher number, called the systolic pressure, is the pressure exerted when the heart contracts and pumps blood through the vessels. The lower number, called the diastolic pressure, is the pressure exerted when the heart relaxes between beats.

Systolic pressure represents the pressure created when the heart contracts and blood surges through the blood vessels.

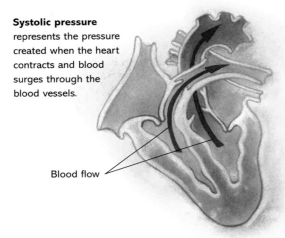

Blood flow

Diastolic pressure represents the pressure created when the heart relaxes between beats.

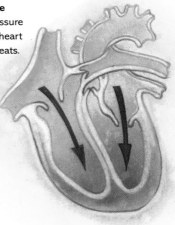

Blood   Vessel wall

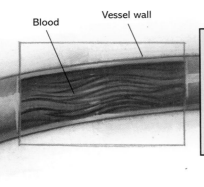

Healthy blood vessel

Healthy blood vessels have elastic walls. When the heart contracts and pumps blood through these vessels, they can expand to accommodate the increased volume of blood.

Narrowed blood vessel

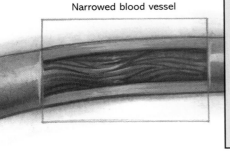

Hypertensive vessel

Blood pressure rises when smaller blood vessels called arterioles become narrowed or lose their elasticity, leaving less room for blood flow and creating more pressure against vessel walls. Medical researchers are not certain what causes the narrowing or loss of elasticity that elevates blood pressure.

Classification of high blood pressure

Physicians classify high blood pressure by its probable health consequences. They consider a systolic pressure of more than 140 or a diastolic pressure of more than 90 serious enough to require treatment. Because blood pressure can vary, physicians never diagnose hypertension on the basis of one reading. They usually obtain at least three separate readings to confirm a diagnosis of hypertension.

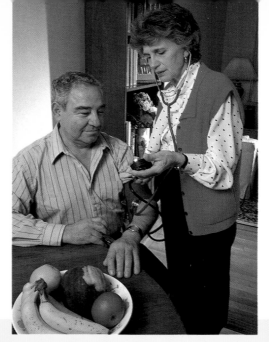

Category	Systolic reading	Diastolic reading	Follow-up recommended
Normal	Less than 130	Less than 85	Check again in two years.
High normal	130 – 139	85 – 89	Check in one year. Many physicians recommend lifestyle modifications at this stage.
Hypertension			
Stage 1	140 – 159	90 – 99	Modify lifestyle. Begin drug treatment if lifestyle modifications are not effective within six months.
Stage 2	160 – 179	100 – 109	Begin drug treatment and modify lifestyle.
Stage 3	180 – 209	110 – 119	Begin drug treatment and modify lifestyle.
Stage 4	More than 210	More than 120	Immediate medical evaluation and treatment with drugs. Modify lifestyle.

Source: Joint National Committee on Detection, Evaluation, and Treatment of High Blood Pressure.

lying condition successfully, the high blood pressure associated with it disappears. In some cases, pregnancy or the use of oral contraceptives also can boost blood pressure temporarily.

Blood pressure rises and falls as the heart beats. Two blood pressure readings are taken to reflect this variation. Pressure against artery walls peaks when the heart contracts and pumps blood through the arteries. This reading is the *systolic* (pumping) pressure. Blood pressure is lowest between heartbeats, when the heart is at rest. This reading is the *diastolic* (resting) pressure.

A nurse, physician, or other health care professional measures blood pressure rapidly and painlessly using an instrument called a *sphygmomanometer*, from Greek words meaning *pulse* and *measure*.

The nurse wraps the sphygmomanometer's rubber cuff around the patient's arm above the elbow and pumps air into the cuff. As the cuff inflates, it compresses the main artery in the arm, momentarily interrupting blood flow down the arm.

The nurse then gradually releases the air in the cuff, placing a stethoscope over the artery, just below the cuff, to listen for the distinct sounds blood makes as it starts to flow again through the artery. These sounds continue until the pressure in the artery is greater than the pressure in the cuff.

When the first sound of rushing blood is heard, the nurse notes the position of a needle on a pressure gauge attached to the cuff. The needle's position at that moment is recorded as the systolic pressure. The diastolic pressure is recorded just after the final sound is heard. The numbers recorded for systolic and diastolic pressure represent how high in millimeters that amount of pressure would lift a column of mercury, a measurement abbreviated as mm Hg. Some blood pressure cuffs have a glass tube that contains a column of mercury. Others use a gauge that responds to air pressure but is calibrated to correspond to a mercury column reading.

There is no ideal blood pressure reading, and for many years, doctors disagreed over the point at which blood pressure was high enough to warrant treatment. Today, most concur that a reading of 140/90 (140=systolic, 90=diastolic) or greater in an adult constitutes hypertension. A reading of less than 130/85 is deemed normal, and a systolic reading from 131 to 139 is considered the high end of normal. Medical researchers believe that a measurement under 120/80 is best for avoiding hypertension-related damage to the heart and blood vessels. Some people have far lower than normal blood pressure. Most of the time, low blood pressure presents no problem, and only rarely is it a sign of an underlying disease.

Blood pressure readings are not static. They tend to fluctuate during the day as levels of physical activity, excitement, and nervousness vary. Even a few cups of coffee can raise blood pressure, as can the anxiety of having blood pressure measured in a doctor's office—a phenomenon termed "white coat hypertension." Measurements taken just minutes apart can vary by 10 to 20 mm Hg. However, if blood pressure readings stay abnormally high for sustained periods, they become a medical concern.

In 1993, a special panel of hypertension experts—the Joint National Committee on Detection, Evaluation, and Treatment of High Blood Pressure (JNC)—proposed the classification for high blood pressure now in use. Until 1993, the early stages of hypertension had been classified as mild or moderate. The JNC panel felt that many people disregarded a diagnosis of mild hypertension because the term conveyed little urgency. Instead, the JNC recommended that high blood pressure be classified by stages, with the first elevated level called Stage 1 rather than mild. The panel also added a category called high normal to include people with systolic readings between 130 and 139 and diastolic readings between 85 and 89. People in this range, the panel said, are at definite risk for developing hypertension.

Study after study has confirmed the relationship between hypertension and increased health risks. One of the largest studies followed about 350,000 middle-aged men (none with a history of heart attack) at 22 medical centers across the nation, starting in the mid-1970's. The researchers found that the higher the men's blood pressure, the greater was their chance of dying prematurely from cardiovascular disease. Men with a systolic blood pressure over 140 had a much higher risk of early death than men with readings under 130. But perhaps just as significant, even those men with high normal systolic pressures between 130 and 139 had twice the risk of dying of heart disease as those with readings from 110 through 119.

Hypertension is sometimes called "the silent killer," because it can cause so much damage while producing no symptoms. The symptom-free nature of the disease makes regular blood pressure screening important for everyone, especially since treatments are widely available and effective.

A 1993 study found that individuals who received treatment for their hypertension had a 40 percent lower risk of a stroke, compared with people whose hypertension was not treated. The death rate from cardiovascular disease also was 21 percent lower in the treated group. The study, conducted by researchers at Harvard Medical School in Boston and Yale University School of Medicine in New Haven, Connecticut, analyzed data from 17 clinical trials involving hypertension patients.

Because such an immense number of men and women have high blood pressure, no one should assume he or she is immune. Nevertheless, researchers have found that some people are at greater risk than others because of their background or lifestyle. In general, the older or more overweight you are, the higher your blood pressure is likely to be. If one or both of your parents have hypertension or if you are African American, you have a higher-than-average chance of becoming hypertensive. Smokers and people who drink alcohol in excess also are prone to hypertension. (For more information on risk factors, see WHO'S AT RISK on page 144.)

Despite the seriousness of hypertension, treatment for the disorder is effective, and the benefits from treatment are substantial. Even modest reductions in blood pressure can improve health. Studies show, for example, that lowering systolic blood pressure readings by just 3 mm Hg could cut the annual death rate from stroke in the United States by 8 percent. According to the American Heart Association, however, many Americans with hypertension receive inadequate treatment or no treatment, because they do not realize that they are ill.

The consequences of high blood pressure

If left untreated, elevated blood pressure can damage blood vessels in several areas of the body and lead to serious health problems.

Stroke
High blood pressure can damage vessels that supply blood to the brain, eventually causing them to rupture or clog. The interruption in blood flow to the brain is known as a stroke.

Eye damage
Prolonged high blood pressure can damage delicate blood vessels on the retina, the layer of cells at the back of the eye. If the damage, known as retinopathy, remains untreated, it can lead to blindness.

Heart attack
High blood pressure makes the heart work harder to pump sufficient blood through narrowed *arterioles* (small blood vessels). This extra effort can enlarge and weaken the heart, leading to heart failure. High blood pressure also damages the coronary arteries that supply blood to the heart, sometimes leading to blockages that can cause a heart attack.

Kidney failure
Prolonged high blood pressure can damage blood vessels in the kidney, where wastes are filtered from the bloodstream. In severe cases, this damage can lead to kidney failure and even death.

Damage to artery walls

Artery walls are normally smooth, allowing blood to flow easily. Over time, high blood pressure can wear rough spots in artery walls. Fatty deposits can collect in these rough spots, clogging arteries and raising the risk of a heart attack or stroke.

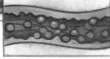

Rough artery walls

Clogged artery

143

Who's at risk

No one should assume he or she is immune to high blood pressure. But medical experts concur that several factors can raise a person's risk. Some of these factors are under our control, but others, such as age and heredity, are not.

Generally, the chances of developing high blood pressure increase as one ages. According to medical researchers, the prevalence of hypertension rises from 21 percent of Americans in their 40's to 54 percent of Americans in their 60's.

Hypertension often runs in families. Thus, people have a greater chance of becoming hypertensive if either one or both of their parents have high blood pressure.

Race also plays a role in a person's risk for hypertension. African Americans on average have about twice the risk of developing high blood pressure as Caucasians. Researchers have also found that hypertension is more likely to develop at an earlier age and be more severe in African Americans.

Neither sex is more vulnerable to hypertension, but in general, more men than women develop hypertension in young adulthood and early middle age. From age 55 to 75, the risks for men and women are about equal. Thereafter, women are more likely to become hypertensive.

Lack of physical activity also increases the risk of developing hypertension, according to medical experts. One study of about 3,000 mostly middle-aged men concluded that the average *systolic* (pumping) pressure of those judged to be fit was lower by almost 10 mm Hg, on average, compared with those who were unfit. *Diastolic* (resting) pressures were also lower by about 6 mm Hg in the fit group. Another study followed the exercise habits of 15,000 men. The study showed that men who did not engage in vigorous physical activity, such as running, singles tennis, swimming, or handball, were 35 percent more likely to have high blood pressure. (Blood pressure is measured by how far it moves a column of mercury in millimeters, abbreviated as mm Hg.)

Those who drink alcohol excessively may also find themselves in the hypertensive range. Studies have shown that women who consume more than 10 drinks a week have systolic readings 3.9 mm Hg higher than nondrinking women. Studies also show that heavy drinking raises blood pressure in men. Research shows that from 5 to 7 percent of hypertension cases in the United States are related to consuming three or more alcoholic drinks a day.

As body weight increases, blood pressure often rises as well, probably because extra weight puts additional demands on the heart for blood. Many studies have shown that overweight individuals have two to six times the risk of becoming hypertensive as people whose weight falls within the recommended range for their height and age. About 20 to 30 percent of cases of high blood pressure are tied to obesity, according to the American Heart Association.

Excess sodium, a chemical in salt, can play a critical role in hypertension. The body needs a small amount of salt to function normally, but the average American consumes far more sodium than required, according to the American Heart Association. In people who are sensitive to sodium, excess salt raises blood pressure by increasing the amount of fluid retained in the bloodstream. Salt can also constrict the blood vessels, further contributing to hypertension. However, only about half of the people with hypertension are sufficiently sodium sensitive that their blood pressure rises when their salt intake increases. And salt appears to have little effect on people whose blood pressure is not already elevated.

Nevertheless, short-term studies have shown that moderate sodium restriction can reduce systolic and diastolic measurements by an average of 4.9 and 2.6 mm Hg, respectively, in people with high blood pressure. Some groups seem to gain even greater benefits from reducing their salt intake, particularly older people and African Americans.

Some evidence suggests that stress plays a part in raising blood pressure. A few studies in the 1970's and 1980's suggested that people in stressful jobs, such as factory workers and air traffic controllers, may have a higher risk for hypertension. And several studies reported in the early 1990's showed that those adolescents and medical students whose blood pressure rose more dramatically in response to short-term stressful situations, such as examinations, were more likely to have elevated blood pressure later in life than were their peers whose blood pressure remained closer to normal. But according to hypertension experts, there is no clear evidence that reducing stress can significantly lower a person's high blood pressure. [R. T.]

Because there is no cure for essential hypertension, treatment involves controlling the disease. The JNC advises lifestyle modifications, such as losing weight or exercising, as the first line of treatment. According to the committee's report, changing daily habits may bring high blood pressure under control without medication in about 25 percent of patients, especially those with only moderately elevated pressure. These strategies can also help prevent hypertension in people with normal blood pressure.

One of the most important lifestyle changes is weight loss, because excess weight puts an extra burden on the heart. Doctors advise those who need to lose weight to reduce their calorie intake. Physicians also recommend that hypertensive people minimize their salt intake, because salt appears to raise blood pressure in people who are sensitive to the sodium in it. The American Medical Association recommends consuming less than 0.2 ounces (6 grams) of sodium chloride daily.

Exercise is another key lifestyle recommendation. Regular physical activity not only helps people shed excess weight, but it also appears to lower blood pressure directly, even if the activity is only moderately strenuous. A brisk, 30-to-45-minute walk three to five times a week can help bring hypertension under control, according to hypertension experts. Physicians recommend that people who are middle-aged or older and have been sedentary for a long time see a physician before beginning an exercise program.

Many studies have shown that cutting back on excessive alcohol use can also reduce blood pressure. Whatever a person's blood pressure, health experts warn against consuming more than two drinks per day. Reducing alcohol consumption may raise blood pressure in the short term, but it drops within a few days.

Smoking contributes to heart disease, and it may decrease the effectiveness of antihypertensive drugs. Research shows that cigarette smoking causes a temporary rise in blood pressure, probably by raising the amount of the heart-stimulating hormone adrenaline in the bloodstream. Although there is no persuasive evidence that quitting smoking lowers blood pressure for more than short periods, people with high blood pressure have a greater chance of complications, including coronary heart disease, if they smoke. Cigarette smoking also appears to contribute to atherosclerosis by injuring artery walls.

Although stress may contribute to hypertension, researchers have not yet demonstrated conclusively that stress management lowers blood pressure. About half the studies on the subject have shown improvements in blood pressure levels from biofeedback, meditation, or relaxation techniques, but evidence for long-term benefits is inconclusive. Nevertheless, physicians counsel, reducing the demands and anxieties surrounding work and other everyday activities improves overall well-being and may possibly lower blood pressure.

The 1993 JNC report suggested that doctors evaluate the effect of lifestyle changes on a patient's blood pressure reading after three to six months. If these approaches fail to bring pressure below 140/90 mm Hg, physicians may prescribe antihypertensive drugs, while urging patients to continue with lifestyle improvements.

Although experts concur that lifestyle adjustments are worth trying, some critics contend that few people are able to maintain the changes indefinitely and that such changes are often unlikely to reduce blood pressure enough to avoid the use of medications. Many doctors believe that if a person's blood pressure is very high (180/110 or above), drug treatment should begin immediately in conjunction with lifestyle approaches.

A study of about 900 men and women with high blood pressure concluded in 1993 that drug treatment combined with lifestyle changes is the most effective treatment for hypertension. The researchers divided study participants into six groups, five of which received a drug from one of the major classes of antihypertensive medications. The remaining group took a *placebo* (inactive substance). Physicians also counseled all participants on lifestyle modifications, such as increasing exercise, controlling weight, quitting smoking, and reducing salt and alcohol consumption.

After four years, blood pressure readings had fallen for all groups, but patients who combined drugs and lifestyle changes recorded the biggest declines. Whereas the drug groups collectively experienced an average drop in systolic and diastolic pressures of 15.9 and 12.3 mm Hg, respectively, the lifestyle-only group registered average decreases of only 9.1 and 8.6 mm Hg. Those taking medications also reported feeling better overall than the placebo group. The study was conducted by researchers from the University of Minnesota in Minneapolis and the National Heart, Lung, and Blood Institute in Bethesda, Maryland.

A growing number of drugs are available for treating hypertension, and physicians may prescribe a combination of drugs. Antihypertensive drugs fall into seven categories: diuretics, beta-blockers, ACE inhibitors, angiotensin II antagonists, calcium channel blockers, sympathetic inhibitors, and vasodilators.

Diuretics remove excess water and sodium from the body by increasing the amounts lost in urine. This action reduces the volume of fluid in the blood vessels, thereby lowering blood pressure. Because diuretics cause frequent urination, patients should take them in the morning rather than just before bed.

Beta-blockers and sympathetic inhibitors work by interfering with nerve signals. Beta-blockers curb nerve signals that normally increase the speed and force of the heartbeat and constrict the blood vessels. As a result, the heart slows and pumps less blood with each beat, and blood pressure drops. Sympathetic inhibitors also dilate the blood vessels by blocking nerve signals.

Angiotensin-converting enzyme (ACE) inhibitors and angiotensin

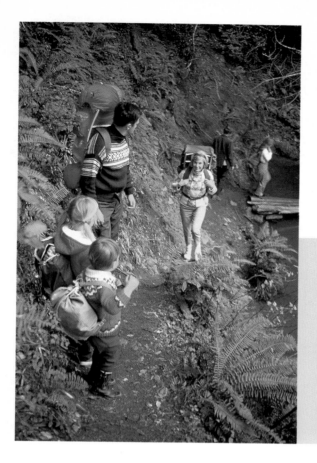

Controlling high blood pressure: Lifestyle changes

Many physicians recommend lifestyle modifications that can help lower blood pressure in patients in the early stages of hypertension. If these measures fail to lower blood pressure sufficiently after a few months, then physicians usually prescribe drugs.

- Losing weight.

- Increasing physical activity.

- Reducing sodium intake.

- Quitting smoking.

- Reducing alcohol consumption.

- Reducing dietary fat and cholesterol.

Source: Joint National Committee on Detection, Evaluation, and Treatment of High Blood Pressure.

II antagonists limit the actions of angiotensin, a protein that raises blood pressure by constricting the muscles in vessel walls. ACE inhibitors interfere with the body's production of angiotensin. Angiotensin II antagonists block the effect of angiotensin on blood vessels.

The remaining drugs work in different ways. Calcium channel blockers prevent calcium molecules from entering muscle cells, where they cause muscles to constrict. Vasodilators also relax muscles in blood vessel walls, allowing the vessels to dilate.

Regardless of how they work, all antihypertensive drugs carry some risk of side effects. Diuretics, for example, may cause weakness, muscle cramps, and impotence (loss of sexual function). Beta-blockers may worsen such medical conditions as Type II (adult-onset) diabetes and asthma. ACE inhibitors can cause rashes, itching, and coughing in some people, and calcium channel blockers can cause swelling of the ankles, headaches, and palpitations. Relatively few people experience serious side effects from their medication, however, and physicians can minimize or eliminate side effects by adjusting the dosage, prescribing a different drug, or by using combinations of drugs in smaller doses.

Controlling high blood pressure: Drugs

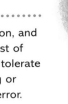

Many types of drugs are available to treat hypertension, and physicians may prescribe a combination of drugs. Most of the drugs have side effects. Because patients usually tolerate some drugs better than others, finding the right drug or combination of drugs is often a process of trial and error.

Drug class	Examples Generic (brand) name
Angiotensin-converting enzyme (ACE) inhibitors lower blood pressure by interfering with the body's production of *angiotensin*, a chemical that causes blood vessels to *constrict* (narrow).	Captopril (Capoten) Lisinopril (Prinivil, Zestril) Enalapril (Vasotec) Benazepril (Lotensin)
Angiotensin II receptor antagonists lower blood pressure by blocking the effect of angiotensin on blood vessels, allowing them to remain *dilated* (expanded).	Losartan (Cozaar)*
Beta-blockers lower blood pressure by blocking nerve impulses to the heart, causing it to slow down and pump less blood.	Propranolol (Inderal) Metoprolol (Lopressor) Atenolol (Tenormin)
Calcium channel blockers lower blood pressure by inhibiting the passage of calcium into muscle cells in the walls of blood vessels, thereby preventing the vessels from constricting.	Diltiazem (Cardizem, Dilacor) Nifedipine (Adalat, Procardia) Amlodipine (Norvasc) Verapamil (Calan, Isoptin, Verelan)
Diuretics lower blood pressure by ridding the body of excess fluids and salt that can increase the volume of blood and increase the pressure inside blood vessels.	Chlorthalidone (Hygroton) Hydrochlorothiazide (Esidrix, Oretic) Indapamide (Lozol)
Sympathetic inhibitors lower blood pressure by blocking nerve impulses that constrict blood vessels, allowing the vessels to remain dilated and reducing the resistance to blood flow through them.	Clonidine (Catapres) Doxazosin (Cardura) Guanabenz (Wytensin) Prazosin (Minipress) Terazosin (Hytrin)
Vasodilators lower blood pressure by relaxing muscles in the walls of blood vessels, allowing them to dilate. They are usually used with diuretics or beta-blockers.	Hydralazine (Apresoline) Minoxidil (Loniten)

*Only drug in this class.
Source: The Joint National Committee on Detection, Evaluation, and Treatment of High Blood Pressure.

GROUP A STREP INFECTIONS
and their complications

Many of the more common diseases caused by streptococcus bacteria result from infection with a subgroup known as group A streptococcus. Most strep A infections involve only a bad sore throat or unpleasant skin condition. But some infections that go untreated have serious consequences—consequences that can usually be avoided by prompt treatment with antibiotics.

Condition	Symptoms	Intervention	Potential consequences
Strep throat	Sudden onset of severe sore throat; fever; swollen and tender lymph nodes in neck.	Penicillin or other antibiotic.	If untreated, may lead to a middle ear infection, rheumatic fever, or kidney inflammation. Infection may spread to nearby tissue.
Scarlet fever	Severe sore throat; fever; scarlet-colored rash that starts on the neck and spreads over the body. White coating may appear on tongue and peel off to reveal a strawberry color.	Antibiotics.	If untreated, may lead to rheumatic fever or kidney inflammation.
Rheumatic fever	*Inflammation* (pain and swelling) in large joints, such as shoulder, elbow, hip, or knee; fever; rapid pulse. In rare cases, pea-sized lumps appear under skin.	Antibiotics; bed rest for up to several months; aspirin or other drugs to reduce inflammation in joints and to lower fever.	Scarring of heart valves.
Kidney inflammation	Mild cases may produce no symptoms. In some cases, puffiness occurs around the eye, blood pressure becomes elevated, or blood appears in urine.	Treatment of symptoms. In advanced cases, kidney dialysis may be necessary to remove wastes from blood.	In rare cases, may lead to kidney failure and a potentially fatal condition called uremia, in which body wastes build up in blood.
Impetigo	Pus-filled blisters that break and leave sores covered by yellow crust.	Antibiotics taken by injection or orally or applied as ointment to infected areas; frequent cleansing of the sores.	
Erysipelas	Itchy red patches, usually on the face, form an area with raised edges. Fever, headache, sore throat may occur.	Antibiotics taken by injection or orally; cold packs, aspirin, or topical anesthetics to relieve pain and itching.	If untreated, infection may spread; can lead to death.
Streptococcal toxic shock	Low blood pressure, fever, respiratory problems, sweating, nausea, pale and clammy skin, rapid pulse.	Large doses of antibiotics given intravenously.	Can cause irreversible tissue damage, organ failure, and death.

How group A strep can affect the body

Group A strep infections—and the immune system's response to them—can affect many areas of the body. Whether an infected individual develops any of the complications depends largely on the particular strep A strain and its capabilities, the site of initial infection, and on how well the individual's immune system can fight the infection.

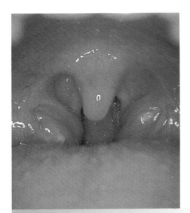

Sore throat
When group A strep bacteria settle in the throat, they cause the infection known as strep throat. As the body fights the disease, the tonsils often become inflamed and the lymph nodes swollen and tender.

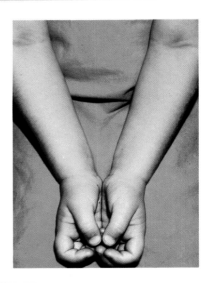

Skin rash
Once in the throat, some strains of strep A bacteria release toxins. The body's response to these toxins produces the scarlet-colored rash characteristic of scarlet fever.

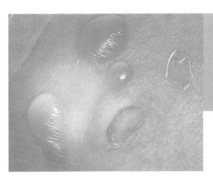

Skin infection
Group A strep bacteria can enter the body through a break in the skin, causing a condition known as impetigo. Pus-filled blisters form on the skin and eventually burst, leaving sores covered with yellowish crust.

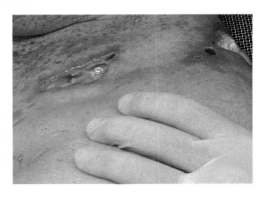

Dying flesh
In very rare instances, an infection with certain strep A strains can destroy flesh. Scientists believe this occurs when enzymes secreted by the bacteria break down proteins in the tissue.

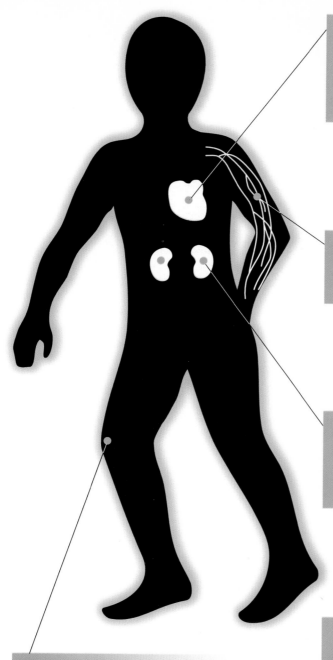

Heart disease
In some cases, inflammation of heart tissue follows untreated rheumatic fever. This condition can damage the heart valves so that they no longer open and close properly. Blood passing through the damaged valves may produce a sound called a heart murmur.

Blood poisoning
In rare instances, strep A bacteria enter the bloodstream, where they multiply rapidly and release toxins. This condition is known as septicemia or blood poisoning.

Kidney disease
In rare instances, tiny particles produced by the immune system in fighting a strep infection become lodged in the glomeruli, parts of the kidney that filter wastes from the blood. As a result, the glomeruli become inflamed, hampering kidney function.

Toxic shock
In rare instances, blood pressure drops dangerously low and fever rises rapidly as the body reacts to strep A toxins. Without prompt treatment, the body goes into shock. Major organs may then fail, with fatal consequences.

Inflamed joints
Joints sometimes become *inflamed* (swollen and painful) as the immune system fights a strep A infection. Scientists believe this condition, which is a symptom of rheumatic fever, results from a misdirected attack by the immune system on the body's own tissue.

155

strain (subgroup) of bacteria and its particular capabilities, the site of the initial infection, and how well the individual's immune system can fight the infection.

When a strep infection begins in the upper respiratory tract, the symptoms of strep throat typically follow, usually from one to four days after exposure to the bacteria. Although strep throat can occur at any age, it occurs most frequently among school-aged children and becomes much less common with age. Symptoms include a fever as high as 104 °F (40 °C) that comes on suddenly, a severe sore throat, and a general feeling of achiness and fatigue. The lymph nodes in the neck often become enlarged and tender, and the throat and tonsils become red and swollen. Some patients, particularly children, also have abdominal pain and vomiting. But others experience milder symptoms.

Scarlet fever was once a widespread and sometimes fatal strep A infection, though today the disease is much less common in the United States and rarely severe. Like strep throat, scarlet fever begins in the respiratory tract. But the bacteria responsible for scarlet fever release a toxin, and the immune system's response to this toxin produces the disease's characteristic scarlet-colored rash. The rash typically begins at the neck and may spread over most of the body except the face, giving a sandpaperlike texture to the skin. After a week or so, the rash fades, and the skin flakes or peels.

In addition to a sore throat and rash, common signs of scarlet fever are a "strawberry tongue" characterized by bright red spots, a flushed face with tiny white lines around the mouth, and fine red lines in the skin creases of the elbows and the groin. People with scarlet fever may not exhibit all of these symptoms, however.

Strep A outside the throat

If strep throat and scarlet fever are not treated, they may have serious consequences, including rheumatic fever and kidney inflammation. Rheumatic fever can follow from one to five weeks after the initial infection, though this happens in only 3 percent of people with an untreated strep throat, most of them children aged 5 to 15, according to studies. Scientists believe the illness is triggered when an immune system that has been fired up to fight a strep infection mistakenly attacks the body's own tissues.

The most common symptoms of rheumatic fever include *inflammation* (pain and swelling) of two or more joints, a red rash, and pea-sized lumps beneath the skin. These symptoms may last from weeks to months. Rheumatic fever can also affect the nervous system and cause Sydenham's chorea, a disorder characterized by involuntary, jerking movements.

If rheumatic fever continues unchecked, the heart tissue can become inflamed. The inflammation may subside without producing any symptoms. But it can result in damage to heart tissue—most often, a scarring and thickening of the heart valves. This condition, known as rheumatic heart disease, can limit some patients' physical activities and shorten their lives.

When the site of the infection is the skin, group A strep can cause impetigo. Impetigo is more common in warmer climates and in areas where hygiene is poor and living conditions are crowded, and it is most frequently seen among children and young adults.

The most common sites of impetigo are the face and the hands. The infection first appears as a rash of tiny, fluid-filled red blisters that break, exposing moist, "weeping" patches of skin. As the fluid dries, it leaves thick, honey-colored crusts.

Strep A bacteria that enter the skin also can cause erysipelas, a disorder that primarily affects the very young and the very old. Symptoms include sudden fever, headache, and itchy, red patches that typically spread across the face and form a tender, inflamed area with raised edges. Blisters can develop in the inflamed area, burst, and then crust over.

Some people with group A strep infections—most commonly strep throat and impetigo—develop an inflammation of the kidney called acute glomerulonephritis. Experts believe that this disease, like rheumatic fever, is triggered by an immune response gone awry. In this case, tiny particles produced by the immune system in fighting a strep infection become lodged in the glomeruli, the parts of the kidney that filter wastes from the blood. As a result, the glomeruli become inflamed or damaged, impairing kidney function.

Mild cases of glomerulonephritis may produce no symptoms. When symptoms do occur, they usually begin from 6 to 21 days after the initial strep infection. Damaged glomeruli may allow blood cells and protein to leak into the urine, turning it the color of tea. Puffiness or swelling, especially around the eyes, is common, and blood pressure may become elevated.

Symptoms usually subside on their own, and about 95 percent of patients recover normal kidney function within a month or two. But in a small percentage of the remainder, the disease progresses so quickly that the kidneys fail—an event signaled by the passage of only small amounts of urine. Kidney failure causes wastes usually eliminated in the urine to accumulate in the body, a potentially fatal condition called uremia.

Invasive strep A—the deadliest infection

In invasive strep, the most notorious of group A strep infections, strep A bacteria cause disease in such normally germ-free sites of the body as the lungs, brain, joints, kidneys, bone marrow, and blood. Although it's not always clear how the bacteria gain entry, many cases of invasive group A strep infections begin with a skin infection or upper respiratory tract infection.

Whether a person develops an invasive infection depends partly on whether he or she has been exposed to certain virulent, toxin-producing bacteria. But because individuals differ in their suscepti-

IS IT A
cold, the flu, or strep?

Runny nose, sore throat, headache, that run-down feeling are all symptoms of a variety of different diseases caused by both viruses and bacteria. Though the cold, the flu, and a strep infection all share symptoms in common, there are some important differences.

	Cold	Flu	Strep throat
Onset of symptoms	Within 1 to 4 days of infection	Within 24 to 48 hours of infection	Within 1 to 5 days of infection
Sore throat	Sometimes	Often	Almost always; often with difficulty swallowing; sudden onset
Fever of 100 °F (37.8 °C) or higher	Rare	Often	Almost always
Respiratory symptoms	Runny nose always, cough often	Chest discomfort and cough often, runny nose sometimes	No cough, runny nose rare
Enlarged and tender lymph nodes	Never	Very rare	Often
Muscle aches, headaches	Often	Often	No headache; muscle aches may be severe
Treatment	Over-the-counter medication to relieve symptoms	Bed rest, fluids, over-the-counter medication to relieve symptoms	Antibiotics, over-the-counter medication to reduce fever

bility to the toxins, some people remain well even if they are infected with virulent strep A strains.

Infection with group A strep can develop into septicemia, commonly known as blood poisoning, in which the bacteria multiply in the bloodstream. Although disease-fighting white blood cells usually stop the infection, in people with a weakened immune system, including the very old and people with such illnesses as cancer or AIDS, the bacteria can multiply unchecked.

Symptoms of septicemia include fever, chills, vomiting, and a red rash. If the infection goes untreated, large numbers of circulating bacteria and the toxins they release can bring on streptococcal toxic shock syndrome (STSS). The process begins when the toxins cause holes in the walls of blood vessels, allowing blood proteins and fluid to leak out. Blood pressure in the body then falls, resulting in shock. Some of the signs of impending shock are sweating, faintness, nausea, pale and clammy skin, and a rapid pulse rate.

What health experts find dismaying about STSS is that most of the patients stricken with it are relatively young—under 50—and otherwise healthy. Also alarming is how quickly patients with a seemingly commonplace skin infection or flulike symptoms—such as fever, chills, and a sore throat—develop potentially fatal shock and suffer organ failure and irreversible tissue damage. These symptoms can come on so quickly that patients are often dangerously ill by the time they seek treatment.

About 5 to 10 percent of all people with invasive group A strep infection develop necrotizing fasciitis, the widely publicized "flesh-eating" infection. Sometimes the infection also destroys muscle, a condition called necrotizing myositis. Scientists believe that the death of these tissues results when enzymes secreted by the bacteria break down proteins in the tissue.

Necrotizing fasciitis usually begins with an infection at a break in the skin. Portals for this infection range from extensive wounds or surgical incisions to such seemingly minor breaches in the skin as chicken pox blisters or a scratch from a thorn.

Not all cases of necrotizing fasciitis begin with a skin wound, however. In some instances, the infection begins deep at the site of a bruise or muscle strain, probably "seeded" by group A strep bacteria already in the bloodstream. In other cases, the condition stems from a strep infection at a site other than the skin, such as pneumonia.

Signs of necrotizing fasciitis include fever and an expanding area of redness, swelling, and severe pain at the wound site. That pain may disappear, however, as the destruction of nerves numbs the area. As the disease progresses, often within hours, shock may set in, along with extensive destruction of the infected tissue. In severe cases, the infection can spread as rapidly as an inch every hour.

Researchers say some strains of group A strep pack such a punch because of a toxin the bacteria produce. They believe the toxin may play a role in streptococcal toxic shock by triggering the immune system to release harmful substances.

Diagnosing a strep infection

Because strep infections can so quickly become serious, physicians stress the importance of seeking immediate medical attention once a strep infection is suspected. Physicians typically diagnose mild strep infections on the basis of the flulike ailments that accompany the infection and a number of telltale symptoms that characterize particular diseases. For example, a severe sore throat is typical of strep throat and a red rash and strawberry tongue indicate scarlet fever. To confirm the presence of a strep infection, physicians usually order laboratory tests.

The conventional lab test for group A strep is a throat culture. Doctors swab the mucus in a patient's throat to obtain a sample of any bacteria present. From that sample, technicians grow a larger sample and test it for group A strep. Results of the throat culture are generally available within a day. Another test method looks for strep A *antibodies* (special disease-fighting proteins) to reveal the presence of the bacteria in the throat swab. The antibody test can provide results in minutes. However, many doctors believe that such tests are less sensitive than the culture method, and they advise a follow-up throat culture if the rapid test result is negative.

In the case of more serious strep infections, such as rheumatic fever or acute glomerulonephritis, physicians typically diagnose the condition on the basis of the patient's symptoms, a history of recent strep infection, and results of blood tests that indicate elevated levels of antibodies to group A strep bacteria. For kidney inflammation, diagnostic procedures include a urinalysis, which reveals the presence of blood and protein in the urine, and tests measuring kidney function. In some cases, a physician may perform a biopsy, a procedure in which a sample of the inflamed kidney tissue is taken from the patient and examined under a microscope.

When a patient's symptoms suggest an invasive infection, physicians can confirm the diagnosis by growing a culture of the bacteria from a blood sample. But because these infections are life-threatening, treatment often is started as soon as physicians even suspect the possibility of invasive disease.

Treating a strep infection

Treatment of a strep infection typically begins with a course of antibiotics. Doctors usually prescribe penicillin to treat strep throat or scarlet fever. Patients who are allergic to penicillin receive an alternative antibiotic, such as erythromycin.

Patients with impetigo may also receive an antibiotic ointment to spread on infected skin. Because impetigo is highly contagious, physicians recommend that infected individuals try not to scratch their sores to avoid spreading the infection further. If they touch a sore, they should wash their hands and make sure others do not share the same towels, washcloths, pillowcases, or clothing until the infection clears. Physicians also advise patients to wash infected areas with soap and gently remove the skin crusts, which helps any antibiotic ointment prescribed by the doctor reach the affected areas.

Erysipelas is treated with antibiotics taken by injection or orally. Physicians may also recommend cold packs, aspirin, or topical anesthetics to relieve pain and itching.

Physicians stress the importance of taking the full course of antibiotics to eradicate a strep infection, even though symptoms often subside after a few days. For patients with strep throat or scarlet fever, failure to take the full dosage may result in continued infection and rheumatic fever.

A patient with rheumatic fever requires bed rest and aspirin or other inflammation-reducing drugs to bring down fever and ease joint pain and swelling. Physicians also prescribe antibiotics to wipe

Medical experts are reexamining the uses of antibiotics as more and more bacteria develop resistance to the drugs.

Keeping the Wonder in Wonder Drugs

By Daniel A. Hussar

PLAGUE STRIKES IN INDIA IN 1994. In Russia, diphtheria infects some 15,000 people in 1994, killing about 1,700, and the World Health Organization (WHO) says it expects between 100,000 and 200,000 new diphtheria cases in 1995. WHO, the United Nations agency responsible for tracking disease worldwide, also warns of a possible spread to other countries, and WHO officials call the diphtheria epidemic "the biggest public health emergency in Europe since World War II [1939-1945]." In the United States and other countries, tuberculosis reemerges as a serious threat in the 1990's. Again and again, killers thought to have been vanquished by antibiotics prove that they are still deadly.

Penicillin, introduced in 1941, and other antibiotics that came after it have saved the lives of millions of people who would have succumbed to pneumonia, scarlet fever, and a host of other diseases caused by bacteria. Little wonder that antibiotics were dubbed "wonder drugs" soon after their appearance or that some public health officials—impressed with the effectiveness of wonder drugs and new vaccines—predicted the end of infectious diseases as a major health threat.

Have wonder drugs lost some of their power, as outbreaks around the world would suggest? The ability of microbes to counter the action of antibiotics figures prominently in the resurgence of certain infections, and the growing problem of drug-resistant bacteria had become serious enough by 1995 that some health officials were warning of a possible medical disaster.

To understand the problem, it's helpful to understand what antibiotics are and what they can and cannot do. An antibiotic is a substance produced by a microorganism that is capable of killing other microorganisms or stopping their growth and multiplication. Penicillin, for example, is produced by a mold. Today, many antibiotics are produced artificially in laboratories.

How antibiotics work

Antibiotics are effective primarily against bacteria and the infections bacteria cause. A few antibiotics can fight infections caused by fungi or parasites, but antibiotics are not effective against viruses.

Antibiotics work against bacteria in several ways, but they all impair the functioning of a bacterium's single cell so that the organism either dies or stops reproducing. Each bacterium is encased by a cell wall that gives it shape and protects it from foreign substances. Just inside the cell wall is the cell membrane, a porous structure through which nutrients and other vital substances enter the cell. Antibiotics can kill bacteria by damaging the cell membrane or by interfering with the growth and repair of the cell wall, thereby enabling the cell's contents to spill out or harmful substances to invade the cell. Antibiotics that work in this way include the penicillins and cephalosporins.

Antibiotics that stop bacteria from reproducing interfere with vital chemical processes within the cell, including the replication of DNA, the cell's genetic material. DNA replication is crucial to bacteria's ability to multiply. Once bacteria no longer multiply, the body's disease-fighting immune system can more easily attack and destroy them. Antibiotics that interfere with cell processes include the aminoglycosides and tetracyclines.

Types of antibiotics

Antibiotics vary in the scope of their activity and are categorized according to the infections they fight best. Scientists and health care professionals may initially classify bacterial infections as Gram positive or Gram negative, depending upon the bacteria's ability to absorb a special dye applied in a laboratory. Each group of bacteria has characteristics that influence its sensitivity to different antibiotics. Some antibiotics are most effective against Gram-negative infections, and others work best against Gram-positive infections. Both kinds of antibiotics are said to have a narrow spectrum of action. Antibiotics that work well against many of the bacteria in both classes are said to have a broad spectrum. But not even a broad-spectrum antibiotic can fight all types of bacteria.

The most commonly used antibiotics include penicillin and many of the drugs derived from it, as well as its chemical cousins, the

The author:

Daniel A. Hussar is the Remington Professor of Pharmacy at the Philadelphia College of Pharmacy and Science.

How antibiotics work

Antibiotics work against bacteria in one of three ways—by interfering with the growth or repair of the bacterium's protective cell wall, by damaging the cell membrane just inside the wall, or by blocking essential chemical processes within the cell.

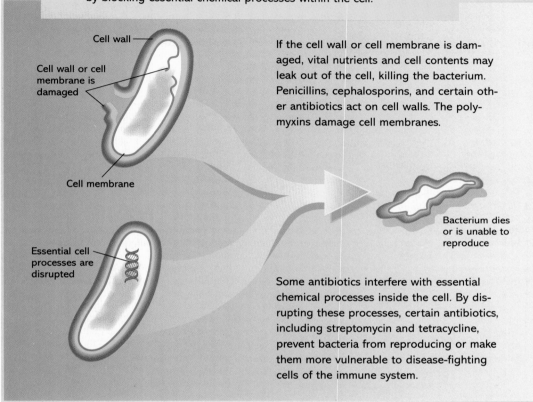

Cell wall

Cell wall or cell membrane is damaged

Cell membrane

Essential cell processes are disrupted

If the cell wall or cell membrane is damaged, vital nutrients and cell contents may leak out of the cell, killing the bacterium. Penicillins, cephalosporins, and certain other antibiotics act on cell walls. The polymyxins damage cell membranes.

Bacterium dies or is unable to reproduce

Some antibiotics interfere with essential chemical processes inside the cell. By disrupting these processes, certain antibiotics, including streptomycin and tetracycline, prevent bacteria from reproducing or make them more vulnerable to disease-fighting cells of the immune system.

cephalosporins. Today, 14 penicillin derivatives are available in the United States—including amoxicillin, ampicillin, and penicillin V—and 21 cephalosporins, including cefaclor and cephalexin. The various antibiotics in each category differ slightly in their chemical makeup to allow each one to work more effectively against certain types of bacteria.

Physicians prefer to prescribe narrow-spectrum antibiotics whenever possible for two reasons. First, extensive use of any antibiotic increases the risk that bacteria will develop resistance to the drug. It's far more dangerous in terms of treating future infections for bacteria to develop resistance to an antibiotic with many uses. Second, by killing so many different kinds of microorganisms, a broad-spectrum antibiotic can upset the balance of microorganisms normally harbored in the human body. These microorganisms perform a number of useful functions, such as aiding in digestion.

It's not always possible to prescribe a narrow-spectrum antibiotic,

Some commonly prescribed antibiotics

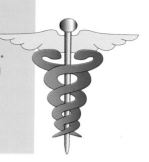

Antibiotics are drugs used primarily to treat infections caused by bacteria. In selecting an antibiotic, physicians consider the site of the infection, the bacteria causing it, and the properties of the antibiotic. Certain conditions, such as a patient's pregnancy, may also influence the choice.

Drug class	Drug name	Action	Used against	Taken
Aminoglycosides	Gentamicin	Prevent production of essential proteins in bacteria.	Many infections, including serious skin and eye and life-threatening infections of the respiratory and urinary tracts.	By injection or as a cream or ointment for certain skin infections.
Cephalosporins	Cefaclor Cefadroxil Cephalexin Cephradrine	Prevent bacterial cell wall growth and repair.	A broad range of infections, including those of the middle ear, respiratory tract, and urinary tract.	Orally or by injection.
Fluoroquinolones	Ciprofloxacin Norfloxacin Ofloxacin	Prevent production of essential proteins in bacteria.	Infections of the urinary tract, intestinal tract, and eye.	Orally, by eye drops, or by injection.
Glycopeptide	Vancomycin	Prevent bacterial cell wall growth and repair.	Serious respiratory tract and other infections that are resistant to other antibiotics.	Usually by injection.
Macrolides	Azithromycin Clarithromycin Erythromycin	Prevent production of essential proteins in bacteria.	A broad range of infections, including those of the respiratory tract and skin. Also used to treat sexually transmitted diseases.	Orally.
Penicillins	Amoxicillin Ampicillin Penicillin V	Prevent bacterial cell wall growth and repair.	A broad range of infections, including those of the middle ear, respiratory tract, urinary tract, and sexually transmitted diseases.	Orally or by injection. Some oral penicillins should be taken at least one hour before or two hours after a meal.
Polymyxins	Polymyxin B	Damage cell membrane.	Skin and eye infections.	Usually as a cream or ointment.
Tetracyclines	Doxycycline Oxytetracycline Tetracycline	Prevent production of essential proteins in bacteria.	A broad range of infections, including minor skin infections, acne, respiratory tract infections, and sexually transmitted diseases.	Usually orally.

Source: *Physician's Desk Reference; Remington's Pharmaceutical Sciences.*

however. There may be no drug specifically targeted at the disease-causing microorganism. Or the precise strain of bacteria responsible for the infection may not be immediately identifiable.

The problem of drug resistance

Health authorities warn against taking antibiotics for every infection. Some mild infections of the middle ear and the sinuses, for example, may clear up on their own. And antibiotics have no effect on colds, which are caused by viruses.

Overuse of antibiotics has created a significant public health problem, infectious disease experts warn. The more antibiotics are used, the more chances bacteria have of adapting to them and developing drug resistance. One way in which adaptation occurs is when a *mutation* (change) in a bacterium's DNA transforms its chemical structure sufficiently to enable the bacterium to withstand an antibiotic's onslaught.

The number of resistant bacteria soars when the less hardy, nonresistant bacteria are killed by an antibiotic and no longer provide competition for resources. The resistant strains can then multiply unchecked and, over time, become the strains that people most commonly encounter. Researchers have found that bacteria can also exchange genetic material, and thus resistant bacteria can transfer their resistance to unrelated strains.

One reason for the rising use of antibiotics has been an increase in the number of infections doctors are treating. For instance, the incidence of middle ear infections, among the most common maladies of young children, has skyrocketed. The number of children treated for middle ear infections soared from 10 million in 1975 to 24 million in 1990, according to statistics from the Centers for Disease Control and Prevention in Atlanta, Georgia. Health officials attribute the rise in part to the proliferation of day-care facilities, where infections can easily spread. New diagnostic techniques have caused a jump in the number of sinus infections treated each year.

Antibiotic resistance has already become a serious problem. Certain strains of the bacteria that cause more than 600,000 cases of gonorrhea in the United States each year have developed resis-

Developing drug resistance

Drug resistance enables bacteria to live despite the presence of antibiotics that would normally kill them. The overuse of antibiotics contributes to drug resistance by killing off drug-susceptible bacteria, thus allowing resistant bacteria to flourish amid far less competition for needed resources.

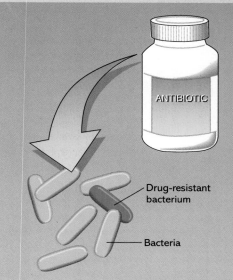

Drug resistance occurs when a bacterium acquires a new gene or a *mutation* (change) in its genetic material that enables it to defend itself against an antibiotic.

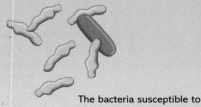

The bacteria susceptible to the antibiotic die, but the resistant bacterium survives.

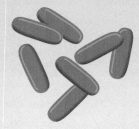

As the resistant bacterium reproduces, a new population of drug-resistant bacteria emerges. Drug-resistant bacteria can also pass genetic material to other bacteria, making them drug-resistant as well.

Tips on taking antibiotics

Antibiotics, like any medication, can be misused, sometimes with serious consequences. The following tips can help prevent unwanted consequences from antibiotic use:

- Take the full course, even if you no longer have symptoms. If you stop taking the antibiotic, some of the tougher bacteria may be left alive to reproduce. These bacteria may develop resistance to the antibiotic.

- Follow the instructions on dosage as well as on how and when the drug should be taken. The body absorbs some antibiotics poorly when they are taken with food.

- Do not share antibiotics with anyone else or take another person's prescription without consulting a physician. You won't receive the full course, nor will the other person.

- Tell your doctor and pharmacist if you have ever had an allergic reaction to an antibiotic. Also tell the doctor about other medications you are taking, to avoid harmful drug interactions.

- Do not use antibiotics that are outdated. Some outdated antibiotics become *toxic* (poisonous).

- Do not pressure your physician to prescribe antibiotics that, in his or her opinion, you do not need. Taking antibiotics unnecessarily may enable bacteria in your body to develop antibiotic resistance.

- If you are pregnant, tell your physician before he or she prescribes antibiotics for you. Some antibiotics can potentially harm a fetus.

- Ask about any potential unpleasant or harmful side effects of the antibiotic you are prescribed and find out what you should do if they occur.

Source: Daniel A. Hussar.

tance to some of the penicillins to which they were previously susceptible and have begun to develop resistance to another class of antibiotics called fluoroquinolones. Certain strains of other organisms have also developed multidrug resistance, including *Streptococcus pneumoniae*, which is responsible for most cases of bacterial pneumonia and many ear infections, and *Haemophilus influenzae*, a common cause of bacterial meningitis. Meningitis is a potentially fatal infection of the spinal fluid and the lining of the brain and spinal cord.

More startling, only one antibiotic—vancomycin—remained effective in 1995 against infections of skin, wounds, and blood caused by certain strains of staphylococcus bacteria. If these bacteria develop resistance to vancomycin as well, deaths from staph infections will undoubtedly soar.

Drug-resistant strains also are part of the recent resurgence of tuberculosis (TB) in the United States, especially in crowded facilities such as hospitals, prisons, and shelters for the homeless. Health officials say that failure to take the full six- to nine-month course of drug treatment is the main cause of drug-resistant TB.

As physicians battle drug-resistant strains, they may be setting the stage for further drug resistance. A four-year survey of 13,351 U.S. physicians, published in January 1995, found that in treating common ailments, such as sinusitis and ear infections, doctors are relying more on the newer, more powerful (and more expensive) antibiotics, such as the cephalosporins, and less on the older antibiotics, such as amoxillin. The researchers noted that increased use of stronger drugs not only raises medical costs but increases the likelihood that bacteria will also develop resistance to these antibiotics.

The possibility of side effects

All antibiotics have the potential to cause side effects. Penicillin, in particular, prompts an allergic response in some people.

Signs and symptoms of an allergic reaction can include shortness of breath, tightening of the air passages, nausea, vomiting, or hives. Because drug reactions can be serious, it's important to call a

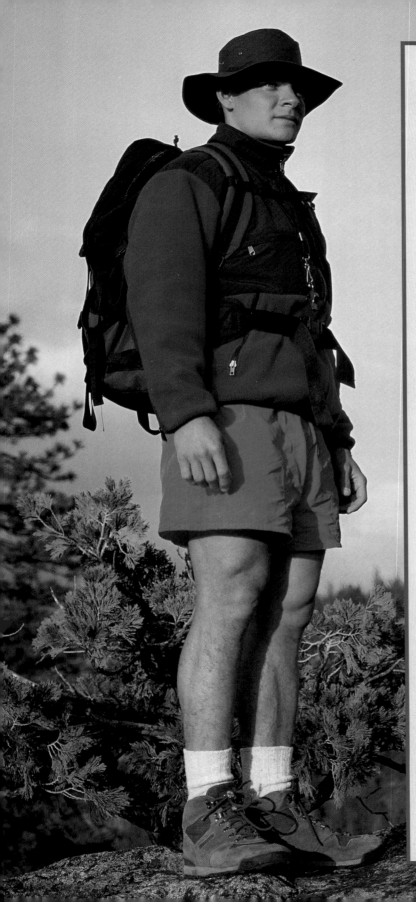

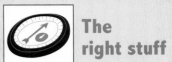

The right stuff

What to wear and what to bring:

Clothes:

- Shirt—polypropylene knit
- Pullover—polyester fleece
- Waterproof jacket and pants set—breathable Gore-Tex or coated nylon
- Hiking shorts—nylon
- Hiking boots—sturdy high-tops
- Socks—thin polypro liner and thick, padded hiking socks
- Hat—broad-brimmed to protect your face from the sun

Daypack with following items:

- Guidebook
- Map
- Compass
- Lunch and snacks—sandwiches, dried fruit, trail mix, bagels
- 1-quart water bottle—lightweight polyethylene
- Water-treatment tablets
- First-aid kit, with instructions
- Utility candle or tube of fire ribbon
- Pocketknife
- Waterproof matches
- Flashlight with fresh batteries
- Whistle
- Space blanket
- Thin polypropylene knit shirt for extra warmth in emergency
- Emergency food, such as powerbars and dried fruit

Additional items that might be needed, depending on weather and location:

- Sunglasses
- Lip balm and sunblock
- Insect repellent

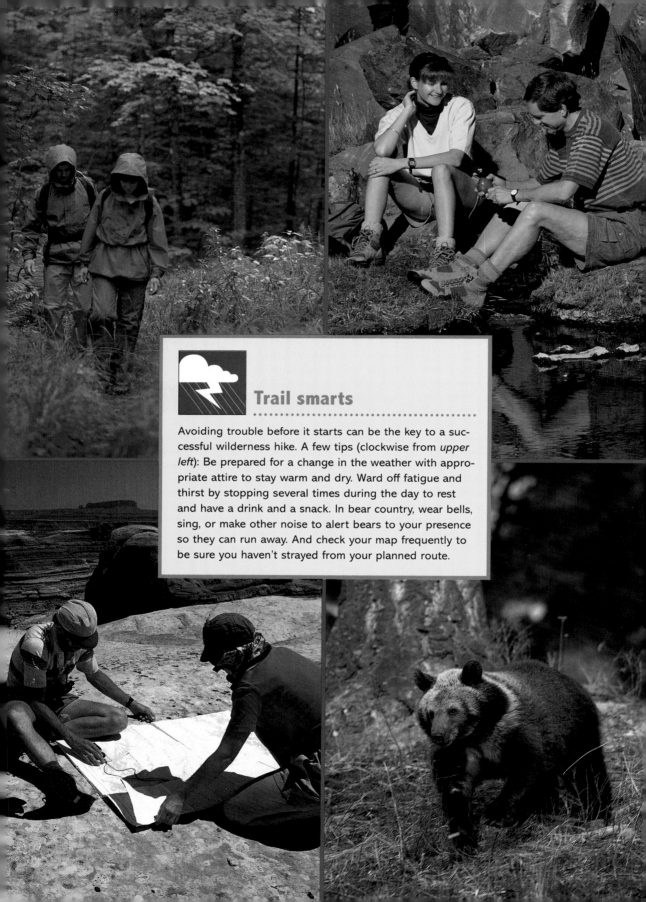

Trail smarts

Avoiding trouble before it starts can be the key to a successful wilderness hike. A few tips (clockwise from *upper left*): Be prepared for a change in the weather with appropriate attire to stay warm and dry. Ward off fatigue and thirst by stopping several times during the day to rest and have a drink and a snack. In bear country, wear bells, sing, or make other noise to alert bears to your presence so they can run away. And check your map frequently to be sure you haven't strayed from your planned route.

difficult to cross? Has ice or snow at higher elevations obscured the trail or made walking treacherous? What is the forecast for the next 24 hours? Are there any special hazards you should be aware of?

Lastly, call a friend to leave word about the starting point of your hike, your planned route, and time you expect to be getting back home. If you do not return on schedule, that person can notify park or forest authorities to look for you.

Some rules for the trail

When hikers end up needing such help, it is often because of foolish actions. Following a few common-sense rules can prevent most problems on a hike.

Assuming you've chosen a hike that's right for your strength and endurance, you should have no trouble avoiding fatigue. Simply walk at a steady, comfortable pace and take frequent breaks for rest and refreshment. Several short time-outs, with snacks of complex carbohydrates such as fruit and granola bars, are better for you than one long stop for a meal.

Remember to drink often, before you're thirsty. Thirst is an early sign of dehydration. Drinking lots of water or other liquids is especially important in hot weather, when there is a danger of getting overheated. But avoid caffeine and alcohol, which speed fluid loss from the body. Drinking alcohol is a bad idea for any hike because it can lead to faulty judgment and it causes the body to lose heat.

Staying warm or cool is also a matter of matching your clothing to the hiking conditions and your exertions. Peel off a layer of clothing before you get drenched with sweat, put on an extra one before you get chilled, and don rain gear while you're still dry.

Taking care of your feet on the trail is also of utmost importance. If you feel one of your boots rubbing your skin and causing an irritation, apply tape or moleskin to the affected spot right away, before a blister forms.

Other rules will help keep you from suddenly discovering that you have lost your way or that a member of the group is missing. Keep everyone together. The two most experienced hikers should take up the first and last positions, with children and beginners between them. If you decide to leave the trail for any reason, take off your pack and place it on the ground as a signal to the others. And at trail junctions, where the path diverges, wait for everyone to catch up before proceeding.

At frequent points along the trail, and especially at junctions, check your map to be certain that you have not veered from your route. Also pay attention to your surroundings: Look for landmarks that can keep you oriented, and note which way streams are flowing.

There are also rules for safety on the trail. Although the hazards one encounters on a hike are usually minimal, certain conditions call for caution.

Be careful crossing streams, and turn back if a stream has been

When things go wrong

Even the most carefully prepared hiker is sometimes faced with an emergency. Knowing how to cope with an unexpected and potentially dangerous situation can prevent a mishap from becoming a calamity.

A fall or other accident is always possible, so you should learn basic first-aid skills before venturing into the wilderness. You need to know how to treat both minor injuries like sprains and more serious threats, such as bleeding.

Two medical problems that you should be prepared to treat are overheating and chilling. If you spot symptoms of either condition in yourself or a companion, take action immediately.

Overheating, or hyperthermia, takes two forms: heat exhaustion and heatstroke. Heat exhaustion comes on slowly and is characterized by weakness and fatigue. Other symptoms include nausea, dizziness, and muscle cramps. Heatstroke is a serious condition that can develop quickly. Sweating stops, the body's heat-regulating mechanism breaks down, and body temperature rises to a life-threatening level. Symptoms typically include rapid pulse, shallow breathing, nausea, and a progressive loss of consciousness.

When a person shows signs of overheating, stop the hike immediately and make the individual rest in the shade and drink lots of cool liquids. If heatstroke seems to be developing, drench the person with the coldest liquids you can find and send for medical help.

Because an accident is always a possibility on the trail, hikers should know how to treat injuries such as sprains, *below left*. In case of a forced overnight stay in the wilderness—whether due to an injury or to getting lost—it's useful to know how to rig an emergency camp, *below right*.

At the opposite extreme is hypothermia, when body temperature drops. The first signs are shivering, lethargy, and low morale. As the condition progresses, the person shivers uncontrollably and becomes confused. The first priority in treating hypothermia is to get the individual out of wind and rain and into dry clothing. Then give the person warm liquids to drink, but nothing containing alcohol. In a serious case, press yourselves against the victim to share body heat.

Another possible situation to be prepared for is getting lost. Should you find yourself off the trail, you can usually retrace your steps. If that isn't successful, however, there may be other options, such as following a compass bearing to a nearby road or following a stream downhill to a settlement. But unless you have complete confidence in your pathfinding abilities, it's usually best to stay put. By remaining in one place, you will make it easier for a search party to locate you.

To increase your chances of being found, spread out a bright-colored object in an opening where it will be visible to searchers and light a smoky fire if you can do so without the risk of starting a forest fire. Every once in a while, blow three blasts—the standard emergency signal—on your whistle.

If you have to spend the night in the wild, find a sheltered spot and rig an emergency camp—a poncho draped over a low branch can serve as a makeshift tent. Wrap yourself and your companions together in a space blanket or poncho and put on all your extra clothing. Sit with some insulation between you and the ground.

To pass the time, sing, tell bad jokes, and munch on your emergency rations. And above all, don't panic. Keep in mind that you left word where you were going, so someone is sure to come looking for you.   [E. D. and E. S.]

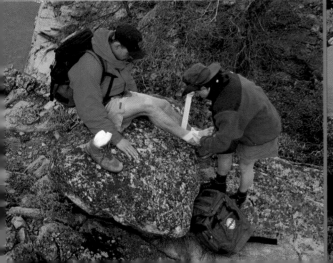

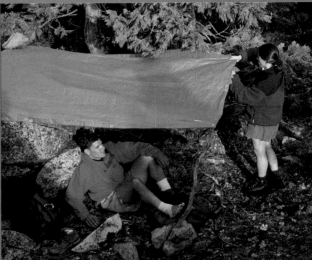

meats and poultry, for example, cannot detect harmful microorganisms, and available laboratory tests are too slow and limited to certify the safety of every shipment of food before its distribution. Besides, there are simply too many places where food can become tainted, including home kitchens, for the government ever to provide a complete shield against food poisoning.

A host of threats, with bacteria heading the list

Many substances can contaminate food. Some of the microbes causing food poisoning are relatively new threats, compounding the prevention problem. A generation ago, most Americans knew that eating undercooked pork could give them a disease called trichinosis and that improperly canned food could cause botulism, a deadly form of food poisoning. But until recently, few people had even heard of campylobacter, listeria, or *E. coli* 0157:H7—bacteria widely recognized as food contaminants only in the 1980's. Similarly, while most cooks know that cracked eggs might be tainted with salmonella bacteria, few may be aware that even flawless eggs can be contaminated, infected by a strain of salmonella within the hen's body.

The microbial sources of food poisoning fall into four categories: infectious bacteria, *toxins* (poisons), parasites, and viruses. Of the four, bacteria are by far the most prevalent threat.

Bacteria can infect food animals and remain in their flesh, or be transferred to the flesh from the intestinal tract, after the animals are slaughtered. The microbes can also enter meats and other foods from water, dirt, or other sources. Thorough cooking almost always kills bacteria, so illnesses from them are typically traced to raw, undercooked, or improperly processed foods, usually of animal origin. But even foods that rarely harbor bacterial contamination can arrive at the table tainted through *cross-contamination,* in which bacteria from one source—such as raw chicken—are transferred to other foods via unwashed hands, utensils, dishes, or cutting surfaces. Moreover, some bacteria that do not usually reside in food can spread by hitching a ride on food prepared by an infected individual.

Once in food, bacteria can multiply rapidly. That is especially true when the food sits out at room temperature.

Salmonella and campylobacter bacteria are responsible for most cases of bacterial food poisoning. The CDC estimates that up to 4 million Americans contract salmonella infections every year, and some 500 die. Salmonella is especially common in poultry; public health studies have indicated that it is present in up to 60 percent of raw chicken sold at supermarkets. The bacteria also thrive in eggs, meats, and unpasteurized milk. The 1994 ice cream-related salmonella outbreak was attributed to cross-contamination: Ice cream mix had been delivered to the factory in a tanker truck that had earlier carried raw eggs.

Campylobacter bacteria rarely kill, but they are the most common bacterial cause of diarrhea in the United States—up to 10 million

Some Leading Causes of Food Poisoning

Food poisoning is a term used to describe illnesses of the gastrointestinal tract (stomach and intestines) brought on by eating contaminated food. The four main contaminants of food are bacteria, *toxins* (poisons), parasites, and viruses.

Bacteria

Cause of poisoning*	Primary sources	Symptoms	Time to onset
Campylobacter jejuni	Undercooked poultry and beef; unpasteurized milk	Abdominal pain, fever, diarrhea	2 to 10 days
Escherichia coli (E. coli) 0157:H7	Undercooked ground beef; unpasteurized milk	Diarrhea, sometimes mixed with blood; abdominal pain; vomiting	1 to 8 days
Listeria monocytogenes	Deli meats; soft cheeses; undercooked poultry, beef, and pork	Headache, fever, vomiting; severe cases can damage the brain or other organs	2 to 6 weeks
Salmonella	Undercooked eggs, poultry, and meat	Abdominal pain, vomiting, diarrhea, fever	5 hours to 3 days
Shigella	Various foods, which are usually contaminated by an infected person with poor hygiene	Fever; vomiting; abdominal pain; diarrhea, often with blood or pus	1 to 4 days

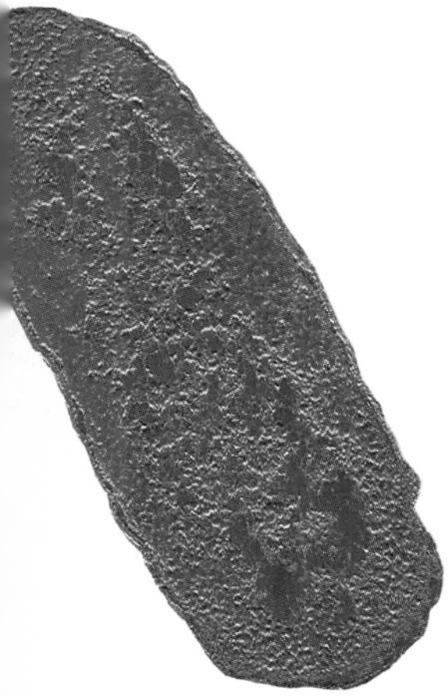

E. coli

*Microbes are shown greatly magnified but not to the same scale.

Critically reviewed by U.S. Centers for Disease Control and Prevention.

	Cause of poisoning	Primary sources	Symptoms	Time to onset
Toxins ▼	*Clostridium botulinum* toxin (botulism)	Improperly canned foods—most often, home-canned vegetables	Double vision; weakness; breathing difficulties brought on by paralysis	4 hours to 8 days
	Clostridium perfringens toxin	Foods left too long at room temperature, especially beef and poultry	Abdominal pain, diarrhea	8 to 24 hours
	Staphylococcus aureus toxin	Foods left too long at room temperature, especially egg or potato salads and pastries	Abdominal pain, vomiting, diarrhea	2 to 8 hours
	Ciguatera toxins	Large reef-dwelling fish, such as grouper, snapper, and amberjack	Abdominal pain, vomiting, diarrhea; nervous system disturbances, such as tingling of hands and feet	2 to 8 hours

Clostridium botulinum

	Cause of poisoning	Primary sources	Symptoms	Time to onset
Parasites ▼	*Trichinella spiralis* (trichinosis)	Inadequately cooked pork or pork products	Abdominal discomfort, muscle pain, fever, swelling of eyelids	7 to 15 days
	Fish-borne parasites	Raw or undercooked freshwater or saltwater fish	Gastrointestinal problems, anemia, liver disorders	Varies, depending on parasite

Trichinella spiralis

	Cause of poisoning	Primary sources	Symptoms	Time to onset
Viruses ▼	Hepatitis A virus	Shellfish from sewage-polluted water; food tainted by infected individual	Fatigue, fever, vomiting, jaundice	2 to 6 weeks
	Norwalk virus and other, related viruses	Shellfish from sewage-polluted water; food tainted by an infected individual	Nausea, abdominal pain, vomiting, diarrhea	Usually within 12 to 48 hours

Hepatitis A virus

cases annually, according to the CDC. Like salmonella, campylo-bacter bacteria frequently infect poultry. Some studies have found that about 80 percent of retail chickens carry this microorganism. Campylobacter infections have also been traced to unpasteurized milk and undercooked meat.

Shigella bacteria infect as many as 1.4 million Americans annually. Although shigella infections are often traced to such foods as potato salad or chicken salad, the microbe can be found in almost any kind of dish, because it enters food during handling. Infected individuals pass shigella bacteria in their feces and can unwittingly spread the microbes to food if they do not wash their hands thoroughly after using the toilet. Shigella outbreaks often are traced to a single food preparer with poor hand-washing habits.

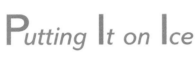

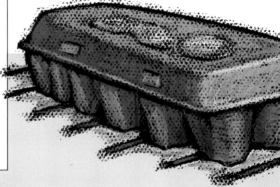

Putting It on Ice

Freezing or refrigeration can prevent most types of bacteria from growing to dangerous levels in foods. Health officials say the following precautions will help keep food safe:

▶ Keep the **temperature** of your refrigerator at 40 to 45 °F (4 to to 7 °C), and keep your freezer cold enough for all foods to remain frozen.

▶ Always obey a food label that says **"Keep refrigerated."** Condiments, such as mayonnaise and ketchup, should be refrigerated after opening.

▶ Store **eggs** in their carton in the main section of the refrig-erator—the temperature on the door shelf is higher.

▶ Wrap **raw meat** and **poultry** in plastic bags to prevent their juices from leaking onto other foods in the refrigerator. To freeze such items, wrap them tightly in plastic, foil, or freezer paper or put them in airtight containers.

▶ Defrost **frozen foods** in the refrigerator rather than on a kitchen counter. The surface of food left on a counter to defrost can serve as a breeding ground for bacteria even before the inside of the food thaws.

▶ Refrigerate **leftovers** as soon as possible after the meal. Divide hot foods into small portions for quick cooling, and allow space around containers for air circulation to keep the refrigerator or freezer temperature from rising. Cover containers tightly to prevent possible transfer of microbes from one batch of food to another.

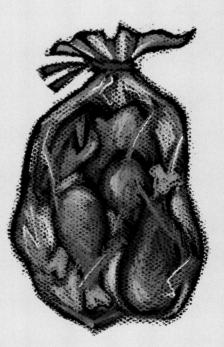

A Cutting Question

▶ Health officials have long recommended plastic cutting boards over wooden ones, on the theory that bacteria can hide and grow in grooves in the wood. A 1993 study, however, yielded a surprising finding: Wood seemed to actually inhibit bacterial growth.

Microbiologists at the University of Wisconsin in Madison smeared salmonella, listeria, and *E. coli* bacteria on various kinds of cutting boards. On plastic boards, the bacteria thrived, but on wooden boards virtually all the bacteria disappeared within three minutes. Even after repeated contaminations over several days, the wooden boards remained germ-free. The researchers speculated that something in the wood had killed the microbes.

But a follow-up study on wood versus plastic cutting boards, conducted in 1994 by the United States Food and Drug Administration (FDA), arrived at a different explanation for this surprising finding. FDA researchers found that bacteria on wooden boards are not killed but instead are drawn into the fibrous surfaces of the wood and trapped there.

The FDA said both wooden and plastic cutting boards are safe for food preparation if used properly. It recommended washing either kind of board with hot, soapy water after using it in cutting up raw meat, poultry, or fish. Here, plastic boards do offer an advantage: Many can be put in the dishwasher.

Such fecal-oral transmission is also responsible for many shigella infections among children in day-care centers or other group settings. Adults who change the diaper of one infected infant and do not wash their hands afterward can transfer bacteria to food—or directly to other children. Left untreated, shigella infections may be fatal to infants.

E. coli infections can also travel person-to-person, but food-borne cases are usually traced to meat or milk from infected cattle. Of the more than 100 strains of *E. coli*, most are harmless. However, the relatively new strain designated *E. coli* 0157:H7—the one responsible for the rash of poisonings from tainted hamburgers in the Pacific Northwest in 1993—has emerged as a leading cause of bloody diarrhea and hemolytic uremic syndrome, a kidney disease that can be fatal. The CDC estimates that 0157:H7 causes about 10,000 to 20,000 infections and 150 to 400 deaths in this country each year.

Other bacteria are involved in smaller numbers of food-borne infections. One that is relatively uncommon but can cause severe symptoms is *Listeria monocytogenes,* most often found in undercooked poultry and seafood, delicatessen meats, and dairy products, such as unpasteurized milk and soft cheeses.

Toxins, parasites, and viruses

Some bacteria cause food-borne illness not by infecting people who ingest them but by producing chemical toxins that poison food. For example, the common bacterium *Clostridium botulinum,* though harmless when ingested, produces *spores* (bacterial "seeds") that can grow in improperly canned foods, releasing a deadly nerve toxin. The contaminated food causes botulism, a disease that can lead to paralysis or death. Fortunately, food-borne botulism is rare—fewer than 40 cases a year in the United States, most of them associated with home-canned foods. Another species of clostridium, *Clostridium perfringens,* which grows in foods left at room temperature, produces a toxin that causes typical gastrointestinal symptoms.

Less well known, but far more common, is toxin poisoning from *Staphylococcus aureus.* Up to half of healthy adults carry staphylococcus bacteria in their noses, on their skin, or in their feces. Introduced to food during preparation, the bacteria grow at room temperature in such foods as cream pastries, custards, mayonnaise, processed meats, and fish.

Not all toxins come from bacteria. Several, for example, are associated with fish and shellfish, which may produce their own toxins or pick up others from contaminated waters. The most common toxin of this type is ciguatera, a chemical that concentrates in the flesh of certain tropical fish. Ciguatera poisoning annually strikes hundreds of Americans, most of them in Florida, Hawaii, and the Virgin Islands, with a variety of symptoms, including diarrhea, muscle aches, and a tingling sensation in the hands and feet.

Food can also be contaminated by microorganisms called parasites. Perhaps the best-known parasitic disease is trichinosis, caused by a tiny roundworm sometimes present in raw pork or game meat. Thanks to improved pork processing and increased public awareness of the need to cook pork thoroughly, trichinosis has declined in recent decades. On the increase, however, are gastrointestinal illnesses from eating raw-fish dishes, such as sushi, that are sometimes infected with parasites.

Viruses do not multiply in food as bacteria do, but they can travel in it—for instance, if an infected person returns a saliva-coated spoon to a serving dish. Many cases of food poisoning are caused by the Norwalk virus and other, related viruses. Much of what is called intestinal flu is probably due to these viruses.

Another viral disease often associated with food-borne transmission is hepatitis A. In many countries, this liver disease typically spreads by way of unsanitary water supplies, but in the United States it tends to be contracted from food prepared by individuals infected

Careful Cooking

Thorough cooking kills most microbes responsible for food poisoning. Health officials offer these guidelines:

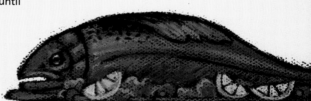

▶ Cook solid cuts of **red meat** until they are medium to well done in the thickest part—no more than light pink in the middle and at least 160 °F (71 °C) as measured by a meat thermometer. (Some experts say at least 165 °F [74 °C] for beef and most other meats.) Ground meat should be cooked until it is well done, with no trace of pink.

▶ **Pork** should also be cooked to the medium to well-done stage—at least 160 °F.

▶ Cook **poultry** until it is well done and the juices run clear, with no trace of pink. A meat thermometer inserted in the thickest part of the breast should read 180 °F (82 °C). If making stuffing, bake it in a pan rather than in the cavity of the bird.

▶ Cook **eggs** until both the yolk and white are firm, not runny.

▶ Cook **fish** until it is opaque throughout and flaky when cut. It should not be translucent, shiny, or rubbery. Allow 10 minutes of cooking for each inch of thickness.

▶ Boil **shrimp** for 3 to 5 minutes, or until the shells turn pink.

▶ Steam **clams** and **mussels** over boiling water until the shells open (5 to 10 minutes). Sauté, bake, or boil shucked oysters until they are plump, about five minutes.

Source: U.S. Department of Agriculture and U.S. Food and Drug Administration.

with the virus. It can also be picked up by eating shellfish, such as raw oysters, from contaminated waters. About 25,000 hepatitis A cases are reported here annually; many more go unreported.

A variety of symptoms

The symptoms of food poisoning depend largely on the microbe or toxin involved. Bacterial infections usually cause gastrointestinal symptoms, such as nausea, vomiting, abdominal cramps, and diarrhea. In severe cases, the diarrhea may contain blood or pus. Victims may also suffer fever, headache, weakness, or fatigue as their bodies fight the infection. The symptoms of bacterial food poisoning begin within a few hours to a few days, depending on the microorganism and the amount ingested.

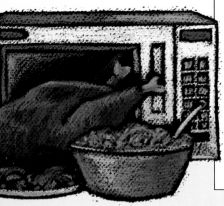

Microwaving Tips

Improper microwaving can leave "cold spots" inside food, where harmful bacteria can survive. To avoid food poisoning when preparing food in a microwave oven, health experts advise following these steps:

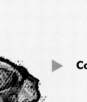

▶ For **packaged foods**, follow the manufacturer's directions for stirring, cooking time, and other procedures. For **home-prepared** recipes, stir the food and turn the cooking vessel several times during heating.

▶ **Cover** food with plastic wrap while it heats so steam can help with the cooking. **Pierce** or **vent** the wrap, but do not let it touch the food.

▶ When cooking **meat**, use a microwave probe to ensure sufficient internal temperature. Alternatively, remove the meat from the microwave oven and check it in several spots with a meat thermometer.

▶ Cook **stuffing** separately from poultry.

▶ Cut **bones** out of roasts before cooking.

Bacterial infections mostly affect the digestive tract because that is where the microbes take up residence. Toxins, however, can spread throughout the body, often producing highly distinctive symptoms. Botulism's hallmarks are double vision, difficulty in swallowing or speaking, and eventual paralysis. Staphylococcus toxin produces many of the same symptoms as a bacterial infection, but often faster and more intensely. Ciguatera poisoning may bring pain, weakness, numbness, tingling, itching, and lack of coordination as well as a range of gastrointestinal symptoms.

The parasitic disease trichinosis can cause diarrhea, fever, and swollen eyelids before progressing to more serious problems in the muscles, the brain, and other organs, depending on where the parasites have traveled in the body. Other parasitic diseases are often marked by severe diarrhea and gastrointestinal symptoms as well as dehydration and weight loss. The hepatitis A virus typically brings weakness, nausea, vomiting, loss of appetite, fever, and *jaundice* (yellowing of the skin and eyes). The Norwalk virus causes diarrhea and vomiting for up to three days.

The severity of a bout of food poisoning varies from one person to the next, depending on the amount of the contaminant ingested and the individual's general state of health. Some people can fight an infection without showing signs of illness. The worst cases, and nearly all deaths from food poisoning, occur in people with a low ability to overcome infection: infants, people over age 60, and people with a weakened immune system, such as those suffering from cancer or AIDS. Death may be caused by organ failure, dehydration from vomiting and diarrhea, or complications and secondary infections.

Treatments for food poisoning

Public health experts say that most cases of food poisoning can be—and are—treated at home without the aid of a doctor. The treatment for the typical case of food poisoning includes clear liquids to replace fluids lost through vomiting and diarrhea and a bland low-fat diet that might include such foods as bananas, rice, apples, and toast. Fever or pain can be controlled with aspirin, acetaminophen (Tylenol), or ibuprofen. Usually, symptoms pass within a day or two. (Parents should note that in children, aspirin can lead to a rare but serious complication of viral infections known as Reye's syndrome. For safety's sake, physicians advise parents to give only acetaminophen or ibuprofen to a child with a fever.)

More serious cases of food poisoning—for example, cases involving repeated vomiting, severe or bloody diarrhea, or a fever that cannot be controlled—may require a doctor's care or a trip to the hospital emergency room. In infants and children, who can dehydrate quickly, a serious case of food poisoning can be particularly dangerous. Doctors caution that a child suffering from multiple bouts of vomiting or diarrhea should receive prompt professional attention.

With botulism, swift emergency care is essential to avoid paralysis or death. Doctors treat food-borne botulism with injections of a special *antitoxin* (substance that neutralizes the toxin). Unfortunately, many cases of botulism are initially thought to be other conditions, such as strokes, which may delay treatment with an antitoxin.

Before treating a patient for a suspected case of food poisoning, a physician may ask a laboratory to test a sample of the patient's stool to identify the specific microbe involved. The doctor may also order blood tests to rule out other diseases and to see what sort of response the body is mounting against the infection. Blood tests will usually reveal the presence of hepatitis A. However, other microbes, and toxins as well, are not always easy to isolate in lab tests, and the illness may pass before the cause is found.

If tests reveal a bacterial or parasitic infection, the doctor may prescribe antibiotics or other drugs to eliminate the microbe. A patient with a severe case of food poisoning or lowered resistance to infection may be hospitalized to receive antibiotics and fluids *intravenously* (directly into the bloodstream) and to be watched, and treated, for signs of organ failure or other possible complications.

Staphylococcus poisoning usually passes within a few hours or days, but the patient's doctor may recommend intravenous fluids in the meantime. Hospitalization is not usually required for hepatitis A.

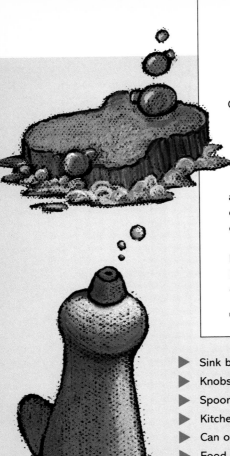

Keeping Clean

Cross-contamination, the transfer of microbes from one food item to another, is a major factor in food poisoning, but health experts say this threat can be minimized by keeping kitchen tools and work surfaces clean. They advise wiping utensils and surfaces regularly with hot soapy water or—even better—a mild bleach solution or commercial disinfectant.

In addition to such obvious microbe breeding grounds as counters, cutting boards, and knives, don't forget these often-overlooked tools and surfaces:

▶ Sink basin, faucet, and sink-drain basket
▶ Knobs and handles on cabinets and appliances
▶ Spoon rests
▶ Kitchen telephone
▶ Can opener blades
▶ Food processor and meat grinder

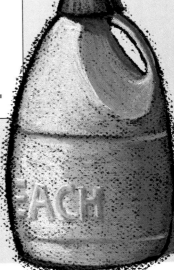

If diagnosed quickly, ciguatera poisoning can be treated with a drug called manitol. Most people with ciguatera poisoning recover completely in two to three weeks, but for others a full recovery can take months or years.

Minimizing the risk of food-borne illness

When food poisoning is confirmed, a doctor may try to determine where and how it happened. But extensive tests of suspect foods are generally done only with highly dangerous diseases, such as botulism or poisoning from E. coli 0157:H7, or when several people are struck simultaneously with the same malady. Although pinpointing the source of an outbreak can be hard, especially if no leftovers are available for testing, determined sleuthing by investigators may identify a food, event, or restaurant as the source of the outbreak. Prompt action by health officials may then eliminate the source of the contamination and help other people avoid being poisoned.

But preventing all such poisonings from occurring in the first place is simply not possible, public health experts say. Given the sheer size of the food industry, no amount of effort by government regulators, food producers, grocers, and restaurant owners can—at least for the time being—completely eliminate food contamination.

Nonetheless, the incidence of food poisoning could probably be greatly reduced if everyone realized the seriousness of the problem and took steps to keep food safe. The person in the best position to prevent most food poisoning is ultimately the one who stores, prepares, and serves food—whether that person is cooking at home or in a restaurant. But many Americans, believing that their food is guaranteed safe, overlook many rules of food safety that were common practice a few generations ago, when people could not depend on refrigeration, chemical preservatives, or government inspection.

Those common-sense rules include buying the freshest products available, storing them properly, cooking them thoroughly, and practicing strict kitchen hygiene. Running a hygienic kitchen means always having clean hands when cooking, keeping raw meats and poultry away from foods that won't be cooked further, and making a concerted effort to keep work surfaces free of contamination.

You can control conditions in your own kitchen, but what happens when you dine out? Health experts advise restaurant-goers to examine an establishment for general cleanliness, a well-trained and well-supervised staff, and foods served properly hot or cold. In short, look for high standards of hygiene and service.

Someday, perhaps, precautions against food poisoning will be less necessary than they are today. The government is refining its food inspection methods, and scientists are experimenting with genetic engineering to increase the resistance of plants and animals to microbes. At the same time, food producers are introducing irradiation technology to kill microorganisms in meats, poultry, and produce.

Still, it is doubtful that any of these developments will ever replace good kitchen hygiene. And in that regard, the experts say, we should all remember what our grandparents told us: Store and cook food properly, clean up after yourself, and wash your hands. There, in a nutshell, is the best advice for preventing food poisoning. • • •

For more information:

These federal agencies provide free food-safety information by telephone, mail, or fax:

- **Food and Drug Administration (FDA)**
  The FDA's Seafood Hot Line provides recorded information 24 hours a day on seafood safety as well as general food safety. Specialists are available to answer questions between noon and 4 p.m. EST. Call toll-free (800) FDA-4010.

- **U.S. Department of Agriculture (USDA)**
  The USDA's Meat and Poultry Hot Line offers recorded food safety information 24 hours a day. Specialists are available to answer questions on weekdays between 10 a.m. and 4 p.m. EST. Call toll-free (800) 535-4555, or (202) 720-3333 in the Washington, D.C., area.

The Hazards of Carbon Monoxide

By Michael Woods

This colorless, odorless, and tasteless gas kills hundreds of Americans in their homes each year and poisons thousands more.

THE SUDDEN DEATH OF FORMER TENNIS STAR VITAS GERULAITIS in September 1994 illustrated the dangers of carbon monoxide, a poisonous gas that kills about 600 Americans every year and injures thousands more. While napping in a friend's guest cottage, Gerulaitis inhaled a fatal amount of carbon monoxide that had seeped from a faulty gas heater. Because carbon monoxide is colorless, odorless, and tasteless, it can build to toxic levels without any warning. And it claims most victims—as it did Gerulaitis—while they sleep.

Malfunctioning furnaces, stoves, kerosene heaters, and other fuel-burning appliances are responsible for about 250 deaths from carbon monoxide poisoning each year, according to the United States Consumer Product Safety Commission (CPSC). An additional 5,000 people require treatment in hospital emergency rooms for poisoning from defective heating devices. Most of these poisonings occur in winter, when people are most likely to use heating devices.

Automobiles left running in closed spaces cause many of the remaining 340 annual deaths from carbon monoxide poisoning. The gas, which is released in automobile exhausts, builds up quickly in closed garages. Fumes also can spread from an attached garage to the rest of the house and harm those family members who are inside.

Carbon monoxide is produced when oil, natural gas, propane, wood, gasoline, and other fuels burn incompletely. (Appliances that use electricity do not produce carbon monoxide.) Fuels burn when they combine chemically with oxygen in the air. If plenty of oxygen is available, the fuel burns completely, and each carbon atom in the fuel combines with two atoms of oxygen, producing harmless carbon dioxide. When the oxygen supply is inadequate, however, each carbon atom combines with only one atom of oxygen, forming deadly carbon monoxide.

Once inhaled into the lungs, carbon monoxide enters the bloodstream and impairs the body's ability to absorb oxygen. It does so by combining with hemoglobin, the substance in blood that carries

House of danger

Carbon monoxide (CO) is a deadly gas produced when fuel burns incompletely due to an inadequate oxygen supply. A typical house has several potential sources of the gas.

A water heater can leak CO through corroded or loosely connected vents.

Furnaces with blocked flues, loose connections, or malfunctioning vents can leak CO.

Automobile exhausts contain CO, and fumes from a car left running in a closed garage can quickly spread to an attached house.

A blocked chimney can divert CO into a home. In tightly sealed homes, deadly fumes can also be drawn back down a clear chimney.

A gas stove can release CO when it is improperly installed or functioning poorly, indicated by a flame that is yellow instead of blue.

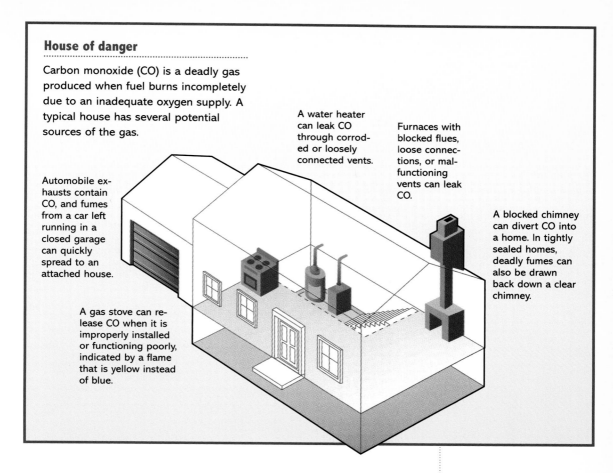

oxygen to cells throughout the body. Carbon monoxide transforms hemoglobin into a substance called carboxyhemoglobin, which cannot carry life-sustaining oxygen.

Concentrations of carboxyhemoglobin in blood are normally around 2 percent, at least in nonsmokers. Smokers inhale carbon monoxide in cigarette smoke and have carboxyhemoglobin concentrations of between 5 percent to 9 percent. When carboxyhemoglobin levels rise to between 10 percent and 20 percent, the shortage of oxygen can produce headaches, nausea, dizziness, and confusion. Blood concentrations between 30 percent and 60 percent can damage the central nervous system and lead to *coma* (prolonged unconsciousness) and death. Carbon monoxide's effects are cumulative, so breathing small amounts over a span of hours can be as deadly as inhaling high concentrations briefly.

Some people are more vulnerable to carbon monoxide damage than others. They include people with cardiovascular or lung disease, who may already suffer from a shortage of oxygen, and infants and fetuses, with their large oxygen requirements for growth and development. Smokers may reach toxic levels faster than

The author:

Michael Woods is science editor of the *Toledo Blade* and the author of many articles on scientific and medical topics.

Colorless, odorless, and deadly

Hundreds of Americans die of carbon monoxide (CO) poisoning every year, and thousands more are treated in emergency rooms. Because CO is colorless and odorless, it cannot be detected with the senses. And CO poisoning is difficult to diagnose because its symptoms are easily confused with those of other ailments.

When CO is inhaled, it travels to the lungs and enters the bloodstream. In the blood, CO takes the place of oxygen on the molecule hemoglobin, which normally transports life-sustaining oxygen to all parts of the body.

Early symptoms of CO poisoning include headache and nausea. As CO in the body increases and oxygen diminishes, vomiting, dizziness, fatigue, and confusion set in.

Breathing and heartbeat grow rapid as the body tries to draw in more oxygen.

When CO replaces more than half the oxygen in the blood, organs that require large amounts of oxygen, such as the heart and brain, may fail, and seizures, unconsciousness, and death may follow.

nonsmokers because they start with higher levels in their body.

The vague nature of early symptoms of carbon monoxide poisoning—headache, dizziness, and nausea—make the condition even more dangerous. Victims may ignore the symptoms, assuming that they arise from a cold, influenza, or fatigue. Physicians, too, may not readily connect such nonspecific symptoms with carbon monoxide poisoning. Fortunately, people with mild carbon monoxide poisoning usually begin to recover when they breathe fresh air or receive an infusion of 100 percent oxygen from paramedics. However, people who survive severe carbon monoxide poisoning may suffer permanent brain damage.

Consumers can do much to prevent carbon monoxide poisoning, says the CPSC. The group recommends having a qualified service technician inspect a home's central heating system and fuel-burning appliances each year. Chimneys and flues on heating devices deserve special attention, because they can divert toxic gases back into the house when blocked.

But even clear chimneys and flues can sometimes reverse the flow of gases. The process, known as backdrafting, occurs because furnaces and other fuel-burning devices use air for combustion, which they draw from outside, through windows, doors, and cracks. Kitchen and bathroom exhaust fans also pull in air from outside. Many of today's homes are weathertight, however, with cracks sealed to reduce energy costs. In cold weather, when windows and doors are shut and exhaust fans are running, replacement air must come from somewhere. It may be carbon monoxide-laden air drawn down the chimney or flue.

Homeowners may want to try a simple test for backdrafting, recommended by the CPSC. First, locate the draft diverter on the furnace or hot water heater. It is a large funnel-shaped collar around the flue pipe. Then, with the furnace or water heater operating and the exhaust fans running, hold a lighted match or stick of incense near the collar. But take care to avoid touching the collar, which is hot and can cause a burn. If smoke is drawn up, the device is operating safely. Smoke that blows down signifies a backdraft.

How a carbon monoxide detector works

Because a carbon monoxide detector can protect your family even when other safety precautions fail, the United States Consumer Product Safety Commission (CPSC) recommends installing a detector in every home. Carbon monoxide detectors cost from $35 to $80 and should be installed in the hall just outside bedrooms, so that they can alert sleepers.

These electronic devices, which look like smoke detectors, operate in one of two ways. Some have a sensor that reacts with carbon monoxide in the air and triggers a loud alarm. Others use a chemically treated disk that darkens when exposed to carbon monoxide. When a beam of infrared light detects a color change, an alarm sounds.

When buying a detector, check the package to make sure that it meets standard 2034. This indicates that the detector has passed safety tests performed by the independent testing organization Underwriters Laboratories. Detectors that meet this standard monitor the air for high carbon monoxide concentrations over short periods and for low concentrations that accumulate over longer periods.

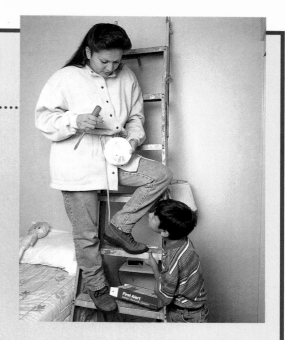

The CPSC recommends against relying on inexpensive detection cards, which have a chemically treated disk that changes color in the presence of carbon monoxide. These cards cost $5 or less, but they only reveal the presence of carbon monoxide if somebody looks at them. Because the devices do not sound an alarm, they provide no protection during the night. [M. W.]

The CPSC suggests several other precautions for preventing carbon monoxide leaks. The group advises people to be on the lookout for loose connections in vents and chimneys; fuel-burning devices that produce soot, unusual odors, or sounds; and furnaces that run constantly or fail to heat properly. The CPSC warns against trying to use a fuel-burning appliance that keeps shutting off. A safety device may be switching off the appliance because it is unsafe to use. The CPSC also underscores the importance of installing and operating fuel-burning devices according to the manufacturer's instructions. Finally, it cautions people to use unvented natural gas or kerosene heaters only in a well-ventilated room and never in a room where someone is sleeping or may sleep.

Other dangerous practices to avoid include using a gas range as an indoor heater; burning charcoal inside the house; leaving a car engine running in an enclosed space; and using fuel-burning equipment inside a tent. These precautions may seem obvious, yet every year hundreds of Americans ignore them and suffer injuries or die as a result.

Knowing what happens when muscles and
skin are injured helps in deciding whether
to apply heat or cold to a minor injury.

Which to Apply:
Heat or *Cold?*

By Rebecca Voelker

S OME OF THE MOST EFFECTIVE TREATMENTS for painful conditions ranging from a twisted ankle to a bout of arthritis may not require a doctor's prescription. Soothing remedies that cost next to nothing are as near as your kitchen faucet and freezer: warm water and ice.

Physicians explain that any type of injury or pain involving soft tissues—skin and muscle—responds to heat and cold. Moreover, the more superficial the injury, the more likely it is to respond.

But how do you decide whether heat or cold works best for a specific condition? To remember which to apply, it may help to understand what happens to the body following an injury and how the body responds to both heat and cold.

When skin and muscles are injured, the body responds by releasing chemical substances that *dilate* (expand) blood vessels and thereby boost the flow of blood into the injured area. These chemical substances also draw additional white blood cells into the area. The increased blood flow serves several purposes. Red blood cells carry oxygen, which injured tissues require to repair themselves and heal. White blood cells help fight infection and also help repair damaged tissues. Applications of heat and cold affect how much blood flows into the injured area.

The action of heat and cold

The application of heat accelerates both the dilation of blood vessels in the injured area and the repair of tissue. Heat also is believed to speed the release of endorphins and serotonin, biochemicals that help fight pain and calm irritated nerves.

The chemical substances that promote healing also produce inflammation: the pain, redness, and swelling that typically accompany an injury. Irritation of nerve endings by the chemicals causes the pain associated with injury. The redness comes from increased blood flow to the area, and the swelling occurs as fluid leaks into the damaged tissue from tiny vessels called capillaries.

Cold has an effect opposite to that of heat. Cold *constricts* (narrows) blood vessels, limiting the amount of blood that reaches the injured area. In this way, cold can help stop bleeding and is therefore the proper treatment for nosebleeds or cuts.

Cold also counters inflammation by reducing blood flow to the area and with it the chemicals responsible for inflammation. Thus,

The author:

Rebecca Voelker is an associate news editor at the *Journal of the American Medical Association.*

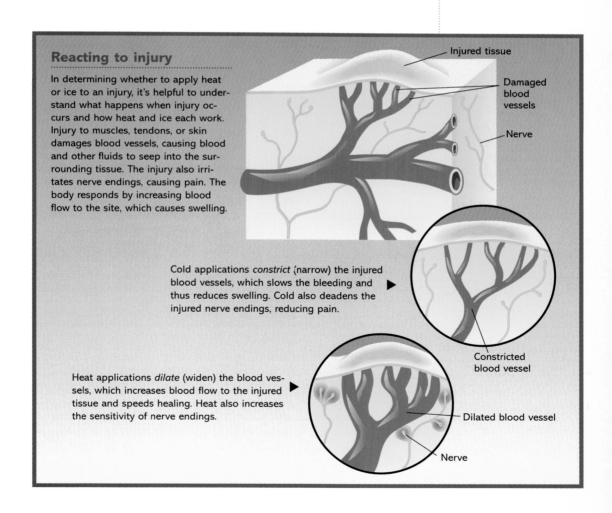

Reacting to injury

In determining whether to apply heat or ice to an injury, it's helpful to understand what happens when injury occurs and how heat and ice each work. Injury to muscles, tendons, or skin damages blood vessels, causing blood and other fluids to seep into the surrounding tissue. The injury also irritates nerve endings, causing pain. The body responds by increasing blood flow to the site, which causes swelling.

Injured tissue

Damaged blood vessels

Nerve

Cold applications *constrict* (narrow) the injured blood vessels, which slows the bleeding and thus reduces swelling. Cold also deadens the injured nerve endings, reducing pain. ▶

Constricted blood vessel

Heat applications *dilate* (widen) the blood vessels, which increases blood flow to the injured tissue and speeds healing. Heat also increases the sensitivity of nerve endings. ▶

Dilated blood vessel

Nerve

cold can alleviate the swelling and pain that accompany inflammation. In addition, the application of cold to injured skin and muscle numbs irritated nerves, thereby relieving pain. In the case of insect stings, constricted blood vessels help prevent the spread of toxins in the area of the bite.

Some simple rules

Experts advise applying the following rule of thumb when deciding whether to apply heat or cold. Apply cold in acute situations—conditions that come on suddenly and involve bleeding or inflammation. Apply heat for conditions that are chronic or prolonged and are accompanied by aches or stiffness.

In some situations, the most effective treatment is cold first—in the acute phase—and then heat during the longer recovery phase. In treating a strained or sprained muscle, for example, physicians recommend applying cold during the first 48 hours after the injury to reduce swelling. This can be done by placing an ice pack on the injured area for several minutes each hour. Physicians advise against immersing the injured muscle in ice water, however, as this can damage soft tissues. After 48 hours, applying heat speeds healing and eases pain.

Joints that are inflamed as a result of arthritis also can benefit from applications of cold and then heat. During the first days of an arthritis flare-up, intermittent cold applications can reduce pain and swelling. After two or three days, heat can help reduce any subsequent stiffness in the affected joints.

Applying heat

Heat stimulates blood flow, which promotes healing, and it is effective in relieving pain and stiffness in joints and muscles. But to avoid swelling and the chance of internal bleeding, heat usually should not be applied within 48 hours of an injury, and it should never be applied to the abdomen when symptoms of appendicitis, such as tenderness and pain, are present. A warm compress can be made by soaking a towel in warm water. A heating pad or hot-water bottle can provide dry heat.

Use	Dry	Moist
Joint pain from arthritis	X	X
Sprains, strains,		
muscle aches		
(after first 48 hours)		X
Skin infections		X
Surgical incisions	X	

Critically reviewed by Mark Stolar, M.D.

Wet or dry?

After deciding which one to apply, the next question is how to apply it. Both heat and cold can be applied in wet or dry form. In general, wet heat and wet cold are more penetrating than their dry counterparts and can therefore be applied for a shorter period.

Soaking in a hot bath, for example, can bring quick relief to someone suffering from a backache or other muscle ache. Similarly, physicians recommend immediately plunging a minor burn under cool running water or placing a towel soaked in water over the burn, to halt further damage to tissue.

In some cases, physicians recommend dry heat, which can be applied with a heating pad, hot water bottle, or heat lamp. When a surgical incision should be kept dry, for instance, the physician may suggest directing a heat lamp at it. In this case, a heat lamp is preferable to other forms of dry heat because it does not come into direct contact with the incision.

Ice, the dry form of cold, can be more effective than cold water in certain situations and easier to apply. For example, ice applied to the side of the nose can quickly constrict the small blood vessels responsible for a minor nosebleed. And an ice collar can help relieve pain and reduce the danger of bleeding following a tonsillectomy.

Whichever way heat or cold is applied—moist or dry—the general idea is to get it as close to the injury site as possible. Various commercial products are available for applications of heat and cold, and a hot or cold compress can easily be made by soaking a towel in warm water or wrapping it around ice.

Insulated ice packs sold in many drugstores efficiently deliver dry cold to injuries on or near the surface of the skin. Other items available include packs containing chemicals that produce a low-temperature liquid when mixed, and gel packs that can be cooled and stored in the freezer between applications.

Some of the gel packs that can be frozen also can be warmed in a microwave oven for heat application. These packs, as well as similar products filled with different materials, provide heat for an hour or so after warming in the microwave.

Always use caution

No matter what method is chosen, physicians warn people to exercise caution. Heating pads that may relieve pain in 10 to 15 minutes can cause burns when allowed to remain in place for an hour or more, especially at a high setting. At the other extreme, ice or cold water applied too long can damage tissues by cutting off the blood supply. And doctors also warn that people with diabetes or any condition in which the hands or feet have lost sensitivity must be especially careful when applying heat or ice.

Perhaps most important, experts emphasize that serious injuries of any kind should receive immediate medical attention from a health care professional. •••

Applying cold

Cold constricts blood vessels, which reduces the supply of blood to the skin. Cold applications are used to control bleeding, reduce pain, and slow the swelling of damaged tissues. A cold compress can be made by wetting a towel or other cloth, or by wrapping a towel around ice.

Use	Ice	Cold water
Minor burns		X
Fever	X	
Headache	X	
Insect bites		X
Hemorrhoids	X	
Nosebleed	X	
Tonsillectomy	X	
Sprains, strains, muscle aches (for first 48 hours)	X	
Swollen eyes, as from allergies		X
Tendinitis	X	

Critically reviewed by Mark Stolar, M.D.

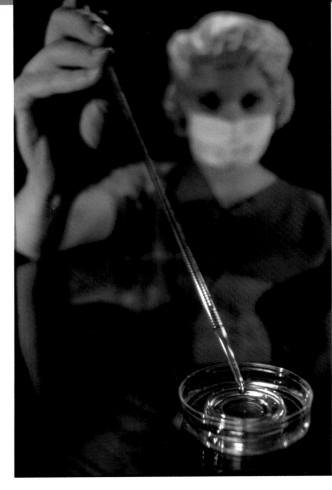

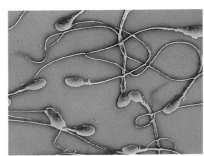

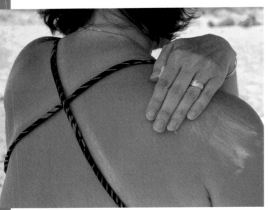

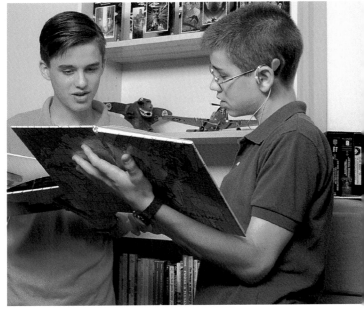

ON THE MEDICAL FRONTIER

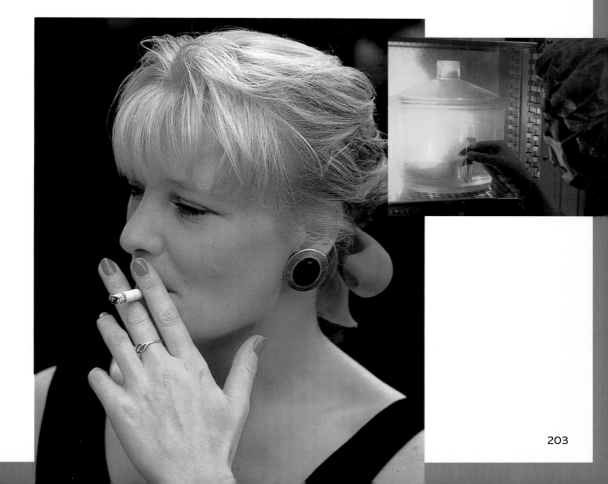

Pregnancy Through Technology

By David Keefe

Advances in reproductive technology have made it possible for many couples who were unable to conceive to realize their dreams of parenthood.

IN EVERY CULTURE AND THROUGHOUT TIME, the birth of a child has been cause for rejoicing, and the inability to have children has been a source of sorrow. Ancient figurines and charms bear witness to prayers offered for fertility long before the beginning of writing. Only in recent decades, however, has medical technology enabled infertile couples to satisfy their longing to have children.

Most fertility specialists define infertility as the failure to conceive during one year of unprotected sexual intercourse. On average, about 25 percent of couples who are trying to conceive succeed each month. By the end of one year, approximately 85 percent have achieved pregnancy. About half of the remaining 15 percent have conceived by the end of the second year. Thus, researchers estimate that infertility affects from 8 percent to 15 percent of couples in the United States.

Since the 1970's, increasing numbers of these couples have sought the help of fertility specialists. In part, this increase reflects improved access to such services. But infertility may also be on the rise in the United States along with a tendency to delay marriage and childbearing, because a woman's fertility declines with age.

Infertility can result from a dysfunction in the woman, in the man, or in both partners. Fertility experts estimate that in about 40 percent of infertile couples, the problem stems from the woman alone; in about 30 percent, from the man alone; and in about 20

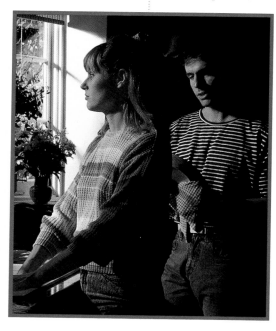

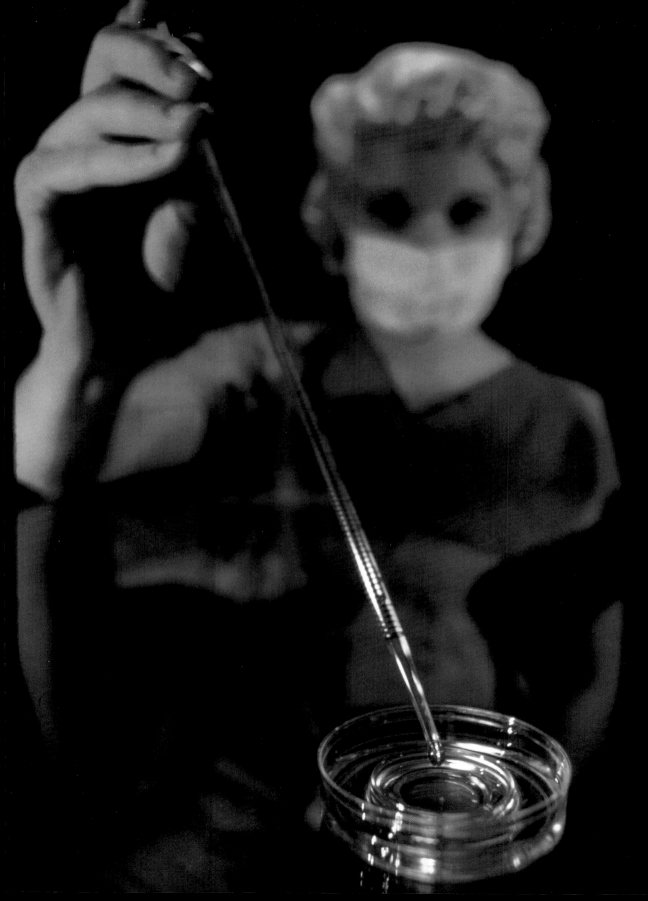

percent, from both partners. In the remaining 10 percent, physicians can find no explanation for the couple's infertility. No matter where the problem lies, treatment may be available.

Glossary

Embryo: The group of cells that forms and grows after a fertilized egg divides.

Gamete intra-fallopian transfer (GIFT): A procedure in which sperm and eggs are placed separately in the woman's fallopian tube for fertilization.

Infertility: Failure to conceive during one year of unprotected sexual intercourse.

In vitro fertilization (IVF): A procedure in which eggs and sperm are united in a laboratory dish.

In vitro fertilization and embryo transfer (IVF-ET): A procedure in which fertilization takes place in a laboratory dish and the resulting embryo is transferred to the woman's uterus.

Zygote: The single cell that results from the union of a sperm and an egg.

Zygote intra-fallopian transfer (ZIFT): A procedure in which a zygote is placed in the woman's fallopian tube.

The author:

David Keefe is assistant professor of obstetrics and gynecology and director of the Reproductive Aging Unit at the Yale University School of Medicine.

To understand the causes and treatment of infertility, it's necessary to know how the reproductive process normally functions. Conception is possible only during the 72 hours or so around ovulation, the time each month when a woman's ovaries release an egg. Each egg is surrounded by a sac called a follicle, which is sensitive to hormones secreted by the pituitary gland at the base of the brain. Beginning in puberty, egg-containing follicles within the ovaries emerge each month and begin to grow, stimulated by the pituitary secretions known as follicle-stimulating hormone and luteinizing hormone. One follicle soon becomes dominant, and it secretes the female hormone estrogen into the bloodstream.

The rising estrogen levels prompt an outpouring of luteinizing hormone from the pituitary gland. This hormone surge causes the egg to break free of its follicle, penetrate the ovary wall, and enter the pelvic cavity. Sticky projections at the end of the nearby fallopian tube reach out, pick up the egg, and move it into the tube. The stage is now set for fertilization by sperm ascending from the vagina.

Sperm are produced continuously in a man's body, beginning after puberty. They develop in the testicles, a pair of glands located behind the penis in a pouch called the scrotum. As sperm mature, they develop a tightly packed nucleus and a long, thin tail, which help them ascend the female genital tract and fertilize an egg. Mature sperm are stored in the epididymis, a coiled tube that sits on top of the testicle. When a man ejaculates, muscle contractions from the scrotum propel the sperm through a tubular extension of the epididymis called the vas deferens. As sperm pass through the vas deferens en route to the penis, secretions from nearby glands mix with them to form semen. Semen protects and nourishes the sperm.

The sperm must pass through the cervix, the entrance to the uterus that lies at the end of the vagina. It is shut tightly with thick mucus during most of the menstrual cycle. However, responding to the increase in estrogen at ovulation, the cervix secretes thinner mucus that sperm can navigate easily. A man deposits tens of millions of sperm in the vagina during intercourse. Between 1 million and 2 million sperm enter the uterus, but only a few thousand reach the fallopian tube, where an egg awaits fertilization. When a sperm fertilizes an egg, the resulting cell is called a zygote.

The single-celled zygote grows by dividing about once each day during the first week after fertilization, and it becomes known as an embryo after the first division. By the sixth day, having moved from the fallopian tube into the uterus, the embryo prepares for implantation. Sticky molecules secreted by the *endometrium* (the lining of the uterus) help the embryo become firmly embedded within the endometrium. A substance secreted by the embryo called human chorionic gonadotropin (HCG) helps maintain a hormonal environment favorable to pregnancy. The most widely used pregnancy test measures levels of this hormone in blood or urine.

Problems can arise at any stage in this process. The man's sperm may be defective. The woman may fail to ovulate, or her fallopian tubes may be blocked. Abnormalities in her cervical mucus or uterus may keep sperm from reaching the egg or prevent implantation of an embryo. Hormone disorders also can cause problems.

Age can also be a factor in the woman's fertility. Egg production begins before birth. The eggs reach a maximum number of more than 7 million in a female fetus's fifth month of development, and they begin disappearing in large numbers almost immediately. This loss continues until the last eggs perish shortly after menopause, the cessation of menstruation. More than 99 percent of a woman's eggs are absorbed by her body and never participate in ovulation.

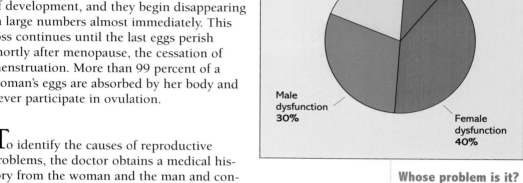

To identify the causes of reproductive problems, the doctor obtains a medical history from the woman and the man and conducts a physical examination of both partners. The physician also requests some tests of reproductive functioning. Questions that the physician may ask the woman in taking a medical history include:

- How long has the couple tried to conceive?
- How often and when does the couple have intercourse?
- How long and how often does the woman menstruate?
- Does she have excessive facial or body hair, acne, cold intolerance, hair loss, or nipple discharge? These symptoms suggest a hormone disorder.
- How strenuously does she exercise or diet, and is she under psychological stress? Intense exercise or dieting and sustained stress can affect ovulation and the regularity of menstrual cycles.
- Has she had any sexually transmitted diseases (STD's) or abdominal or pelvic surgery? STD's and surgery can leave scar tissue that interferes with the egg's passage to the fallopian tube.
- Does she use tobacco, alcohol, caffeine, or other drugs? These substances, if used in excess, can impair reproductive ability.

The information uncovered by the history and physical examination determines the tests the doctor requests for the woman. Because each test must be done at a specific time of the menstrual cycle, one month is typically set aside as a "study cycle" for gathering information instead of attempting conception.

The first test discovers if and when the woman ovulates. One method involves measuring body temperature each morning at the

Whose problem is it?

About 85 percent of couples conceive within a year of trying. Many couples who fail to conceive in that time seek the help of a specialist to find the cause of the problem. Infertility can result from a reproductive problem in the woman, in the man, or in both partners. In some cases, physicians can find no cause for a couple's infertility.

Male reproductive system

Sperm produced in the testicles travel through the vas deferens. There they are mixed with fluid from the seminal vesicles to create semen, which is released through the urethra. Various malfunctions in this process can prevent a man from impregnating a woman.

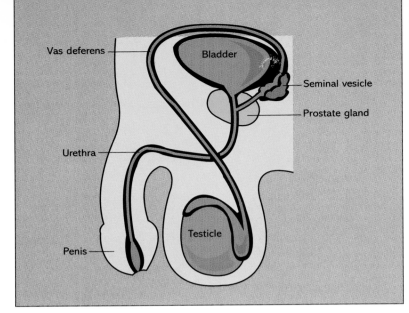

Organ	Function	What can go wrong	Possible treatment
Testicle	Produces sperm	Produces too few sperm, abnormally formed sperm, or sperm not vigorous enough to reach and penetrate an egg.	Sperm can be concentrated in the laboratory and inserted directly into a woman's uterus or used to fertilize eggs that are then inserted into the uterus.
Vas deferens	Transports sperm	Transport of sperm prevented by blockage.	Surgery can sometimes remove the blockage, or sperm can be taken from the testicles and used to fertilize the eggs.
Penis	Ejaculates sperm	Fails to become or remain erect; impaired ejaculation.	Counseling may help if the problem is psychological; a medical or surgical procedure, if the problem is physical.

same time, because a woman's temperature rises slightly just after ovulation. The physician may recommend using a highly sensitive thermometer specially designed for this task. A woman can also use a home test kit that detects the preovulatory rise in luteinizing hormone, which shows up in the urine.

If a woman does not menstruate or menstruates infrequently, treatment with the hormone progestin should induce a menstrual period. If no period follows, even after further treatment with progestin and estrogen, menstrual flow may be blocked, for example, by adhesions within the uterus. Adhesions occur when normally separate uterine tissues grow together, usually after infection or surgery.

Obstructions may also occur in the fallopian tubes. To look for these and to determine if the uterine cavity is normal, the doctor uses a hysterosalpingogram. In this procedure, a harmless substance is injected into the uterus that makes the uterus visible in an X ray. The doctor then examines the X-ray images for abnormalities.

The doctor also may test the receptivity of the woman's endome-

Female reproductive system

Eggs released from the ovaries pass through the fallopian tubes to the uterus. If an egg is fertilized by a sperm in the fallopian tube, it develops into a rapidly growing embryo that travels to the uterus and attaches to the uterine lining. Various malfunctions in this process can prevent a woman from becoming pregnant.

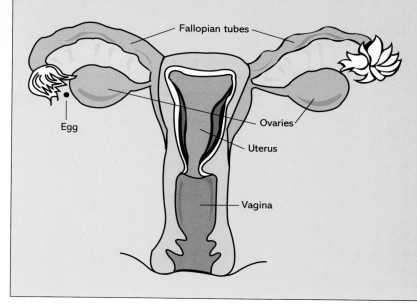

Organ	Function	What can go wrong	Possible treatment
Ovary	Produces and releases eggs	Eggs fail to mature or be released.	Drugs can stimulate ovulation.
Fallopian tube	Receives egg and sperm for fertilization	Tube blocked as a result of infection or structural abnormality.	Surgery can sometimes remove blockages or fertilized eggs can be inserted directly into the uterus, bypassing blockage.
Uterus	Receives fertilized egg and carries fetus to full-term baby	Implantation of fertilized egg prevented by various abnormalities; mucus at the entrance to the uterus can damage sperm.	Surgery often can repair abnormalities.

trium. This test requires a biopsy, a tissue-sampling procedure that can be performed in the doctor's office. The doctor removes a small sample of the uterine lining, and a laboratory doctor examines the tissue under a microscope for evidence of a hormone imbalance.

If the woman does ovulate, the physician may use a post-coital test. For this test, the woman goes to the doctor after having intercourse. The doctor removes mucus from her cervix and examines it under a microscope to see how many sperm are moving within it. If the sperm wriggle in place, antibodies to sperm may be present. Antibodies are immune system molecules that detect and immobilize any substance foreign to the body. In this event, the woman's— or even the man's—immune system has identified the sperm as foreign and mounted an attack against them.

In women in their late 30's or older, doctors check levels of follicle-stimulating hormone. Secretions of this hormone rise as the number of eggs and follicles in a woman's ovaries dwindle, so the test provides a rough idea of how plentiful her eggs are. A scarcity of eggs makes it highly unlikely that the woman will conceive.

If these assessments reveal no explanation for the couple's infertility, the doctor will probably recommend more invasive procedures. A surgical technique called laparoscopy enables the physician to examine the fallopian tubes, ovaries, uterus, and other pelvic structures for abnormalities. The physician performs the procedure using a laparoscope—a metal tube with lenses, a light system, and a channel for surgical instruments—which is inserted into a small incision at the navel. In a procedure known as hysteroscopy, the physician views the uterine lining by inserting a hysteroscope, a device similar to the laparoscope, through the vagina into the uterus.

Tests of the man's fertility are as important as tests of the woman's fertility. At the initial evaluation, the man also provides a medical history. Questions the physician typically asks include:
- Has he fathered any children in the past?
- Has he had any illnesses, especially mumps, diabetes, or sexually transmitted infections, which can damage reproductive organs? Has he been exposed to toxic chemicals or radiation, which can damage sperm? Does he smoke, drink alcohol, or use other drugs?
- Has he ever injured his testicles or exposed them to excessive heat, for example, through regular hot tub use or prolonged sitting? Sperm form only within a certain temperature range.

In the physical examination, the doctor evaluates such features as hair distribution, testicle size, and the penis, looking for unusual

Analyzing sperm

The most important evaluation of male fertility is the semen analysis. A laboratory technician examines a semen sample with a high-powered microscope that produces images on a screen, *left*. Normal sperm, *top right*, should be mobile and plentiful in the semen. Deformed sperm, *bottom right*, can result in infertility.

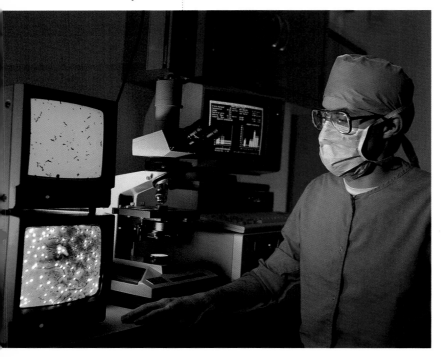

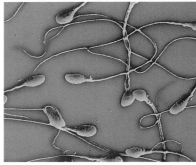

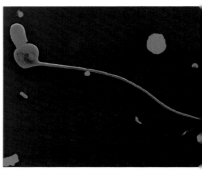

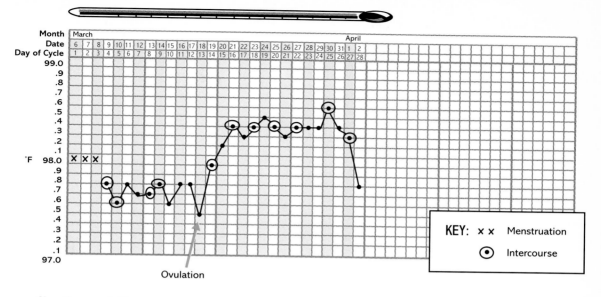

Month	March																								April		
Date	6	7	8	9	10	11	12	13	14	15	16	17	18	19	20	21	22	23	24	25	26	27	28	29	30	31	1	2
Day of Cycle	1	2	3	4	5	6	7	8	9	10	11	12	13	14	15	16	17	18	19	20	21	22	23	24	25	26	27	28

Ovulation

KEY: x x Menstruation

⊙ Intercourse

Charting ovulation

The most common cause of infertility in women is the failure to *ovulate* (release an egg). One way a woman can determine if and when she ovulates is by taking her temperature each morning before getting up—and noting the number on a calendar. Body temperature rises slightly just after ovulation, and a specially calibrated or highly sensitive thermometer can detect this rise. A woman can also find out if she ovulates by using a home urine test that measures levels of a hormone released just before ovulation.

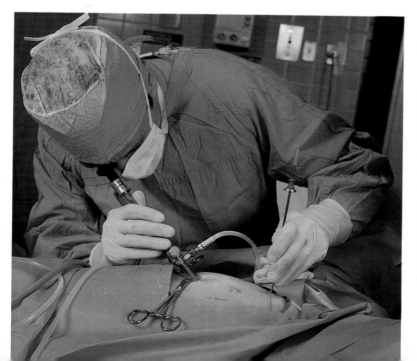

Investigating surgically

A surgical technique called laparoscopy enables the physician to examine a woman's pelvic structures for abnormalities and in some cases to correct them. The physician performs the procedure using a laparoscope—a metal tube with lenses, a light system, and a channel for surgical instruments—which is inserted into a small incision at the navel.

211

In vitro fertilization

Many cases of infertility can be treated by carrying out part of the reproductive process outside the body in a glass test tube or laboratory dish, a procedure known as *in vitro* (in glass) fertilization. The three major types of in vitro fertilization differ in the stage at which the transfer to the woman's body takes place. Transfer to the fallopian tubes requires surgery, whereas transfer of an embryo to the uterus can be done with a syringe.

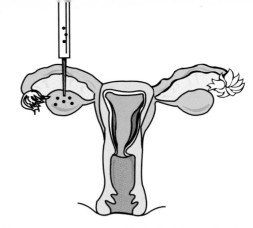

The woman receives drugs that stimulate the ripening of eggs in her ovaries. Just before ovulation, a physician removes the ripe eggs from her ovaries.

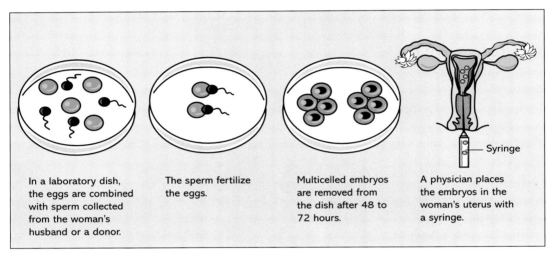

In a laboratory dish, the eggs are combined with sperm collected from the woman's husband or a donor.

The sperm fertilize the eggs.

Multicelled embryos are removed from the dish after 48 to 72 hours.

A physician places the embryos in the woman's uterus with a syringe.

Syringe

In vitro fertilization and embryo transfer (IVF-ET)

In IVF-ET, several eggs are removed from a woman's ovaries and mixed in a dish with her partner's sperm. If fertilization occurs and the fertilized eggs divide, the resulting embryos are transferred to the woman's uterus. This technique is helpful if the woman's fallopian tubes are blocked, the man's sperm are abnormal, or no cause can be found for the couple's infertility.

A laboratory incubator keeps the eggs and sperm at the proper temperature for fertilization, which usually occurs within hours.

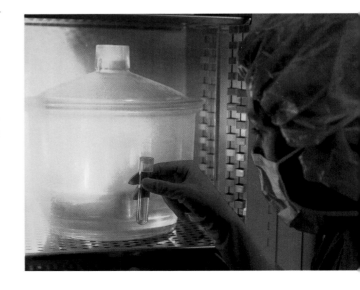

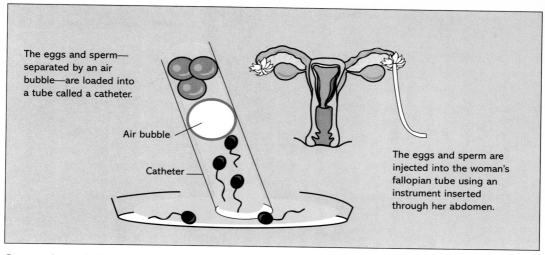

The eggs and sperm—separated by an air bubble—are loaded into a tube called a catheter.

Air bubble

Catheter

The eggs and sperm are injected into the woman's fallopian tube using an instrument inserted through her abdomen.

Gamete intra-fallopian transfer (GIFT)

In GIFT, *gametes* (eggs and sperm) are placed separately in the woman's fallopian tube. GIFT is used in cases where the woman's fallopian tubes are normal and doctors cannot determine why fertilization does not occur.

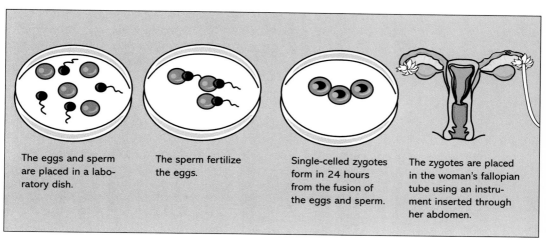

The eggs and sperm are placed in a laboratory dish.

The sperm fertilize the eggs.

Single-celled zygotes form in 24 hours from the fusion of the eggs and sperm.

The zygotes are placed in the woman's fallopian tube using an instrument inserted through her abdomen.

Zygote intra-fallopian transfer (ZIFT)

In ZIFT, *zygotes* (fertilized eggs) are created by mixing eggs and sperm in a laboratory dish. Zygotes are then placed in the fallopian tube to begin development into embryos. ZIFT, unlike GIFT, allows the doctor to make sure that fertilization has occurred, an advantage in cases where a woman's body appears to produce *antibodies* (immune-system cells) that damage or kill sperm.

features or any signs of insufficient male hormones. After the interview and examination, the man undergoes the critical evaluation of male fertility—semen analysis.

For the semen test, the man provides a specimen of his semen, which a technician examines under a microscope. Semen normally contains at least 20 million sperm per milliliter, of which about 60 percent demonstrate normal *motility* (movement) and about 60 percent have a normal shape. Although doctors are not sure how many sperm are needed for fertility, they do know that higher sperm counts are associated with increased fertility. In some cases, absolutely no sperm appear in the semen, a condition called *azoospermia*. Azoospermia may result from damaged sperm-producing mechanisms in the testicles or from obstruction of the ducts.

More tests may be necessary to identify the source of a problem with sperm production. One test measures levels of various hormones, including the male hormone testosterone, because inadequate testosterone can lower sperm production. If an obstructed vas deferens is suspected, the doctor can view the duct using X rays.

Once physicians identify the cause or causes of infertility, couples can consider various treatment options. One of the most treatable causes of infertility is abnormal ovulation. There are several methods of inducing ovulation in premenopausal women. One of the most common involves administering a drug called clomiphene citrate. The drug is a weak estrogen compound that triggers ovulation by boosting the production of pituitary hormones.

In some women, a malfunctioning adrenal gland interferes with ovulation, and treatment with an adrenal hormone can help induce ovulation. In other cases, excess production of the milk-stimulating hormone prolactin prevents ovulation. This condition may cause a discharge from the nipple and can usually be corrected with a drug.

Some women cease ovulating as a result of extreme weight loss, strenuous exercise, or stress, all of which can disrupt the hormones that stimulate the ovaries. The condition usually goes away on its own, once the cause is eliminated. But some of these women require treatment with the hormone gonadotropin to initiate ovulation.

If a woman's ovaries receive inadequate stimulation from pituitary hormones, hormone treatment may help her become pregnant. The treatment can cause a number of eggs to ripen in follicles, and doctors must monitor hormone levels carefully to limit the chances of a multiple birth, which occurs in about 10 to 15 percent of cases.

Adhesions can be treated surgically during a diagnostic laparoscopy, as can endometriosis—a disease in which cells from the endometrium grow outside of the uterus. Endometriosis can hinder fertility by damaging the ovaries or fallopian tubes. While the woman is under anesthesia, the surgeon inspects the pelvic area and abdomen and cuts away adhesions or endometrial growth, most often using a *laser* (high-energy light beam), scissors, or electrical knife.

Success rates

In vitro fertilization requires an investment of time and money. The first attempt does not always succeed, and the couple may need to repeat the procedure several times before they achieve a successful pregnancy—or give up. The procedures are also expensive, with a single attempt costing on average about $7,000 to $10,000 in 1995.

Type of procedure	Total performed in 1992	Success rate (deliveries per retrievals)
IVF-ET	29,404	17 percent
GIFT	5,767	26 percent
ZIFT	1,993	23 percent

Source: *Fertility and Sterility*, 62: 1121-1128, 1994.

Abnormalities inside the uterus, including adhesions and growths called fibroids, can be removed during hysteroscopy.

When the man is infertile, some simple steps may solve the problem. The most common obstacles to male fertility—low sperm count and low motility—can be bypassed by collecting the man's sperm and injecting it directly into the uterus. This procedure, called intrauterine insemination, ensures that a good concentration of sperm reaches the uterus. In other cases, varicose veins in the scrotum disrupt sperm formation by raising the temperature in the testicle. Doctors can correct the problem in a minor surgical procedure. A blocked vas deferens, perhaps from an infection, can also be surgically corrected. If these procedures fail to restore sperm production, the couple may consider using donated sperm.

In cases of unexplained infertility, with no diagnosed defect to correct, doctors try instead to increase the overall efficiency of the reproductive process. The woman receives drugs so that her ovaries release additional eggs and her hormonal levels are favorable for pregnancy. The physician then injects her husband's sperm into her uterus. The objective is to increase the number of sperm and eggs available for fertilization. From 15 to 18 percent of couples conceive from a single treatment, and repeated attempts may be necessary.

If these approaches fail, couples may consider more technologically advanced techniques. The first procedure usually considered is *in vitro* fertilization. In vitro, which means *in glass*, refers to the glass laboratory dish or test tube in which fertilization occurs.

Before the procedure, the woman receives drugs to stimulate her follicles. Just before ovulation, the doctor removes a number of eggs from their follicles within the ovaries. Eggs are most often retrieved in one of two ways: through laparascopic surgery or with a needle guided by high-frequency sound waves known as ultrasound. Using laparoscopy, the surgeon inserts a thin needle into the abdomen toward the enlarged follicles, from which the fluid that contains an egg is removed. Using images produced by ultrasound, the surgeon guides a long, thin needle through the vagina into the ovary and then into each of the ripe follicles, removing the fluid with the eggs.

An *embryologist* (specialist in caring for eggs and embryos) uses a microscope to search the follicular fluid for eggs. Also at this time, a technician concentrates sperm collected from the man by washing away the semen and removing less active sperm. The embryologist then mixes the eggs with the vigorous sperm in a laboratory dish. A laboratory incubator keeps the eggs and sperm at the proper temperature for fertilization. Fertilization usually occurs within hours, and by the next day there should be several zygotes.

About 48 to 72 hours after fertilization, the physician transfers the developing embryos into the woman's uterus. The technique most often employed delivers the embryos through the vagina and cervix, using a narrow, flexible tube called a catheter. Usually, about three or four embryos are placed in the uterus to increase the chances of a pregnancy. This procedure, in vitro fertilization and embryo transfer (IVF-ET), is useful if the woman's immune system attacks sperm or if she has tubal adhesions or endometriosis, conditions that prevent the eggs from reaching the uterus through the fallopian tubes. IVF-ET can also help overcome severe sperm abnormalities in the man.

If the woman has defective eggs or no eggs, the IVF-ET technique may be used with eggs obtained from a donor. Before the man's sperm fertilize the donated eggs, the woman is given hormone treatments to prepare her endometrium for the resulting embryo.

When the woman has normal fallopian tubes, the couple may choose between two other reproductive technologies that follow nature's model more closely. In both techniques, the transfer occurs in the fallopian tubes. In zygote intra-fallopian transfer (ZIFT), the sperm fertilize eggs in a laboratory dish. The single-celled zygotes are then transferred to the fallopian tube using laparoscopy. In theory, the fallopian tubes provide a more natural environment for the growth of an embryo. The procedure also enables the embryos to enter the uterus at the customary time.

In gamete intrafallopian transfer (GIFT), the eggs and sperm, which are known also as gametes, are placed in the fallopian tubes separately before fertilization. A technician washes the semen from the sperm, as with IVF-ET, and then loads the most active sperm into a catheter. Eggs are also loaded into the catheter, separated from the sperm by a bubble. The physician then delivers the contents of the catheter to the woman's fallopian tube by means of laparoscopy. If all goes as anticipated, a sperm fertilizes an egg in the fallopian tube, and an embryo then proceeds to the uterus.

Of the three procedures, GIFT follows nature's course most closely. Many doctors prefer ZIFT over GIFT, however, because it allows them to confirm that fertilization has occurred prior to the transfer. Both ZIFT and GIFT have a drawback, compared with IVF-ET, in that the transfer requires laparoscopic surgery under general anesthesia. Thus, they carry all the risks—and costs—of surgery.

The most common unintended effect from assisted reproductive technologies is multiple births. These occur because fertility drugs can prompt the release of several eggs at the same time. In addition, the assisted reproductive technologies involve the transfer of several embryos, eggs, or zygotes to the uterus. As many as 30 percent of assisted pregnancies result in multiple births—about 25 percent in twins and 3 percent in three or more births.

Pregnancy rates following in-vitro fertilization average about 20 percent each month. Success rates from assisted-reproductive technologies vary greatly from clinic to clinic, owing in large part to the different criteria clinics use in accepting couples for treatment. All clinics have found that the older the woman, the smaller the chances of success. Women whose follicles respond poorly to hormone stimulation also have low pregnancy rates. Some clinics that report high success rates exclude women in these two categories.

Evaluation and treatment for infertility can be uncomfortable, time-consuming, and expensive, thereby placing serious emotional strain on a couple. Whether the couple pulls together or draws apart depends on their personalities and their feelings for each other. Friends and family members who already have children may fail to comprehend the infertile couple's pain, leaving the couple feeling isolated. Insurance companies may deny coverage, or provide only limited coverage, for infertility services, adding to the couple's burden. In spite of these hurdles, many couples are committed to pursuing every available option. Their tenacity reveals the depth of their longing to have children and so complete their family.　●●●

For more information:

The American College of Obstetrics and Gynecology (ACOG)
409 12th Street SW
Washington, DC 20024-2188

The American Society for Reproductive Medicine
1209 Montgomery Highway
Birmingham, AL 35216

Resolve, Incorporated
5 Water Street
Arlington, MA 02174

Cochlear Implants:
Delivering Sound to the Deaf

By Carol A. Turkington

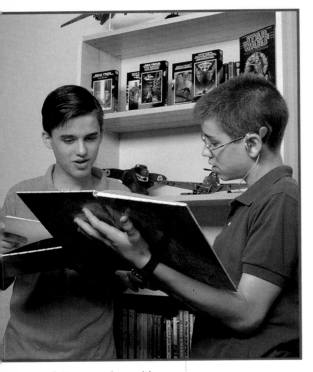

A teen-age boy with a cochlear implant, right, listens to his friend as the two look over some books.

Cochlear implants can help some profoundly deaf people hear. But experts stress that the implant is not for everyone.

FOUR-YEAR-OLD AMY, dressed in ballet slippers and tutu, stands in front of the mirror, smiling at her reflection. The world slips away as she sways to the music, lost in her dreams of becoming a ballet dancer.

Last year, the realization of those dreams seemed all but impossible when Amy became deaf following a serious ear infection. Today, with the aid of a special electronic device, Amy's dream may come true.

Amy is one of a growing number of children who have been fitted with a cochlear implant, a new and controversial treatment for hearing loss. Unlike hearing aids, which merely amplify sound, the implant actually functions in the same way as the structure called the cochlea in the inner ear and helps send sound from the ear to the brain. For Amy and others, the cochlear implant can offer the means of hearing speech and sounds from the environment—something that no other hearing device can offer.

Despite the benefits the implant seems to offer, hearing specialists and members of the deaf community continue to debate whether these benefits outweigh the inherent risks and limitations of the device. First of all, the device is surgically implanted, and the procedure, like any major surgery, carries with it some risk. Second, manufacturers can offer no promises on how well a person will hear with an implant. In addition, after receiving the implant, some people end up feeling alienated from the deaf community while, at the same time, not feeling fully a part of the hearing world.

Even so, the device's potential ability to restore some hearing has a strong appeal for many people. Significant hearing loss affects more than 15 million Americans, making it the most common physical disability in the United States. Hearing loss can result from a defect in the *auditory* (hearing) nerve or parts of the middle or inner ear. The most frequent cause of deafness involves damage to hair cells, tiny structures in the cochlea. The hair cells help us hear by stimulating the auditory nerve, which transmits sound signals to the brain. Hair cells can be destroyed by many means, including infection, trauma, loud noise, the aging process, or birth defects. When hair cells fail to function, the auditory nerve remains unstimulated and deafness results. The cochlear implant by-passes the damaged hair cells and helps establish some degree of hearing by stimulating the hearing nerve directly.

All cochlear implants consist of the same basic equipment. A microphone, worn behind the ear, picks up sound and routes it along a wire to a speech processor that can be worn in a small shoulder pouch, a pocket, or on a belt. The processor amplifies sound, filters out background noise, and turns sound into *digital* (numeric) signals before sending it to a transmitter worn behind the ear. A magnet holds the transmitter in place through its attraction to the receiver-stimulator, a part of the device that is surgically attached beneath the skin to the skull. The receiver picks up digital signals forwarded by the transmitter and converts them into electrical impulses. These impulses flow through *electrodes* (electrical conductors) contained in a narrow, flexible tube that has been threaded into the cochlea. As many as 22 electrodes, depending on the type of implant, carry the impulses that stimulate the auditory nerve and thus send a signal to the brain. The brain then interprets the signals as specific sounds.

Before an individual can receive an implant, specialists at an implant clinic conduct a careful evaluation. Extensive hearing tests determine how well the candidate hears with a hearing aid. Currently, the Food and Drug Administration (FDA), which regulates the device, limits the implant to people with severe to profound hearing loss. The FDA has imposed this limitation because the implants are so expensive—a minimum of $25,000 for the evaluation, surgery, and postoperative therapy—and because results cannot be predicted.

Implant candidates first undergo a trial with powerful hearing aids. If the hearing aids fail to improve hearing adequately, a physician then performs a physical examination and obtains an X-ray image called a CT scan to evaluate whether the candidate's inner ear is suitable for an implant. Some patients have a cochlea that has

Glossary

Auditory nerve: The nerve that carries sound in the form of electrical impulses to the brain, which interprets the impulses as sound.

Cochlea: A snail-shaped structure in the ear that contains the nerve endings that transmit sound as electrical impulses to the auditory nerve.

Cochlear implant: Electronic device that helps restore hearing through stimulation of the auditory nerve.

Hair cells: Tiny structures in the cochlea that stimulate nerve fibers in response to sound waves.

The author:

Carol A. Turkington is a free-lance medical writer.

How we hear

Hearing is a complex process. It involves the conversion of sound into electrical impulses and the transmission of these impulses from the ear to the brain. The process begins when sound, which consists of vibrations that travel in waves, enters the ear and strikes the paper-thin eardrum, causing it to vibrate. A chain of three small bones called ossicles in the middle ear then conducts this vibration to fluid that fills the passages of the snail-shaped cochlea. The cochlea contains more than 15,000 tiny structures called hair cells.

As the three small ear bones vibrate, they create waves in the fluid of the cochlea, which in turn cause the hair cells to vibrate. When the hair cells move, they generate electrical impulses in the auditory nerve. The nerve transmits the impulses to a part of the brain that perceives and interprets electrical stimulation as sound.

Most hearing problems stem from damage to the hair cells. When the hair cells fail to function, the auditory nerve remains unstimulated, and hearing loss results.

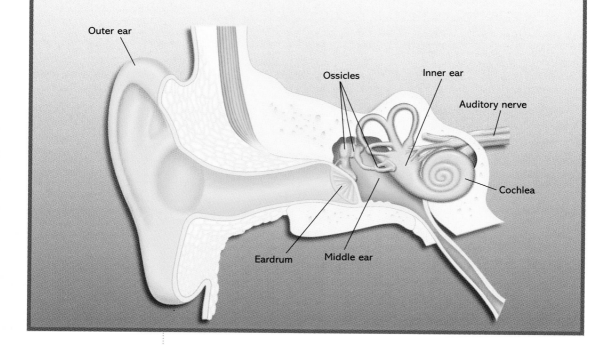

Outer ear

Ossicles

Inner ear

Auditory nerve

Cochlea

Eardrum

Middle ear

been left permanently scarred by infection or disease. Such patients may make poor candidates for an implant. The physician also screens for the presence of an ear infection, which can adversely influence the surgery's outcome, and determines whether the patient can safely undergo general anesthesia. Finally, a physician may order a psychological evaluation to learn about a patient's expectations. Patients should be highly motivated and have a realistic understanding of what an implant can and cannot do. A patient who passes this careful evaluation is eligible for an implant.

Implanting the device involves major surgery, during which the surgeon makes an incision behind the ear and opens the mastoid bone, the ridge on the skull behind the ear. The surgeon then places

How the cochlear implant works

A cochlear implant is an electronic device designed to restore some degree of hearing in people with severe to profound hearing loss. Unlike hearing aids, which merely amplify sound, the implant functions like the cochlea in the inner ear. Through a series of external and internal devices, the implant stimulates the auditory nerve with electrical signals that are transmitted to the brain and interpreted as sound.

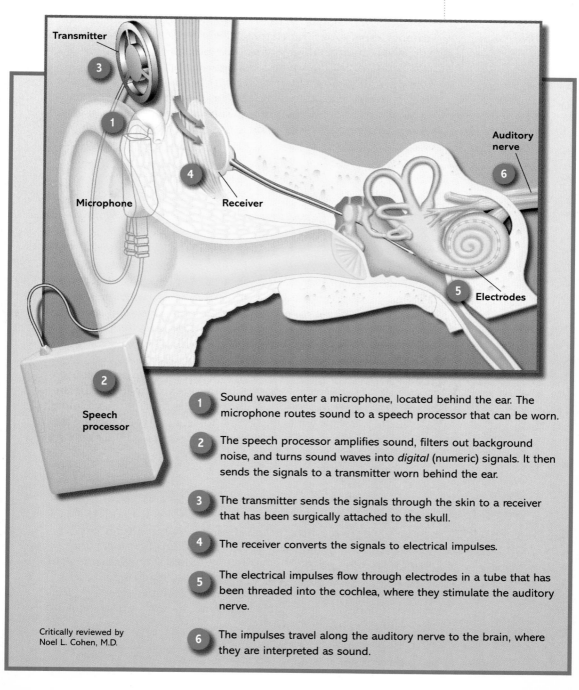

Transmitter

3

1

Microphone

4

Receiver

Auditory nerve

6

5

Electrodes

2

Speech processor

1 Sound waves enter a microphone, located behind the ear. The microphone routes sound to a speech processor that can be worn.

2 The speech processor amplifies sound, filters out background noise, and turns sound waves into *digital* (numeric) signals. It then sends the signals to a transmitter worn behind the ear.

3 The transmitter sends the signals through the skin to a receiver that has been surgically attached to the skull.

4 The receiver converts the signals to electrical impulses.

5 The electrical impulses flow through electrodes in a tube that has been threaded into the cochlea, where they stimulate the auditory nerve.

6 The impulses travel along the auditory nerve to the brain, where they are interpreted as sound.

Critically reviewed by
Noel L. Cohen, M.D.

the receiver-stimulator in the mastoid bone and gently threads the electrodes into the cochlea. The operation takes about three hours, and the hospital stay usually lasts only a day or two.

After a month or so, when the surgical wounds have healed, the patient returns to the implant clinic to be fitted with the external parts of the device—the speech processor, microphone, and transmitter. A clinician tunes the speech processor, setting levels of stimulation for each electrode from soft to loud. An important training period then begins, during which the implant recipient learns how to interpret the sounds heard through the device. The length of the training period varies from days to years, depending on how well the patient can interpret the sounds heard through the device.

The sounds heard through a cochlear implant differ somewhat from the sounds normally relayed to the brain and have been described as robotlike or cartoonlike. This difference occurs because the implant's 22 or fewer electrodes cannot possibly match in complexity the workings of approximately 15,000 hair cells. Nonetheless, cochlear implants have significantly improved the communication skills of many deafened adults.

The majority of profoundly deaf patients who receive an implant are able to discern medium and loud sounds, including speech at comfortable listening levels. Many recipients use sound clues from the implant in combination with reading a speaker's lips and watching for other facial cues. According to clinical trials evaluated by the FDA, almost all adults improve their communication skills when using the implant along with lip reading, and some can understand spoken words without lip reading. More than half of adult recipients who lost their hearing after they learned to speak can understand some speech without lip reading after a cochlear implant, according to physician Noel L. Cohen, an ear, nose, and throat specialist at New York University in New York City. About 30 percent can understand spoken sounds well enough to use the telephone.

Children who were born deaf or who lost their hearing before acquiring speech have the most difficulty in learning to use the implant. Recent research suggests, however, that most of these children are able to learn spoken language and understand speech using the implant, and many are able to attend regular schools rather than traditional schools for the deaf.

Unfortunately, it's impossible to predict who will benefit from a cochlear implant and to what extent. Many factors affect how a person responds to the device. In general, the later in life a person experiences deafness and the shorter the duration of deafness, the more speech the person is likely to understand through the implant. Someone with a healthy auditory nerve is also likely to fare better than a person with a damaged auditory nerve. Finally, good postoperative training can make all the difference in how well an implant recipient comprehends sounds.

The benefits of cochlear implants

The Food and Drug Administration (FDA) regulates medical devices to ensure their safety and effectiveness. The FDA bases its approval of a device such as a cochlear implant on information gathered in clinical trials. Although no cochlear implant can restore normal hearing, FDA clinical trials have demonstrated that implants can benefit people with hearing loss in a number of ways. These demonstrated benefits are listed below.

Children*

- Children are able to detect conversational-level environmental sounds, including speech, at comfortable listening levels.
- Some children can identify everyday sounds, such as car horns, doorbells and birds singing, from a set of alternatives.
- Many children can identify words from a set of alternatives without lip reading.
- Some children exhibit improved lip reading.
- A few children can recognize speech without lip reading.
- After training and experience with the device, many children demonstrate improvements in speech.

Adults**

- All can hear conversation and environmental sounds at comfortable listening levels.
- Almost all showed improved lip reading.
- Almost all improve their communication abilities when using the implant in conjunction with lip reading.
- More than half can understand speech through the implant alone (without lip reading).
- Some have a limited ability to use the telephone.

*The words *few, some,* and *many* represent the following percentage of children who participated in the FDA clinical trials:
  Few—greater than 5 percent and equal to or less than 34 percent.
  Some—greater than 34 percent, less than 52 percent.
  Many—equal to or greater than 52 percent.
**Represents adults who became deaf after learning language and oral speech.
Source: Cochlear Corporation.

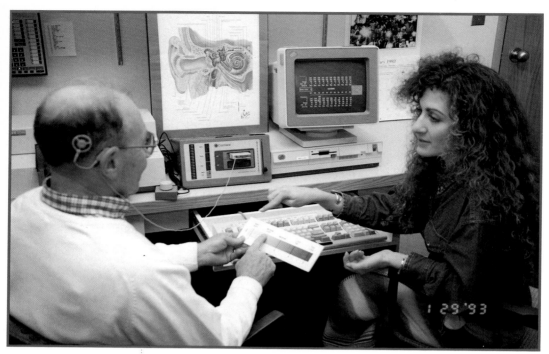

An audiologist, right, tests the hearing of a man with a new implant. The audiologist measures how well the patient can hear a range of sounds from soft to loud.

In general, the cochlear implant interferes little with the everyday activities of the person who wears one. Rechargeable batteries for the device are typically replaced daily. The external parts of the device should be protected from moisture and should be removed before swimming. And appropriate protective head gear should be worn during sports.

The risks and complications of cochlear implant surgery are few, but prospective patients should consider them seriously. Some patients experience dizziness after the surgery, and paralysis of the face has occurred in a few instances. As with any major surgery, there is a risk of infection at the site of the operation. Furthermore, researchers are uncertain about the long-term effects of electrical stimulation on the nervous system. Damage to the implant's internal components can also occur—through a blow to the head, for example—rendering the device inoperative.

The FDA requires that implant candidates, besides being severely to profoundly deaf, experience no significant benefit from hearing aids. In addition, candidates must be at least 2 years old, the age at which hearing specialists can verify the severity of a child's deafness and evaluate whether the child can benefit from a hearing aid.

Before the FDA approves a new implant, it gathers information on the safety and effectiveness of the device through long-term clinical trials. The FDA also monitors the frequency of adverse reactions to the implant and the rate of implant failure. Some forms of the device are still undergoing investigation in clinical trials.

Critics of the implant say that its cost is too high considering that its effectiveness cannot be predicted. The use of implants in children is particularly controversial. Some critics charge that parents who seek the operation for a deaf child are, knowingly or not, sending the child a message that deafness is unacceptable. These critics also feel that parents have no right to impose an implant on a child who will then belong neither to the deaf community nor to the hearing world. Proponents argue that the device is of considerable benefit to the majority of people who have one and that there is nothing wrong with trying to improve communication skills in deafened adults and children.

Experts stress the implant is not for everyone and that potential candidates should become well informed before making a decision on obtaining an implant. Meanwhile, research on improving the efficiency of cochlear implants continues. • • •

Where to get help

For additional information on cochlear implants, hearing loss, and deafness, the following organizations and support groups can be of help.

- **Alexander Graham Bell Association for the Deaf,** 3417 Volta Place NW, Washington, DC 20007 (202/337-5220, V/TTY).

- **American Speech-Language-Hearing Association,** 10801 Rockville Pike, Rockville, MD 20852 (800/638-8255, 301/897-5700, V/TTY).

- **Cochlear Implant Club International,** P.O. Box 464, Buffalo, NY 14223-0464 (716/838-4662, V/TTY).

- **National Association of the Deaf,** 814 Thayer Avenue, Silver Spring, MD 20910 (301/587-1788, V; 301/587-1789, TTY).

- **National Information Center on Deafness,** Gallaudet University, 800 Florida Avenue NE, Washington, DC 20002 (202/651-5051, V; 202/651-5052, TTY).

- **Hearing Loss Link,** 2600 W. Peterson Avenue, Suite 202, Chicago, IL 60659 (312/743-1032, V; 312/743-1007, TTY; 312/743-5490, FAX).

- **Self Help for Hard of Hearing People,** 7910 Woodmont Avenue, Suite 1200, Bethesda, MD 20814 (301/657-2248, V; 301/657-2249, TTY).

V - voice; TTY - text telephone; V/TTY - voice and text telephone.

The battle waged on so many fronts has
not been won, but there have been gains
and the arsenal of weapons is expanding.

Are We Winning the War on Cancer?

By Steven I. Benowitz

I N SEPTEMBER 1994, the National Cancer Advisory Board warned
the United States Congress that the war on cancer, formally declared in 1971 by President Richard M. Nixon, had stalled. The
board, made up of leading experts in cancer treatment and research,
said that unless the war's strategy were changed so that every cancer
patient had access to treatment and unless the latest laboratory findings were quickly brought to the patient's bedside, cancer would become the nation's leading killer by the year 2000, surpassing heart
disease. Moreover, the board warned in its report, one American in
three would develop cancer during his or her lifetime, and one in
five would die of the disease. It was a grim prognosis, especially
since more than $23 billion had been spent on cancer research since
the assault began.

Yet these sobering statistics obscure much of the ground scientists
have gained in the cancer war. Promising new therapies, improved
drugs and surgical techniques, and better diagnostic tests for certain
cancers have given many cancer patients longer, better lives. And research scientists are gaining a greater understanding of how the disease begins and behaves.

Cancer experts also note that a major change has occurred in the

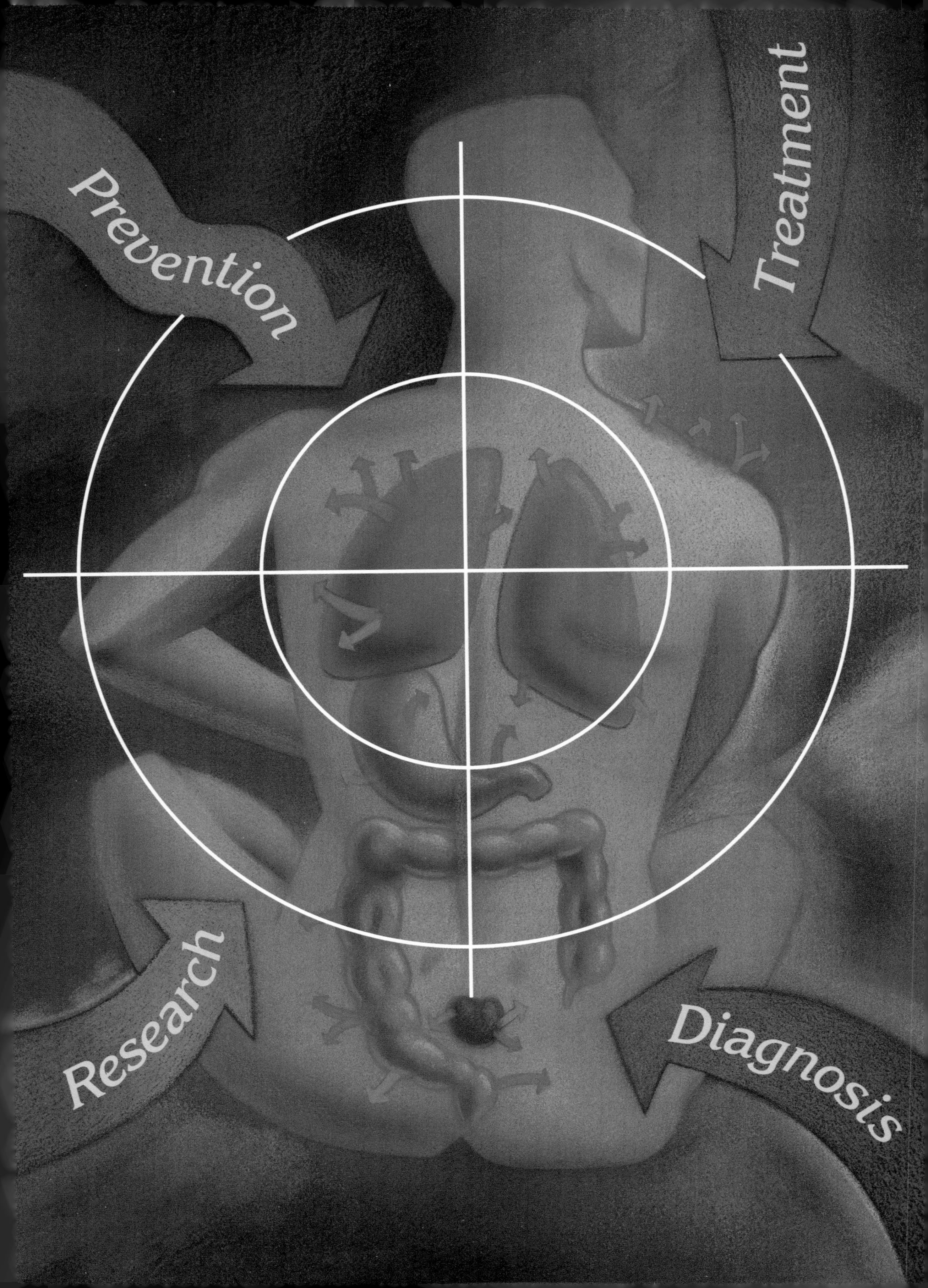

Prevention

Treatment

Research

Diagnosis

A continuing war

The war on cancer was formally declared in 1971, when President Richard M. Nixon signed the National Cancer Act. At the time, expectations ran high that an all-out assault, backed by the government's resources, would result in a quick victory. But cancer has proven to be a complex and elusive enemy.

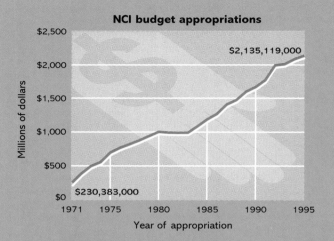

NCI budget appropriations

$2,135,119,000

$230,383,000

Millions of dollars

Year of appropriation

Expenditures on the war

The budget for the National Cancer Institute (NCI), the largest of the federal government's National Institutes of Health, has risen from $230 million in 1971 to $2.1 billion in 1995. In all, the NCI has spent more than $23 billion on cancer research.

culture of cancer. Doctors and patients discuss the disease and the treatment options far more openly today than in the past. And most important, a diagnosis of cancer, once the most dreaded disease of all, for many patients no longer means a sentence of death or unmanageable pain.

The war on cancer officially began with Nixon's signing of the National Cancer Act on Dec. 23, 1971. The act was significant for several reasons. First, it provided funding to establish a number of medical centers dedicated to clinical research and cancer treatment under the oversight of the National Cancer Institute (NCI), today the largest of the federal government's National Institutes of Health. Second, the act created an organizational structure that enabled cancer researchers and doctors to share findings, exchange ideas, and promote public education. Third and perhaps most important, the act gave the research community a green light—and the funding—to pursue research on cancer at the molecular level.

At the time the act was signed, it was widely believed by members of Congress and other public officials that by putting the government's considerable resources behind an all-out assault on cancer,

The author:

Steven I. Benowitz is a free-lance science writer

228

Rising cancer incidence and mortality

The number of new cancers diagnosed in the United States has risen from 320 for every 100,000 people in 1973, the first year NCI tallied the statistics, to 405 per 100,000 in 1991, the latest year available. Cancer deaths have risen far more slowly, from 162 deaths per 100,000 people in 1973 to 173 per 100,000 in 1991.

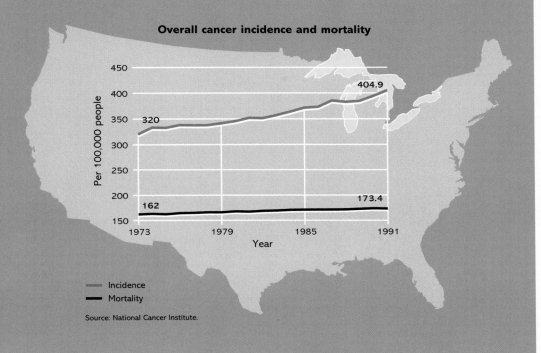

Overall cancer incidence and mortality

Per 100,000 people

320 · 404.9

162 · 173.4

1973 · 1979 · 1985 · 1991

Year

— Incidence
— Mortality

Source: National Cancer Institute.

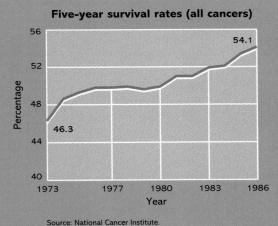

Five-year survival rates (all cancers)

Percentage

54.1

46.3

1973 · 1977 · 1980 · 1983 · 1986

Year

Source: National Cancer Institute.

Improved cancer survival

The percentage of people alive five years after starting cancer treatment has risen steadily since 1973. Of those first treated in 1973, 46 percent were alive in 1978. Of those first treated in 1986, 54 percent were alive in 1991. The five-year survival rate is also known as the cure rate.

More Americans die of lung cancer than of any other cancer. Although more men than women develop lung cancer and die of it, rates among women are still rising while men's rates have begun to fall. The disparity arises because women took up smoking in large numbers years after men, and their lung cancer rates do not yet reflect the overall drop in smoking rates since the 1960's.

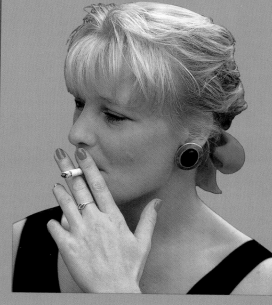

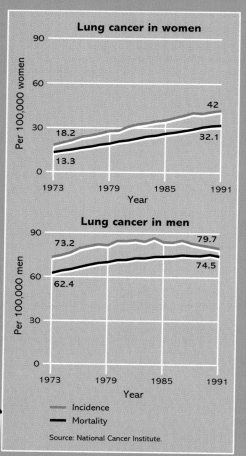

Lung cancer in women

Per 100,000 women

18.2
13.3
42
32.1

1973   1979   1985   1991
Year

Lung cancer in men

Per 100,000 men

73.2
62.4
79.7
74.5

1973   1979   1985   1991
Year

— Incidence
— Mortality

Source: National Cancer Institute.

a cure would be found relatively quickly, perhaps even in time for the 1976 bicentennial of the nation's founding. Confidence in the ability of scientists, to accomplish near miracles fostered such beliefs. After all, American space scientists had landed a man on the moon in 1969. Few people expected that cancer would turn out to be so complex. "The problem was that science had the technology for the moon landing. We didn't have the same basic knowledge of cancer," says Peter Greenwald, the director of the NCI's Division of Cancer Prevention and Control.

Cancer—the uncontrolled proliferation of cells—is a disease of the genes. For cancer to develop, something must go awry in a gene, or more likely in several genes. Most often, these cancer-causing genes direct cell growth or development.

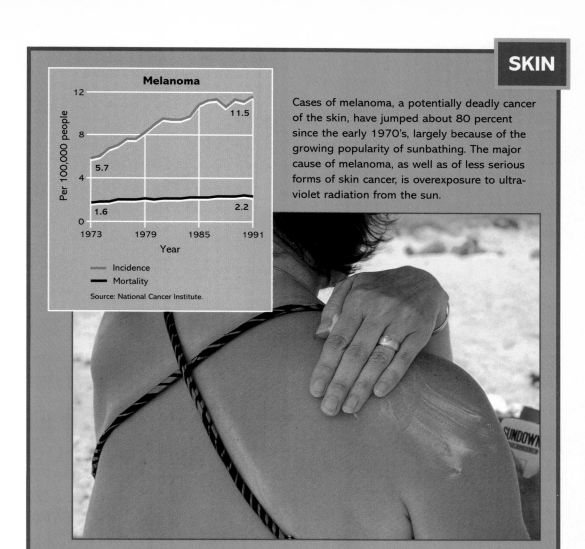

Melanoma

Per 100,000 people

12

8

4

0

5.7

11.5

1.6

2.2

1973   1979   1985   1991

Year

—— Incidence
—— Mortality

Source: National Cancer Institute.

Cases of melanoma, a potentially deadly cancer of the skin, have jumped about 80 percent since the early 1970's, largely because of the growing popularity of sunbathing. The major cause of melanoma, as well as of less serious forms of skin cancer, is overexposure to ultraviolet radiation from the sun.

Years of research on the ways in which cells turn cancerous have shown that cancer tumors are not the same. For example, the structure of tumor tissue varies from site to site, and tumors develop differently, depending on the site. Tumor research has convinced some scientists that cancer may actually be as many as 150 different diseases. While it's difficult to assess the progress of a war fought on so many fronts, statistics on cancer incidence, deaths, and survival rates provide one key measure of just how well the war is going.

The NCI and the American Cancer Society (ACS) compile data on the number of cases of each type of cancer—breast, lung, prostate, and so on—diagnosed each year; on the number of cancer deaths by type of cancer; and on the age, sex, and race of cancer patients. From the data on cancer incidence (cases diagnosed per year) and

The incidence of prostate cancer has soared—up by more than 150 percent from 1973 to 1991. The rise is due largely to improved diagnosis through the Prostate Specific Antigen (PSA) test, a blood test that detects aggressive prostate cancers long before symptoms arise, *below right*. Despite rising incidence, the mortality rate from this cancer has remained fairly constant.

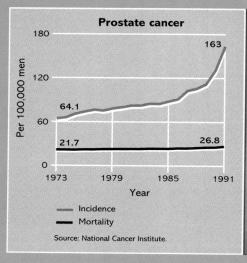

Prostate cancer

Per 100,000 men

180

163

120

64.1

60

21.7   26.8

0

1973   1979   1985   1991

Year

— Incidence
— Mortality

Source: National Cancer Institute.

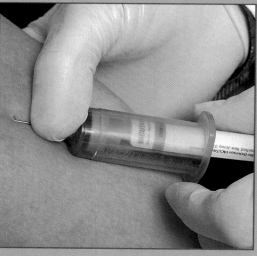

mortality, statisticians can determine the five-year survival rate. This rate, the so-called cure rate, represents the percentage of patients whose cancer has not recurred in the five years following treatment.

The NCI and ACS statistics indicate that, overall, cancer has been on the rise since the war began. In 1971, some 635,000 Americans were diagnosed with cancer, and about 335,000 died of it. In 1995, some 1,252,000 new cases of cancer would be diagnosed (not including 800,000 cases of highly curable and hard-to-track skin cancers), according to the ACS, and 547,000 people would die of cancer. Furthermore, the NCI estimates that the cure rate has improved by only 4 percent since 1971.

The U.S. population, of course, has grown since 1971, and so a rise in the number of cancer cases over nearly a quarter century could be expected and need not necessarily signify a rise in cancer rates. To adjust for population growth and provide a more accurate basis for comparison, the NCI calculates cancer incidence and mortality rates for every 100,000 Americans.

The NCI makes a further adjustment to rates to take into account the aging of the U.S. population. The 1990 census found that people over age 65 constituted the fastest-growing group in the population. Because the genetic changes that lead to cancer generally take place over many years, the longer people live, the greater are their chances of developing cancer. Moreover, much of the gain in American longevity comes from a 30 percent drop in heart disease death rates since 1970. With fewer people dying prematurely of heart disease, more people are living long enough to develop cancer. Thus, an increase in cancer incidence might reflect this increase in longevity. To adjust for the aging of the population, statisticians compare cancer rates among similar age groups. They generally use 1970 cancer rates as the basis for comparison.

Yet even after taking population growth and aging into account, the overall cancer rate per 100,000 people rose from 320 in 1973—the first year the NCI tallied the statistics—to 405 in 1991, the latest data available. Although the percentage of patients alive after five years is up for most cancers, people diagnosed with cancer still tend to die of it and nearly half of them die within five years.

What's causing this rise in cancer statistics? Part of it results from

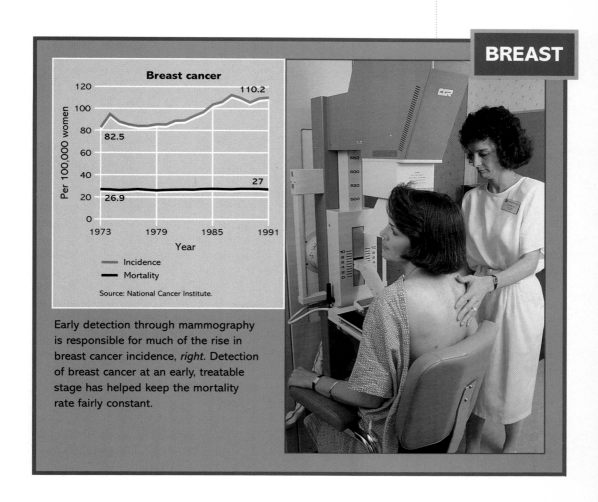

BREAST

Early detection through mammography is responsible for much of the rise in breast cancer incidence, *right*. Detection of breast cancer at an early, treatable stage has helped keep the mortality rate fairly constant.

233

new diagnostic techniques, NCI researchers say. For example, magnetic resonance imaging (MRI), an imaging technique that has become widely available since the 1970's, enables doctors to spot tumors in the brain, liver, and other soft tissues. Previously, these cancers often went undetected, and thus uncounted.

Similarly, reported cases of prostate cancer have skyrocketed as the result of a newly developed and widely used blood test, the prostate specific antigen (PSA) test. The ACS estimated that 244,000 new cases of prostate cancer would be diagnosed in 1995, up from 106,000 in 1990 and 66,000 in 1980. A study reported in 1995 by researchers at the Harvard Medical School and the Harvard School of Public Health in Boston found that the PSA test detects nearly 90 percent of aggressive prostate cancers five years before symptoms arise and that it spots more than half of them a decade before they would otherwise be noticed.

No one knows to what extent early detection of most prostate cancers matters in the long run, however. First, detecting cancer does not mean curing cancer. Second, prostate cancers usually grow slowly, especially in older men, *oncologists* (cancer specialists) note, and many men with prostate cancer die of other diseases before can-

COLON

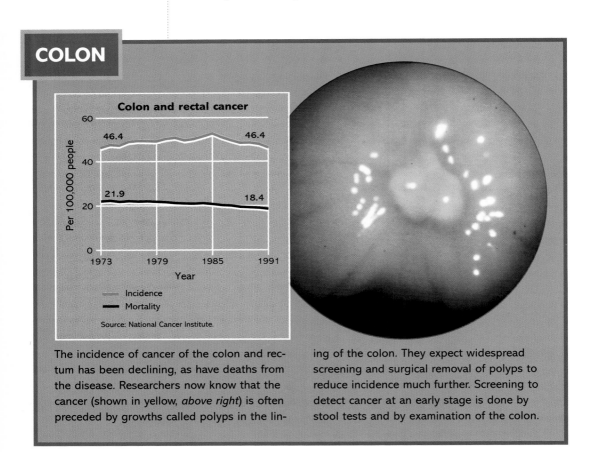

The incidence of cancer of the colon and rectum has been declining, as have deaths from the disease. Researchers now know that the cancer (shown in yellow, *above right*) is often preceded by growths called polyps in the lining of the colon. They expect widespread screening and surgical removal of polyps to reduce incidence much further. Screening to detect cancer at an early stage is done by stool tests and by examination of the colon.

234

cer threatens their life. The NCI has recently begun a large, multi-center national study to determine whether early diagnosis and treatment helps prostate cancer patients live longer. As yet, there are no agreed-upon recommendations for when or whether men should have the PSA test.

Public awareness also contributes to rising statistics. While there has been a slow, steady increase in the incidence of breast cancer since the 1970's, the recorded incidence soared in the mid-1970's after First Lady Betty Ford and Margaretta (Happy) Rockefeller, the wife of former Vice President Nelson Rockefeller, were diagnosed with the disease. Their public statements following their diagnoses prompted large numbers of women to be screened for breast cancer. Cases diagnosed jumped from about 74,000 in 1973 to 90,000 in 1974, the year of Betty Ford's surgery. Public education campaigns by the American Cancer Society have also encouraged women to get regular breast cancer screening through mammograms.

The NCI expects some leveling off before long in breast cancer and prostate cancer rates. The dramatic rise over the last 20 years, NCI researchers have concluded, was due in large part to earlier diagnosis and hence the statistical bulge created should be temporary.

Changes in behavior have profoundly affected rates for some cancers. Cases of melanoma, a deadly form of skin cancer, have jumped nearly 80 percent since the early 1970's, owing largely to the soaring popularity of sunbathing, according to the NCI. Sunbathing has also caused less serious forms of skin cancer to swell in number, up from 115,000 in 1971 to 800,000 in 1995.

The leading cancer killer of both men and women in the United States is lung cancer, exacting a toll estimated at 157,400 lives in 1995. Smoking, the ACS says, is responsible for 87 percent of these cancers. After rising for years, lung cancer incidence among men peaked in 1984 and has dropped steadily since 1988, reflecting a cut in smoking that began years earlier.

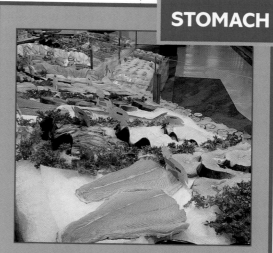

STOMACH

Stomach cancer rates have plummeted in the United States. Scientists generally credit the decline to improved refrigeration and less reliance on food preservation through salting, smoking, and pickling—processing thought to contribute to stomach cancer.

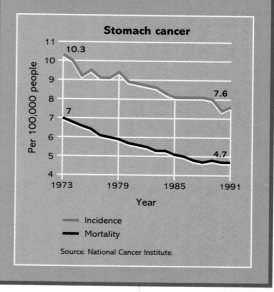

Stomach cancer

Per 100,000 people

11	10.3
10	
9	
8	7.6
7	7
6	
5	4.7
4	

1973 — 1979 — 1985 — 1991

Year

—— Incidence
—— Mortality

Source: National Cancer Institute.

Among women, however, lung cancer cases increased 100 percent from 1973 to 1990, the result, researchers say, of a smoking habit that became widespread after World War II (1939-1945), years after men took up the habit in large numbers. Since 1987, more women have died of lung cancer each year than of breast cancer, which was the major cancer killer of women for more than 40 years, according to the ACS.

Lung cancer accounted for more than a quarter of the 547,000 American cancer deaths the ACS projected for 1995. Indeed, the NCI claims that lung cancer accounts for a large part of the 7 percent overall rise in cancer death rates from 1973 to 1991. If lung cancer is excluded, overall death rates from cancer would have declined by 14 percent from 1950 to 1990, according to the ACS.

Other cancers are on the rise for no obvious reason, according to the NCI. These include kidney cancer, testicular cancer, and non-Hodgkin's lymphoma, a cancer of the lymph nodes.

Not all the war news is grim, however. Some cancer rates are clearly on the downswing, and more drops are anticipated. As cancer experts point out, changes in incidence and death rates nearly always lag behind treatment advances by a decade or so. "We've progressively improved the treatment of cancer patients, reduced some of the incidence, recognized ways to prevent cancer, and made some major breakthroughs in some of the cancers we face," says Robert Young, president of Fox Chase Cancer Center in Philadelphia. Young points out that experts knew practically nothing in the 1960's and the early 1970's about the genetics of cancer and the mechanisms whereby some cancers developed resistance to the drugs used to treat them.

While early diagnosis appears to have raised reported incidence rates of breast and prostate cancers, it has lowered rates of other cancers. Cervical cancer rates have dropped dramatically, owing largely to the Pap smear, a test that detects precancerous changes in cells in the *cervix* (entrance to the uterus). Physicians can then destroy the cells by freezing them, a technique known as cryotherapy, before the

CERVIX

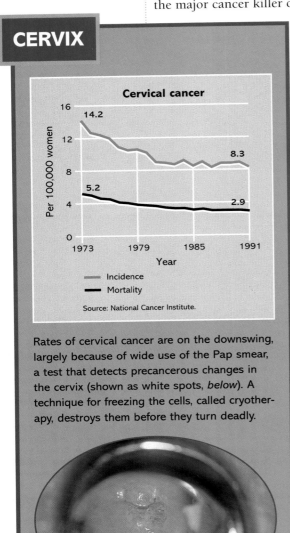

Rates of cervical cancer are on the downswing, largely because of wide use of the Pap smear, a test that detects precancerous changes in the cervix (shown as white spots, *below*). A technique for freezing the cells, called cryotherapy, destroys them before they turn deadly.

cells turn deadly. The incidence of cervical cancer has fallen by 36 percent from 1973 to 1991, and the death rate by 42 percent.

Most experts contend that changes in breast cancer death rates are only now beginning to show up, the result of impressive surgical improvements and drug therapies introduced in the 1980's. In early 1995, the Department of Health and Human Services announced that the death rate from breast cancer among American women fell almost 5 percent from 1989 to 1992, representing the largest short-term decline in four decades.

Changes in breast cancer treatment are among the most dramatic advances in the war on cancer. Most women with breast cancer no longer need undergo a disfiguring radical mastectomy, in which the breast and underlying chest wall muscle are cut away. A long-term study conducted by the NCI from 1976 to 1984 established that lumpectomy—the removal of the cancerous tumor and surrounding tissue—followed by radiation is just as effective as mastectomy in preventing recurrences of breast cancer. And for many women whose breast cancer has spread to nearby lymph nodes, chemotherapy—the use of cancer-killing drugs—has helped prevent recurrence.

Of the major cancer killers in the United States, the battle against colon cancer may be the most winnable, according to many oncologists. Cancers of the colon and rectum rank fourth among the most common cancers in the United States—138,200 new cases in 1995—but second among cancer killers—55,300 deaths.

What makes researchers so optimistic are advances in diagnosing the disease when it is still highly treatable. Growths called polyps in the lining of the colon usually precede colon cancer, and removal of these polyps may greatly reduce the incidence of colon cancer, by as much as 87 percent according to one study. Screening stool samples for blood, a 1993 study showed, can be an effective way to detect large polyps or early-stage cancers. Even more accurate diagnostic procedures—colonoscopy and sigmoidoscopy—provide a view of the colon by insertion into the colon of a lighted tube with a miniature camera at the end. Oncologists also credit higher survival rates among colon cancer patients to improved surgical techniques and better use of chemotherapy and radiation.

Since the early 1970's, colon and rectal cancer death rates have dropped about 20 percent among white Americans, and the NCI expects a more dramatic decline as screening becomes more widespread. At the same time, rates for colon and rectal cancer have risen among African Americans. Experts blame this disparity on reduced access to medical care among blacks and on a lack of preventive health services in general.

Deaths from less common cancers also have fallen. Fewer children are dying of leukemia and bone cancer. Cancer deaths in children have been cut by more than half since 1950, to an estimated 1,600 in 1995 says the ACS, thanks to improved diagnosis and treatment.

Testicular cancer, the most common cancer of young men aged 20 to 35, also ranked as the leading cancer killer for that age group before the war on cancer began. Thanks to a drug called cisplatinum, developed in clinical trials during the 1970's, about 92 percent of the 7,100 new cases diagnosed each year are now cured.

Hodgkin's disease, a cancer of white blood cells, killed more than three-quarters of its victims before the 1970's. Today, with new combinations of chemotherapy drugs, more than three-quarters of the 7,800 cases diagnosed annually are cured.

Stomach cancer, a leading cancer killer worldwide, kills comparatively few Americans today—14,700 deaths in 1995, according to the ACS. Scientists generally agree that better refrigeration and fewer foods cured by smoking, salting, or pickling account for the drop in its prevalence.

Treatment advances have also improved the quality of life for cancer patients. New surgical techniques for treating osteosarcoma, a bone cancer, along with improved use of chemotherapy and radiation, have resulted in more patients leaving the hospital with limbs intact. Patients treated for cancer of the larynx, or voicebox, almost always lost their voice prior to the war on cancer. Today, by combining surgery with radiation and chemotherapy, doctors are saving more voices.

These triumphs in treatment have been tempered by failures, however. The news remains bleak for most patients who have cancers that have *metastasized* (spread) into surrounding tissue or to distant sites. And cancers of the liver, lung, ovary, and pancreas are still very difficult to treat.

Progress in chemotherapy has come mainly from combining existing drugs in new ways, according to oncologist Nicholas Vogelzang of the University of Chicago Medical Center. In many cases, however, drugs that initially work in combating a cancer ultimately lose their effectiveness as the cancer develops resistance to the drug. According to one theory, cancer cells that do not die from an initial dose of drugs may actually develop ways to pump the drug out of the cell before it can take effect. If the cancer comes back, this theory says, it's made up of drug-resistant cells.

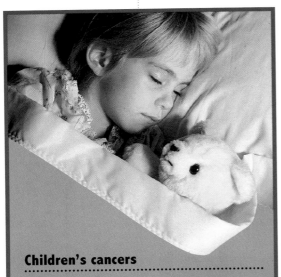

Children's cancers

Although cancer is rare in children, it is the chief cause of death by disease among children aged 1 through 14, according to the American Cancer Society (ACS). The ACS also says that:

- About 8,000 new cases of cancer are diagnosed in children each year.

- Leukemia, a cancer of the blood, accounts for about one-third of those cancers, or 2,600 cases.

- Other common cancer sites in children include the bone, lymph nodes, brain, nervous system, and kidneys.

- Mortality rates for all children's cancers have declined 60 percent since 1950.

- About 1,600 children die of cancer each year, one-third of them from leukemia.

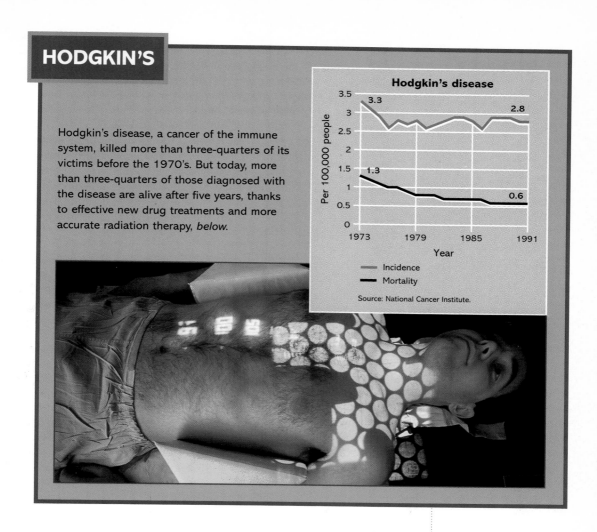

HODGKIN'S

Hodgkin's disease, a cancer of the immune system, killed more than three-quarters of its victims before the 1970's. But today, more than three-quarters of those diagnosed with the disease are alive after five years, thanks to effective new drug treatments and more accurate radiation therapy, *below.*

Hodgkin's disease

Per 100,000 people

3.5
3.3
3
2.8
2.5
2
1.5
1.3
1
0.5
0.6
0

1973   1979   1985   1991

Year

— Incidence
— Mortality

Source: National Cancer Institute.

Many experts predict that the greatest turnaround in cancer will come in prevention, rather than in new treatments. Prevention efforts may involve behavioral changes, including elimination of smoking, avoidance of prolonged exposure to the sun, and improved diet. A number of studies that compared cancer rates in different countries suggest that a diet lower in fat and higher in fruits, vegetables, and fiber might reduce the risk of the four most common cancers in the United States: lung, prostate, breast, and colon. Antismoking campaigns have already begun to bring down lung cancer incidence.

"We need to begin an expanded prevention research effort parallel to the research in cancer treatment begun years ago," says former NCI epidemiologist John Bailar, an outspoken critic of the government's war on cancer. Bailar sees advances coming from research in chemoprevention, which entails giving a drug to prevent cancer. One example is the drug tamoxifen, which is given to some breast cancer patients after surgery to help prevent a recurrence of the disease. Tamoxifen works by blocking the action of the female hormone estrogen, which might promote the growth of any cancer cells remaining in the body. A nationwide trial was underway in 1995 to determine whether the drug can also prevent breast cancer from developing in the first place in healthy women who are at high risk for the disease.

Other researchers are looking to vaccines, not to prevent cancer so much as to bolster the body's natural immune defenses against cancer cells already present. Since the mid-1980's, cancer researcher Malcolm S. Mitchell, now at the University of California at San Diego, has tested vaccines on patients with advanced melanoma. Although only 20 percent of his patients have responded to the therapy, these patients almost certainly would have died without the treatment. Mitchell notes that cancer vaccines are more effective when given in combination with alpha-interferon, a disease-fighting protein produced by the body, which he believes helps the immune system recognize a tumor. Mitchell anticipates testing a vaccine for advanced breast cancer and predicts that advanced cancers of the colon, stomach, and ovary will all be candidates for cancer vaccines.

Steven A. Rosenberg, chief of surgery at the NCI, also believes that progress against cancer will come from strengthening the body's natural immune system responses. In 1986, Rosenberg first tested interleukin-2, a protein produced by the body that helps activate various immune system cells. It is now being tested in several centers around the country against such cancers as kidney, skin, breast, and prostate. Despite potentially severe side effects, the drug has shown some promise in treating advanced cancers in patients in whom all other therapies have failed.

Some of the most astounding advances in the war on cancer have come in identifying cancer-causing genes. Scientists are studying these genes as targets for drugs to treat and prevent cancer, and for screening tests to diagnose people who have a genetic susceptibility for cancer. Although promising, such treatments are decades away.

In 1975, cancer researchers and Nobel Prize winners Michael Bishop and Harold E. Varmus and their colleagues at the University of California at San Francisco introduced the idea that we all carry potential cancer-causing genes called oncogenes. In its normal state, an oncogene controls cell development or cell division, but *mutations* (changes) in the gene—as a result of a virus, chemical, or other factor—can turn off the controls, permitting the cell to multiply wildly and resulting in cancer. By mid-1995, researchers had discovered some 70 of these rogue genes. Researchers have found another dozen or so tumor-suppressor genes that are responsible for suppressing such unchecked cell growth. Cancer can also result if tumor-suppressor genes are omitted or inactivated in the process of cell division.

Many of these cancer-causing genes are targets for drugs. One specific target under scrutiny by scientists is a tumor suppressor named p53. Scientists suspect that a damaged p53 gene may be responsible for more than half of all tumors, including many colorectal, lung, and breast tumors. When functioning normally, p53 works somewhat like a spell-checker, correcting flaws in genetic material that might be the first step on the way to cancer. When p53 malfunctions, these flaws go uncorrected and tumor growth may proceed unchecked. Researchers hope to learn more about the role played by the p53 gene and to devise ways of replacing the defective gene or restoring its ability to function.

Oncogenes and tumor-suppressor genes are not the only targets of gene therapy. Cancer researchers hope to use gene therapy to trick the body's immune system into launching an attack against cancerous cells. Such treatments have had limited successes to date, but most clinical trials are still in the early stages. One recently completed trial that began in March 1993 at the NIH tested the idea of inserting "suicide genes" inside a brain tumor. A herpesvirus gene was inserted into the tumor, making tumor cells with the virus DNA sensitive to the antiviral drug ganciclovir. When ganciclovir was administered, the drug attacked the cells, and tumors shrank in 6 of the first 15 patients who received the therapy.

"The new tools we're getting from molecular biology are promising, but there aren't any magic bullets," says Michael Blaese, chief of the gene therapy branch at the National Center for Human Genome Research. "Drugs that look promising in the test tube and in animal tests take years of development before they can be used in people."

Many experts contend that it is still too early to judge the war's success or failure. "Part of the problem is lack of money for research, and the fact that the government is being streamlined," says Robert Young of the Fox Chase Center. Indeed, only 15 percent of research proposals are funded, down from 25 percent just a few years ago. Young thinks that the most important step in accelerating the pace of cancer progress is for the NCI to fund more grant proposals, which would quickly tap into the pool of ideas in the research community.

The NCI's Peter Greenwald views the war on cancer as ongoing. "In the next several decades, we will see the effects from years of both clinical and basic research," he says, and adds, "I see the war as a steady forward march.   •••

For further reading:

Beardsley, Tim, "A War Not Won." *Scientific American,* January 1994, pp. 130-138.

McAllister, Robert M. and others. *Cancer.* Basic Books, 1993.

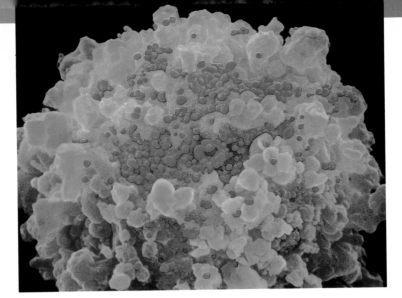

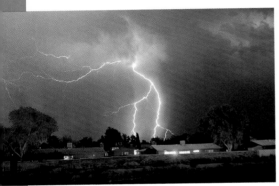

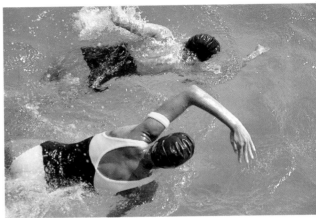

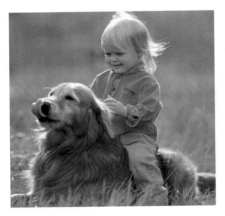

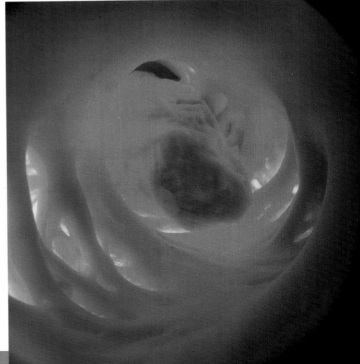

HEALTH UPDATES AND RESOURCES

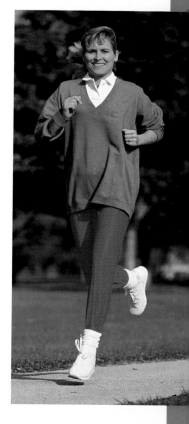

Aging

Two recent studies suggest ways to prevent falls, a frequent cause of serious injury in older people. One study, published in May 1995, focused on exercise. Researchers at Washington University in St. Louis, Missouri, analyzed data from exercise programs involving 2,328 people, most over age 70, at seven health centers and nursing homes. The programs lasted from 10 to 36 weeks and included various combinations of endurance, strength, flexibility, and balance training.

Compared with similar groups of older people who did not exercise, participants were about 10 percent less likely to suffer falls during the next two to four years. Balance training—including exercises based on tai chi, a Chinese martial art—proved especially beneficial, reducing falls by as much as 25 percent.

Another study, published in September 1994, found that a program of preventive strategies can reduce falls among older people who are at high risk for these accidents. Researchers from Yale University in New Haven, Connecticut, monitored 301 adults aged 70 or older, each of whom had at least one risk factor for falling—such as low blood pressure when standing up, use of sedatives, or trouble walking. Half the participants received one or more interventions designed to prevent falls, including instruction in safer ways to walk

or climb stairs, balance training, or changes in medication dosages. The other people received occasional home visits by health care workers but no measures specifically meant to lessen falls.

In the following year, 35 percent of the people in the intervention group suffered falls, compared with 47 percent of the other group. As a bonus, members of the intervention group also turned out to have fewer risk factors for falling at the end of the study than they had at the start.

Older drivers. Age or medical disease may not be valid reasons to prevent older people from driving, according to a May 1995 study.

Researchers from the University of California at Los Angeles tested the driving skills and cognitive abilities of 25 older drivers who had no chronic physical diseases but who did suffer mild mental impairment from either early Alzheimer's disease or *vascular dementia* (mental deterioration as a result of hardening of the arteries or stroke). They also tested 15 older drivers who had diabetes but no mental impairment, as well as 24 physically and mentally healthy older drivers (over age 60) and 16 healthy younger drivers (aged 20 to 35).

While the older drivers who had no mental impairment—regardless of their physical health—scored as well

The wrong medicine
Nearly one-fourth of all Americans over 65 have been given prescriptions for inappropriate drugs, says a 1994 study from Harvard Medical School in Boston. Some drugs should not be given to older patients because they can cause such side effects as confusion, sleepiness, heart problems, or respiratory failure. In most cases, safer alternatives exist, the researchers say.

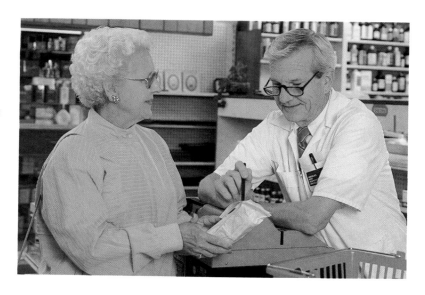

as the young people on the tests, drivers with Alzheimer's or vascular dementia did markedly worse and committed more serious errors, such as turning onto streets marked "Do Not Enter." The researchers suggested that specific testing procedures for evaluating older drivers would be a fairer way to identify unsafe drivers than simply revoking licenses based on age or medical diagnoses.

Exercise for easier sleep. Daily exercise can alleviate nighttime confusion and insomnia in people in the early and intermediate stages of Alzheimer's disease, say researchers at Case Western Reserve University and two hospitals in Cleveland.

In a study published in February 1995, 11 Alzheimer's patients aged 68 to 90 engaged in a four-week program of light exercise, including walking and flexibility movements. The researchers then compared these patients' sleep patterns with those of 11 Alzheimer's patients who did not exercise. The exercisers slept more soundly and exhibited less restless behavior than the nonexercisers.

Better vision, better life? Researchers at Harvard Medical School and Harvard School of Public Health and associated Boston hospitals reported in November 1994 that improved vision after cataract removal may slow a later decline in quality of life. Cataract, a clouding of the lens of the eye, occurs in many people over 65.

The researchers studied a group of patients before and after cataract extraction. One year after surgery, 341 of 420 patients showed improvement in vision-related activity. Compared with the patients who did not demonstrate this improvement, these people also showed less severe declines in most measurements of general health status, including mental health, physical and social function, vitality, and pain.

Protecting bones with estrogen. Women using estrogen replacement therapy to prevent hip and wrist fractures should start the therapy early in menopause and continue indefinitely, according to a study published in January 1995. A team led by research-

Reducing the risk of dangerous falls

Failing eyesight and strength along with slower reflexes put older people at risk of falling. A four-year study by researchers at Yale University in New Haven, Connecticut, found that a combination of techniques can reduce the risk of falling by nearly a third. The recommendations:

- Reevaluate with a physician the need for more than four prescription drugs at any one time. Taking too many drugs can have unintended side effects, which may increase the risk of a fall.

- Make sure that hearing aid and eyeglass prescriptions are up to date and correct.

- Remove household hazards, such as loose rugs, and add safety devices, such as grab bars or rails on stairs and bathtubs.

- Learn safe techniques for getting in and out of a bed or a bathtub.

- Receive strength and balance training. Some simple exercises, such as leg lifts or standing on tiptoe while leaning against a kitchen counter, can make older people steadier on their feet.

Sources: *New England Journal of Medicine,* Sept. 29, 1994; *Medical Tribune,* Oct. 20, 1994.

ers at the University of Pittsburgh in Pennsylvania studied 9,704 women 65 years and older.

The researchers found that women currently on estrogen therapy had a lower risk for nonspinal fractures than those who had never used estrogen. The benefit to wrists and hips was greatest among current users who had started estrogen within five years of menopause and had taken it longer than 10 years. The therapy was particularly effective in reducing hip fracture among women over age 75. Women who had stopped the therapy, however, showed no substantial benefit, no matter when they first started estrogen or how long they had taken it.   • Rein Tideiksaar

In WORLD BOOK, see AGING.

As expected, fewer new cases of AIDS were reported to the United States Centers for Disease Control and Prevention (CDC) in 1994 than in 1993. The CDC had expanded the definition of AIDS in 1993, which meant that more people infected with the AIDS-causing HIV (human immunodeficiency virus) were classified as having progressed to the disease. The CDC said the new definition was the primary reason behind the jump from 47,572 new cases in 1992 to 106,618 new cases in 1993.

Although the number of new AIDS cases dropped to 80,691 in 1994, the CDC reported that, overall, AIDS increased in the United States at about the same rate as it had in 1993. The new cases in 1994 represented 18 percent of the total number of cases (441,528) reported since 1981, when the CDC began tracking the disease.

Women at high HIV risk. In 1994, almost 18 percent of new AIDS cases occurred among women (14,081 cases), up from 7 percent (534 cases) 10 years earlier, the CDC reported in February 1995. Although the CDC said that nearly 60 percent of the new cases in 1994 could be attributed to the expanded AIDS definition, the 1994 rate of infection represented a threefold jump from 1985, and the rate was rising more rapidly among women than among men. In 1994, more than 40 percent of new HIV infections among women resulted from contaminated needles used to inject illegal drugs. Another 38 percent had had sexual intercourse with a partner who was at risk for HIV infection or AIDS, who was known to be HIV-positive, or who had AIDS.

HIV and donor sperm. Women who underwent artificial insemination prior to 1986 have an increased risk of HIV infection, according to a March 1995 report by researchers at the Los Angeles County Department of Health Services. Artificial insemination is a reproductive technique typically used to overcome infertility. In the technique, *semen* (sperm-containing fluid) from a donor or from a woman's partner is placed in the woman's uterus. Fertility clinics began screening donor semen for HIV in 1986.

The California researchers conducted two types of studies at five fertility clinics that kept detailed records of sperm donors and recipients. In one study method, the researchers first identified HIV-infected women who had reported having the insemination procedure. They then identified infected donors and other women who had received sperm from those donors. In the second method, the researchers identified an HIV-infected

HIV battleground
From the first day of infection, HIV, the AIDS-causing virus (red), multiplies in the body's immune cells (green), destroying them in the process, according to two studies reported in January 1995. Researchers had previously thought that, after a brief infectious period, HIV remained relatively dormant until something triggered its proliferation months or years later.

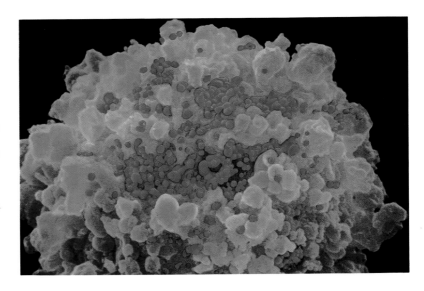

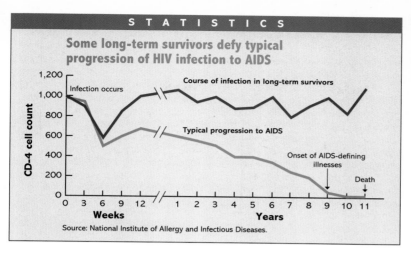

STATISTICS

Some long-term survivors defy typical progression of HIV infection to AIDS

Course of infection in long-term survivors

Infection occurs

Typical progression to AIDS

Onset of AIDS-defining illnesses

Death

CD-4 cell count

1,200
1,000
800
600
400
200
0

0   3   6   9   12   1   2   3   4   5   6   7   8   9   10 11

Weeks   **Years**

Source: National Institute of Allergy and Infectious Diseases.

An estimated 5 to 10 percent of HIV-infected people defy the typical progression to AIDS and remain healthy. According to studies reported in January 1995, long-term survivors have low blood levels of HIV, and their infection-fighting CD-4 cells mount a strong response to the virus as it replicates. The researchers speculate that some combination of a weakened HIV strain and a strong immune response may account for long-term survival.

donor, and they then located the recipients of his sperm. In all, the researchers identified 230 women who had been inseminated with semen from five HIV-infected donors. Of these women, 199 consented to HIV-testing, and 7 tested positive for HIV.

Even though reports of HIV infections through donor insemination prior to 1986 have been uncommon, researchers believe that some women may unknowingly be HIV-positive and could be candidates for therapy. For that reason, they said there was an "urgent need" to consider testing donors and recipients involved in artificial insemination prior to 1986.

HIV-infected baby recovers. In March 1995, researchers at the University of California at Los Angeles announced that a boy infected at birth with HIV had no trace of the virus by the time he was 1 year old, even though he had received no treatment. Blood tests showed that he was still free of HIV at age 5.

The scientists used sophisticated techniques to confirm that the child was HIV-positive 19 days after birth and 51 days later. The tests found no trace of HIV at 12 months of age and thereafter. The California researchers said the boy's case suggests that the immune system may be able to fight off the AIDS virus naturally. Such evidence would be significant for vaccine research.

The researchers noted that this was the first documented case of re-

covery from HIV infection. Earlier, unconfirmed reports have described cases in which the virus was cleared from the body. But blood samples may have been contaminated in the laboratory, or other errors may have affected those test results.

HIV and health care workers. The risk to patients of becoming infected with HIV from HIV-infected health care workers is very small, according to a CDC study reported in May 1995. The CDC researchers evaluated HIV test results for 22,171 patients who had been treated by 51 HIV-infected health care workers. No evidence was found of worker-to-patient transmission of HIV. None of the patients of 37 out of the 51 health care workers tested positive for the AIDS virus. Although 113 patients of the other 14 health care workers were HIV-positive, laboratory follow-up tests and other evidence indicated that the health care workers were not the source of infection.

New therapy for HIV patients. Early results of a study reported in March 1995 show that a new treatment bolsters the weakened immune systems of patients infected with HIV who have not yet progressed to full-blown AIDS. The therapy, developed at the National Institute of Allergy and Infectious Diseases, involves a protein called interleukin-2 (IL-2), which the body makes to boost its response to infection.

The researchers reported that once every two months the patients in the study were attached to an infusion pump that provided a continuous dose of IL-2 for five days. Six of the 10 patients in the study responded to the treatment with a 50 percent or greater rise in T-cells, disease-battling white blood cells. After as much as $3\frac{1}{2}$ years of therapy, there were no signs that the effectiveness of the treatment was declining. Side effects of treatment included reductions in blood pressure as well as flulike symptoms that persisted in some patients for about two weeks after the IL-2 infusion.

It was not clear whether the treatment could help patients resist AIDS-related infections or whether the therapy would lengthen life span. The IL-2 treatments had no effect on patients who already had AIDS when the study began.

AZT research. AZT (also known as zidovudine), the first drug approved to fight HIV directly, loses its effectiveness after about two years of treatment. This was the conclusion of a multicenter study reported in August 1994 by the AIDS Clinical Trials Group. AZT is used to slow the progression to AIDS in patients infected with HIV.

The study involved 1,565 patients who were infected with HIV but had no symptoms of AIDS. They were divided into two groups—one receiving AZT and the other a *placebo* (an inactive substance). The patients taking 500 milligrams of AZT each day for as long as $4\frac{1}{2}$ years experienced a significant slowing of the progression toward AIDS for two years. Thereafter, however, they faced the same risks of progression to AIDS as the placebo group.

Another study found that when patients received AZT in combination with an experimental new drug called 3TC (or lamivudine), their immune system showed greater improvement than it had when either drug was administered alone. Why this occurred remained unclear, the researchers said when they reported their findings at the American Society for Microbiology meeting held in Washington, D.C., in February 1995.

New HIV test. University of Pittsburgh scientists reported in April 1995 that they had developed a test that can help determine how rapidly a person infected with HIV will develop AIDS. The new test measures the amount of genetic material from the AIDS virus present in the blood.

The 62 HIV-positive men who participated in a study of the test all knew approximately when they had been infected. Those with persistently elevated blood levels of HIV genetic material in the two years following infection had a high risk of developing AIDS or a significant immune system impairment within a few years. The men with consistently low levels of the genetic material had only a small chance of becoming ill. The new test may be a more accurate predictor of the progression of the disease than any other existing test.

Vaccine research. Research continued in 1995 on the development of an AIDS vaccine, but the availability of such a vaccine was still expected to be years away. In October 1994, an advisory panel to the World Health Organization, an agency of the United Nations, approved full-scale clinical trials of two experimental vaccines. Both vaccines had already undergone testing for safety and immune system response. The final phase was designed to evaluate the vaccines' ability to prevent HIV infection and was not expected to begin until 1996.

Investigators at St. Louis University School of Medicine and other centers reported in August 1994 that a genetically engineered vaccine stimulated the production of antibodies capable of attacking some strains of HIV. They tested the vaccine on 57 volunteers aged 18 to 60 who were not infected with HIV. The volunteers received either the active vaccine in varying doses or a placebo. In 33 of the 48 volunteers who received the vaccine, two doses triggered production of antibodies capable of neutralizing HIV-infected cells. Three doses triggered such a response in 46 volunteers. None of the volunteers had any serious adverse reaction to the vaccine.   • Richard Trubo

See also SEXUALLY TRANSMITTED DISEASES. In WORLD BOOK, see AIDS.

Drug use among students in the United States rose in 1994, according to a major annual survey by the University of Michigan in Ann Arbor. The most pronounced rise was in marijuana use. One in three high school seniors reported smoking marijuana at least once during 1994, a 4 percent increase over 1993, and one in four sophomores reported smoking it, a 6 percent increase over 1993. Among 8th-graders, 13 percent said they had smoked marijuana during the year, up from 9.2 percent. Still, overall drug use was well below the peak years of the late 1970's and early 1980's, researchers said.

The most widespread increases in drug use occurred among 8th-graders. They reported heavier use of hallucinogens, cocaine, crack, heroin, and steroids. Tenth-graders used more hallucinogens, cocaine, and barbiturates, and 12th-graders used more hallucinogens.

Past surveys have shown that perceptions about drugs affect drug use. For example, an increased perception that a drug is harmful tends to reduce its use. Disapproval of drug use by peers has a similar effect. Since 1992, there has been a gradual but significant decline in the perceived risks of drug use, particularly among 8th- and 10th-graders. The Michigan researchers said that the 1994 survey reflects these changing attitudes.

Binge drinking on campus. Binge drinking among college students is especially prevalent among residents of fraternity and sorority houses and on residential campuses in the Northeast and North Central regions of the nation, according to researchers at the Harvard School of Public Health in Boston. They reported the findings of their study in December 1994.

The study defined binge drinking as consuming at least five drinks in a row for men and at least four in a row for women. Students at traditionally black colleges and women's colleges had the lowest rates of binge drinking. Overall, older students were less likely to binge than younger students.

The researchers mailed questionnaires to over 25,000 students on 140 campuses nationwide, and 17,592 were returned. The goal was to learn the extent of binge drinking and the resulting health and behavioral consequences. Establishing a trend was not a goal, as there has been no previous large-scale study of the problem.

Nearly 45 percent of all the respondents reported having gone on at least one drinking binge, and 20 percent said they were frequent binge drinkers. The more frequent the binge drinking, the more likely the students were to engage in risky behavior, including having unplanned and unprotected sex, getting into trouble with campus police, damaging property,

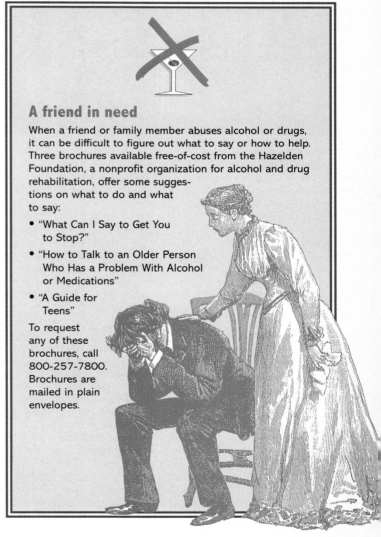

A friend in need

When a friend or family member abuses alcohol or drugs, it can be difficult to figure out what to say or how to help. Three brochures available free-of-cost from the Hazelden Foundation, a nonprofit organization for alcohol and drug rehabilitation, offer some suggestions on what to do and what to say:

- "What Can I Say to Get You to Stop?"
- "How to Talk to an Older Person Who Has a Problem With Alcohol or Medications"
- "A Guide for Teens"

To request any of these brochures, call 800-257-7800. Brochures are mailed in plain envelopes.

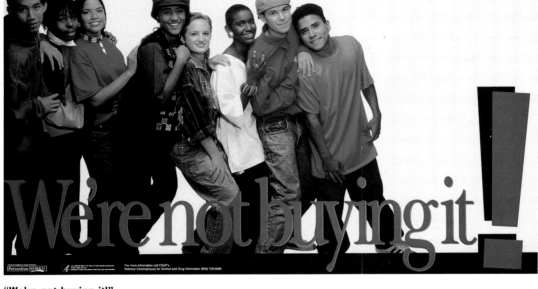

ALCOHOL

We're not buying it!

"We're not buying it!"
Educational material from the Center for Substance Abuse Prevention, including the poster above, stresses the importance of peer influence in preventing teen-age drinking. The center, a federal information clearinghouse, is offering the materials to parents and groups concerned with underage drinking. For information, telephone the center at 800-729-6686 or 800-487-4889.

injuring themselves, or driving while drinking. Still, less than 1 percent of the respondents said they had a drinking problem.

Ritalin and cocaine. In 1995, scientists from the Department of Psychiatry at the State University of New York in Stony Brook began investigating a drug used in the treatment of attention deficit disorder (ADD), a form of hyperactivity often found in substance-abusing families. The concern among scientists has been that ritalin, the drug most commonly prescribed in the United States for the treatment of ADD, appears to resemble cocaine in its action in the brain.

The New York researchers investigated the actions of ritalin in human brains and of cocaine in baboon brains. The researchers found that both drugs enter the brain with similar rapidity and that both act on dopamine, a *neurotransmitter* (chemical messenger) in the brain. Previous research has shown that dopamine is involved in the "high" that results

from narcotics. The drugs appeared to differ, however, in the rate at which they cleared the brain and in the duration of the high. Although ritalin was cleared from the brain more slowly than cocaine, it produced a shorter high. The scientists used this finding to support the continued use of ritalin. They concluded that because ritalin stays in the brain longer than cocaine, youths would be less likely to take repeated doses of it.

Spending saves money. For each $1 spent on treatments for drug and alcohol abuse in California, $7 was saved, mainly through a reduction in crimes to obtain money for drugs. Smaller savings came from reduced health care costs, especially to treat drug-related emergencies. These findings were reported in October 1994 by the University of Chicago's National Opinion Research Center, which conducted an evaluation of the California Department of Drug and Alcohol Programs.

The study covered 83 treatment

programs run by the California agency. These ranged from group homes, the most expensive to operate, to short-term outpatient services, the least expensive. The researchers interviewed 1,857 randomly selected drug abusers who were addicted to alcohol, cocaine, or heroin at the time they entered treatment. When treatment ended after 15 to 24 months, those who had been interviewed initially were interviewed again.

In comparing the data, the scientists found that the overall crime rate among study participants had fallen by 72 percent. The researchers cited two reasons for the drop. First, the people no longer needed money to buy drugs, and second, they had the support of new friends and counselors who encouraged more ethical behavior. The group's emergency room admissions also fell by a third.

The California agency said the findings were important because California jails were filling with drug users at a cost to taxpayers of $20,000 per year for each person jailed. However, some critics said that not all the savings could be attributed to the treatment programs. They said many people give up drugs or alcohol on their own, especially as they mature. In addition, critics pointed out, most people entering treatment programs are highly motivated to give up their addiction. Therefore, the success rate of the study could not be assumed to apply to all drug abusers.

Children, drugs, and values. Several studies in 1994 and 1995 confirmed that families have an important influence on whether children use drugs. A two-year study of seventh-graders was reported in September 1994 by scientists at Louisiana State University Medical Center in New Orleans. The study found that a positive parent-child relationship was associated with low alcohol and drug use when the children entered their teens.

Positive relationships meant parents spent time with their children and communicated with them on a give-and-take basis, both talking and listening. When the parents listened to their children with empathy, the adolescents appeared less likely to be disruptive or to choose friends who might exert an undesirable influence on them.

The researchers concluded that parents should be advised to focus on developing a good relationship with their children rather than on screening friends. Instead of criticizing a child's lifestyle, the parents should discuss the child's likes and dislikes. This kind of interaction, the researchers said, helps the child develop critical thinking skills, thus reducing the influence of peers.

Another study, reported in April 1995, looked at the influence of parental beliefs. Researchers from the University of Nevada, Las Vegas, gave questionnaires to children in treatment for drug problems and to their parents. Children without drug problems and their parents also filled out questionnaires. The questions concerned attitudes about work, religious faith, education, and the family.

The values of both groups of parents differed very little. But the children in drug treatment held far different beliefs from the parents and from the children not in treatment. These findings suggest that parents of at-risk youths were less able to transmit their attitudes and beliefs to their children. The researchers concluded that there is a need for parent training in communication skills as part of drug prevention programs.

Pathways to drug abuse. A study of adoptees reported in January 1995 confirmed a hypothesis that there are two independent biological pathways to drug abuse. One pathway leads directly from an alcohol-abusing biological parent. The second, less direct pathway, involves a biological parent with an antisocial personality disorder. This disorder is characterized by aggressive behavior and such antisocial acts as lying and stealing.

The study by psychiatrist Remi Cadoret and colleagues at the University of Iowa in Iowa City focused on 95 men who had been given up for adoption to any of four adoption agencies in Iowa within a few days of birth. The adoptees were between 18 and 45 years of age at the time of the study. They had at least one biological parent known through hospital or prison records to abuse drugs or alcohol or to have an antisocial personality disorder. They were matched for age and adoption agency with 102 men who did not have a biological parent with such problems.

Using standardized psychiatric questionnaires, researchers conducted separate interviews with the adoptive parents and the adoptees. The questions they asked concerned the adopted child's development, any diagnosis or treatment for drug abuse, as well as any serious "disturbance" in the family, such as divorce, separation, or mental illness.

Cadoret and colleagues analyzed the hospital and prison records to diagnose the problems of the biological parents. They also analyzed the questionnaires of the adoptive parents and adoptees. The information was coded so that the scientists did not know into which group a study subject fell.

Statistical analysis of the data indicated that having an alcoholic biological parent increased the risk of substance abuse in offspring. Having a biological parent with an antisocial personality disorder increased the likelihood first of aggressive behavior in an adoptee and eventually of drug dependence. "Disturbed" adoptive parents also contributed to drug dependence.   • Gayle Hamilton

In WORLD BOOK, see ALCOHOLISM; DRUG ABUSE.

Allergies and Asthma

Most infants and young children who experience bouts of wheezing are suffering from temporary conditions that will not lead to asthma later in life, pediatrician Fernando D. Martinez and his colleagues at the University of Arizona College of Medicine in Tucson reported in January 1995. The investigators further concluded, however, that in a substantial minority of cases, early wheezing may lead to asthma, either because there is a genetic predisposition or because the lungs have been damaged by illness.

Physicians have long known that asthma runs in families and that genetic factors seem to play a role.

They have also observed that some infants and children who suffer attacks of wheezing following colds or other respiratory tract infections develop asthma when they get older. But it was not known to what extent these factors might be interrelated or how asthma might sometimes develop in response to environmental influences, such as exposure to cigarette smoke.

Martinez and his associates studied more than 800 children from birth to 6 years of age and noted how many suffered attacks of wheezing during that time. They also noted factors that could have contributed to

Car fumes blamed for many asthma attacks
Urban smog, caused largely by automobile exhaust fumes, is implicated in the rising incidence of asthma attacks in many big cities, physicians meeting in London said in September 1994. The doctors said that someone suffering from mild asthma caused by an allergy is particularly at risk in a smoggy environment. Such individuals may develop more severe asthma symptoms.

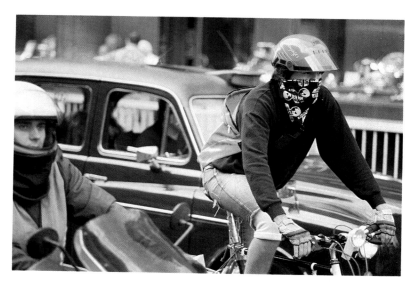

the children's wheezing, including respiratory illnesses, allergies, and mothers who smoked.

At the age of 6, the children were assigned to four categories, according to their medical history: those who had never suffered wheezing attacks (51 percent), those who had wheezing episodes only briefly in very early childhood (20 percent), those who had no problem in infancy but began wheezing later (15 percent), and those who had persistent wheezing that began in infancy and continued up to age 6 (14 percent).

The researchers identified a number of risk factors associated with wheezing attacks. In the group with persistent wheezing during their first six years of life, risk factors included having a mother who smoked and suffering from nasal inflammations apart from ones caused by colds. Wheezing of late onset was found to be associated with having a mother with asthma and suffering from nasal inflammations in the first year of life. Temporary early wheezing was associated only with maternal smoking.

In addition, allergies were more prevalent in the two groups of children with wheezing at age 6 than in the group that had never wheezed.

The investigators concluded that although many children may experience wheezing brought on by cigarette smoke or respiratory illnesses, most of these children (60 percent) will stop wheezing by the age of 6. The researchers speculated that early wheezing may often be caused by the relatively small airways in younger children's lungs. After a few years, as airways enlarge, wheezing ceases.

But in some cases, children who wheeze later develop asthma. Why?

The investigators said further research would be needed to determine how asthma develops. They added, however, that their findings showed that asthma is not a simple disease but rather can be caused in several ways. For example, the finding that many children with wheezing had allergies suggested that allergic sensitivities that crop up during the first year of life may contribute to the later development of asthma. They also concluded that chronic respiratory illnesses in the first years of life

The truth about asthma

Asthma has become one of the most common chronic conditions, affecting at least 10 million Americans—including 3 million children. Yet myths about asthma persist. Here are some of the more damaging ones:

* *Myth: Asthma is a psychological condition.* Asthma has nothing to do with a troubled childhood, improper mothering, or emotional problems. As with many physical illnesses, however, asthma can become worse with stress.

* *Myth: Children grow out of asthma.* Asthma often goes into remission when children reach their teens, but symptoms may reappear at any age.

* *Myth: Asthma doesn't require medical treatment.* Most people with asthma require medical intervention to prevent or treat attacks.

* *Myth: Moving to Arizona will help.* Some asthmatics benefit from a change of climate, but others are exposed to new allergens that trigger their asthma.

* *Myth: Asthma doesn't kill anyone anymore.* About 5,000 Americans die of asthma each year. Most of those deaths could be avoided with proper medical care.

For answers about asthma, call Allergy and Asthma Network/Mothers of Asthmatics, Inc., toll-free at 1-800-878-4403.

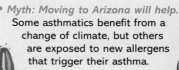

may sometimes damage the lungs and set the stage for asthma.

Controlling dust mites. Dust mites, microscopic organisms that are common in most homes, are a major cause of asthmatic attacks. They can also cause eczema, a skin disorder that produces itching and inflammation. These problems are caused by *allergens* (irritating proteins) in the mites' bodies or in their feces. Several studies reported in late 1994 and early 1995 discussed ways that people with asthma or a susceptibility to eczema can protect themselves from mites.

Mites often infest bedding and mattresses. Laundering is an effective way of getting rid of mites in bed linens. Previously, only washing with hot water was recommended, but allergy experts in Kirchelm-Bolanden, Germany, noted that warm water (about 85 °F [30 °C]) works just as well if a mite-control agent containing the chemical benzyl benzoate is added to the water. As for mattresses, investigators at the Royal Hospital for Sick Children in Bristol, England, reported that special water-proof covers work well in keeping mattresses almost free of mites.

Dust mite allergens collect in house dust and settle with it on flat surfaces, furniture, and carpeting. Frequent and thorough house cleaning can help cut down on the allergens.

Tannic acid, a chemical found in tea, can *denature* (alter) the proteins in mite allergens so they no longer cause allergic responses, according to researchers at the University of Virginia Health Science Center in Charlottesville. They sprayed carpets with commercial solutions containing 1 percent and 3 percent concentrations of tannic acid and found that both were effective at denaturing mite allergen proteins.

The University of Virginia investigators also reported that a common household insecticide, Raid Flea Killer, eliminated dust mites in carpets. They concluded that many such products would work equally well, though none penetrate well into pads underneath carpets, which also harbor mites. Therefore, they said, the best solution may be to remove carpeting from the home.

Asthma and chronic heartburn. Gastroesophageal reflux (GER), better known as heartburn, is a common ailment that can worsen a patient's asthma. Moreover, recent research shows that heartburn may actually cause many asthma attacks. In April 1995, physician William G. Simpson of the University of Kentucky College of Medicine in Lexington reviewed findings about chronic GER and how it can be treated.

Simpson reported that physicians have found that treating asthma patients with drugs called histamine receptor blockers is effective in preventing episodes of heartburn and alleviating asthma. Although these drugs relieve GER within days, they can take up to 12 weeks to ease asthma symptoms.

Simpson also reviewed the effectiveness of surgery for GER. There are several operations for correcting the condition, and doctors have reported that the surgical procedures have ended or markedly alleviated asthma symptoms in anywhere from 34 to 77 percent of their asthma patients.

Several other measures can also help relieve GER-related asthma, Simpson found. They include elevating the head of one's bed a few inches, eating small amounts of food several times a day, abstaining from food and drink for two to three hours before bedtime, and using antacids.

Cat and dog dander. Protein particles shed from the skin and fur of cats and dogs, known as dander, are a common allergen in homes. Dander floats for long periods in the air and collects in curtains, toys, and upholstery. Washing a pet frequently has been shown to reduce dander, and grooming the animal with an *emollient* (softening agent) may cut it even further.

In March 1995, researchers at Eindhoven University of Technology in Eindhoven, the Netherlands, reported that using a grooming emollient on cats' fur reduced the level of dander shed by the cats. They did not test the emollient on dogs, but it seemed likely to work just as well in reducing canine dander.

Neutralizing apple allergens. Many people have an allergic reaction to apples, experiencing an irritation of the lips and mouth and a tight feeling in the throat. The same people have less of a problem with cooked apples, however, because heat denatures the allergen proteins.

In March 1995, researchers at Drechsteden Hospital in Dordrecht, the Netherlands, demonstrated that heating apples for 1 minute in a microwave oven has the same effect. They found that microwaving denatures the offending proteins without affecting the texture or flavor of the fruit.　　• Dominick A. Minotti

In WORLD BOOK, see ALLERGY; ASTHMA.

Research reported in late 1994 and early 1995 gave strong support to a theory that several forms of arthritis are triggered by infection in people who are born with a defective gene that renders them susceptible to the diseases. Although the cause of most forms of arthritis is unknown, doctors have suspected that common infections, which are harmless to people with a normal gene, play an important role in rheumatoid arthritis (RA), systemic lupus erythematosus (SLE), and ankylosing spondylitis (AS).

Rheumatoid arthritis. Researchers at the University of California at San Diego reported in May 1995 findings about genes in patients with RA. The researchers focused on the gene that determines a person's *leukocyte* (white blood cell) type. The gene produces a protein—called HLA, for human leukocyte antigen—that appears on most of the body's cells.

All proteins consist of a long string of building blocks called amino acids. The investigators noted that more than 90 percent of patients with severe RA have in their HLA protein a specific sequence of five amino acids. They then looked for this sequence elsewhere in nature, and they found it in a protein produced by the bacteri-

Filling holes in knees

Some people with knee injuries may benefit from an experimental treatment described by doctors in Sweden in October 1994. The surgery is meant to repair small holes in knee cartilage, which can lead to osteoarthritis if untreated. The surgeon first takes a sample of healthy cartilage cells from elsewhere in the knee. These cells multiply in a laboratory culture for two to three weeks and are then mixed with liquid to form a suspension. Next, the surgeon removes a small piece of tissue from the leg and sews it over the hole to form a flap. Finally, the surgeon injects the suspension of cultured cells beneath the flap, where—if all goes well—they form new cartilage. Defective cartilage appears on the left; repaired cartilage appears on the right.

Source: *New England Journal of Medicine,* Oct. 6, 1994.

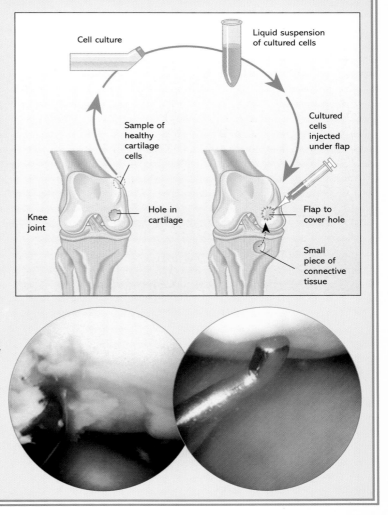

Cell culture

Liquid suspension of cultured cells

Cultured cells injected under flap

Sample of healthy cartilage cells

Knee joint

Hole in cartilage

Flap to cover hole

Small piece of connective tissue

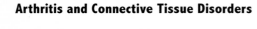

Hot tip for arthritis patients

Arthritis patients can now soothe their aching joints with a cream derived from hot peppers.

Capsicum, a key constituent of these spicy vegetables, along with its components capsicum oleoresin and capsaicin, are classed as counterirritants—substances that provide pain relief by creating a distracting sensation on the skin surface. In addition to producing a passing feeling of warmth, capsaicin seems also to have a chemical effect on the body's mechanism for transmitting pain signals. Drug researchers add that for maximum relief, patients may need to apply the drug every four to six hours for two to six weeks.

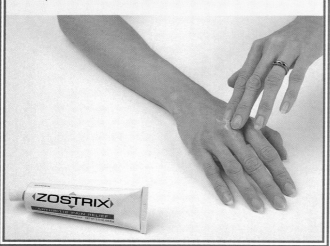

um *Escherichia coli (E. coli),* present in the human digestive tract.

The body's immune system, which identifies and attacks foreign substances, sees the proteins on cells as labels that indicate whether the cells belong in the body. Since the immune cells do not normally react to the body's own proteins, cells of people with RA should not react to the *E. coli* protein, which contains the same amino acid sequence as their own cells. Yet the investigators found that both blood and joint fluid cells from RA patients reacted vigorously to the *E. coli* protein. Moreover, the patients' cells did not react to a modified version of the *E. coli* protein that lacked the sequence of five amino acids.

The investigators theorized that

some people's immune cells become sensitized to the *E. coli* protein when the bacterium enters their bloodstream, perhaps through an intestinal infection. Their immune cells then start reacting to that infection. If their own body cells carry the same key sequence of five amino acids, their immune cells then may mistakenly attack these body cells as well. This triggers the disease known as RA. These findings suggest that in the future a vaccine based on the five amino acids might be developed to prevent or treat RA.

Systemic lupus erythematosus. In April 1995, researchers reported that certain small portions of bacterial DNA (deoxyribonucleic acid, the molecule genes are made of) stimulate immune cell activity in mice that are particularly prone to SLE. The mice, like human SLE patients, have immune cells that are constantly active. The investigators, from the University of Iowa College of Medicine in Iowa City and the U.S. Food and Drug Administration in Bethesda, Maryland, sought to find out what causes this unusual activity. They theorized that the bacterial DNA might also be responsible for the same immune cell response in lupus patients.

The investigators also found that the bacterial DNA had no such effect in normal mice. Normal mice, they discovered, coat the bacterial DNA with chemical substances called methyl groups, but SLE-susceptible mice do not. The investigators suggested that disease-prone mice—and, presumably, people—are born without the ability to coat the bacterial DNA. Because the bacterial DNA is found everywhere, the cells of these mice and people remain constantly active, resulting in SLE.

Ankylosing spondylitis. Bacteria commonly found in the intestine may trigger AS, an arthritic disease that causes the bones of the spine to fuse together, in people with a particular HLA type. This finding was reported in December 1994.

One of the first clear clues that genes may make a person susceptible to a type of arthritis was a 1973 discovery that AS occurs almost exclusively in people with the HLA type known as B27. Still, the reason for the link between AS and the person's HLA type remained unclear.

By a technique called transgenics, which involves transferring genes from one species to another, it is now possible to make one animal take on some characteristics of another. Researchers at the University of Texas Southwestern Medical Center in Dallas and the University of Wisconsin in Madison studied transgenic rats that carried the human gene for B27 HLA. These transgenic rats develop a disease similar to human AS.

By delivering baby transgenic rats surgically and maintaining them in a sterile environment, the scientists were able to keep the baby rats from coming into contact with normal bacteria. These "germ-free" transgenic rats did not develop AS. The investigators then exposed the rats to bacteria that normally inhabit the intestine. The rats developed AS.

The investigators concluded that both the human gene B27 and common intestinal bacteria are necessary for AS to occur. This finding offers hope for a future vaccine to prevent the disease in susceptible people.

A new therapy for RA was described in October 1994 by researchers at the Kennedy Institute of Rheumatology in London. Because RA involves uncontrolled inflammation in the joints, one approach to treating RA is to block, at a very early point, some step crucial to the development of inflammation. Most available treatments are crude, however, and block many steps of inflammation at once. Because inflammation is one way the body fights infection, this leaves patients susceptible to disease.

The London researchers treated RA patients with an antibody to tumor necrosis factor alpha, or TNFa, a molecule essential to the early stages of inflammation. The antibody blocks TNFa's ability to initiate inflammation.

The researchers divided 73 patients into three groups. One group received a high dose of the antibody; a second, a low dose; and the third, no treatment. After four weeks, 80 percent of the people who received the high dose, and almost half of those who took the lower dose, experienced significant improvement in their RA. But only 8 percent of the untreated patients improved. Those whose disease later recurred responded equally well to another round of the new treatment.

Because the TNFa antibody is expensive and inconvenient—it must be given by injection—this treatment is not likely to be widely used. However, these results demonstrate that it is possible to develop specific and safe therapies targeted to early stages of inflammation.   • Michael D. Lockshin
In WORLD BOOK, see ARTHRITIS.

Birth Control

A vaccine to prevent pregnancy won international attention in 1994. Progress continued toward another contraceptive vaccine in 1995.

Contraceptive milestone. The first successful effort to vaccinate women against pregnancy drew praise when a research group led by G. P. Talwar of the National Institute of Immunology in New Delhi, India, announced their results on August 30, 1994. Talwar's team had produced and tested a vaccine that blocks implantation of fertilized eggs in the lining of the uterus.

The vaccine works by causing the body to produce *antibodies* (immune system cells) that destroy a hormone called human chorionic gonadotropin (HCG). This hormone is produced by an embryo, the group of cells that forms and grows after a fertilized egg divides. HCG is essential for implantation of the embryo in the uterus.

The researchers said that the vaccine stimulates antibody production for only a few months, and so women would require booster shots to remain protected. Family planning authorities anticipated opposition to the vaccine from people who define conception as the beginning of pregnancy and feel that the vaccine induces abortion. Talwar, however, denied that the vaccine causes abortions, saying that evidence showed the anti-HCG effect occurs before implantation of

Birth Control

RU-486 clinical trials
Studies on the safety and effectiveness of the abortion drug mifepristone, commonly known by its trade name RU-486, began in the United States in November 1994. A doctor dispenses the drug, which ends pregnancy by making the lining of the uterus unreceptive to the embryo.

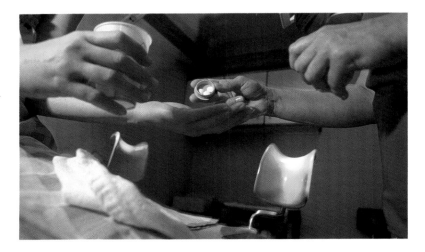

RU-486 clinical trials
Studies on the safety and effectiveness of the abortion drug mifepristone, commonly known by its trade name RU-486, began in the United States in November 1994. A doctor dispenses the drug, which ends pregnancy by making the lining of the uterus unreceptive to the embryo.

the egg, the point that most medical professionals define as the beginning of pregnancy. Research continued, however, on other vaccines, including one that would prevent the union of egg and sperm.

On July 7, 1995, researchers at Duke University Medical Center in Durham, North Carolina, announced the discovery of a protein in sperm that may lead to a new birth control vaccine or drug. The protein, called zona receptor kinase (ZRK), triggers a reaction that dissolves the outer shell of an egg, thereby allowing a sperm to enter. Further research may lead to a vaccine for women that would act against ZRK or a drug for men that would inactivate ZRK.

Birth control sponge gone. The manufacturers of the Today sponge, once a popular birth control device, removed the product from the market in January 1995. Whitehall-Robins Healthcare said they had stopped making the sponges because they could not afford to upgrade their production plant to meet standards set by the Food and Drug Administration (FDA). In 1994, the FDA said that the plant did not meet FDA guidelines for clean water and air.

The sponge, introduced in 1983, was a polyurethane disk, saturated with spermicide, that fit over the cervix. It was available without a prescription, could be inserted as long as 24 hours before intercourse, and had no significant side effects.

Abortion pill. In October 1994, the Population Council, a nonprofit research organization in New York City, began clinical trials in the United States of the abortion drug mifepristone, often called by its trade name RU-486. By mid-November, thousands of women had called to volunteer for the trials. At 12 to 20 testing sites across the nation, 2,100 women were to be accepted.

Mifepristone has been on the market since 1988 but only in some European countries and China. In early 1994, the French makers of RU-486 donated the U.S. patent rights for the drug to the Population Council, which sought FDA approval to market the drug. The French makers declined to enter the U.S. market because of the American controversy over abortion.

RU-486 can be used to end a pregnancy during the first three months. A pregnant woman takes two doses of pills three days apart, under a doctor's supervision. Most women experience nausea, headaches, and weakness after the first dose. The second dose causes strong uterine contractions that result in the expulsion of the fetus. Two weeks later, the woman returns to the doctor for a follow-up examination.

Proponents of RU-486 say that the drug offers women a less invasive option than a surgical abortion. A surgical abortion, however, takes only about 15 minutes, followed by a one-day recovery.   • Mary Carvlin
In World Book, see Birth control.

A new drug to treat sickle cell anemia was found so effective that a study of it was halted in January 1995, five months earlier than scheduled. The drug, hydroxyurea, is the first effective treatment for the disease. Sickle cell anemia is a hereditary blood disorder that in the United States affects about 72,000 African Americans.

About 8 percent of African Americans carry one abnormal gene for sickle cell disease. This means they have a condition called sickle cell trait but not the disease. To develop sickle cell anemia, a person needs two abnormal genes, one from each parent.

People with sickle cell anemia have abnormal hemoglobin, the substance in blood that transports oxygen and gives blood its red color. When their red blood cells are exposed to oxygen, they become stiff and sickle-shaped. These rigid, sickled cells can become trapped in tiny blood vessels, reducing the supply of oxygen to the surrounding tissues. In addition, red blood cells are destroyed as the blood circulates through the body.

The reduced blood flow can bring on painful attacks known as crises, which require hospital treatment. Sickle cell patients can also develop life-threatening problems involving the heart, brain, kidneys, or lungs.

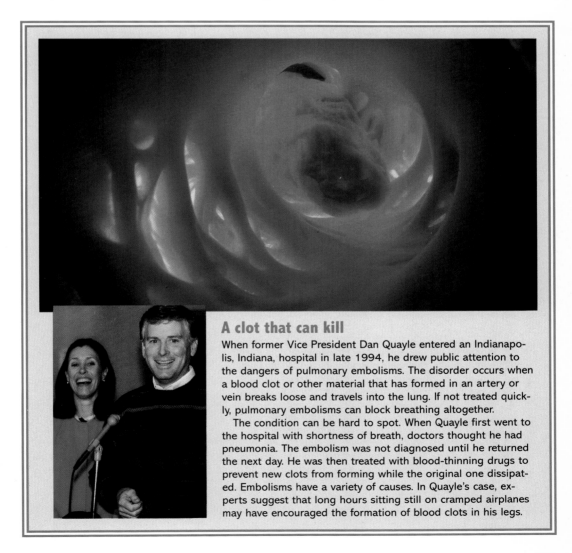

A clot that can kill

When former Vice President Dan Quayle entered an Indianapolis, Indiana, hospital in late 1994, he drew public attention to the dangers of pulmonary embolisms. The disorder occurs when a blood clot or other material that has formed in an artery or vein breaks loose and travels into the lung. If not treated quickly, pulmonary embolisms can block breathing altogether.

The condition can be hard to spot. When Quayle first went to the hospital with shortness of breath, doctors thought he had pneumonia. The embolism was not diagnosed until he returned the next day. He was then treated with blood-thinning drugs to prevent new clots from forming while the original one dissipated. Embolisms have a variety of causes. In Quayle's case, experts suggest that long hours sitting still on cramped airplanes may have encouraged the formation of blood clots in his legs.

In 1992, the National Heart, Lung, and Blood Institute, part of the National Institutes of Health (NIH), began testing hydroxyurea as a treatment for sickle cell anemia. The study involved 299 patients at 21 medical centers in the United States.

The researchers found that hydroxyurea reduced by 50 percent both the frequency of crises and the number of hospital admissions for complications of the disease. Patients receiving hydroxyurea also required half as many blood transfusions as patients who received a *placebo* (substance with no active ingredients).

Hydroxyurea does not cure sickle cell anemia. Instead, it increases the production of fetal hemoglobin, a form of hemoglobin normally produced by fetuses but not by adults. Fetal hemoglobin typically constitutes about 1 percent of the hemoglobin in adults. The increased levels of fetal hemoglobin prevent the red blood cells of sickle cell patients from becoming rigid and blocking blood flow.

Patients treated with hydroxyurea must take the drug daily for the rest of their life. Frequent blood count monitoring is needed to establish an appropriate dose. In addition, researchers have found that long-term use of the drug may increase a person's risk of developing leukemia. For this reason, the researchers who conducted the study and the NIH have recommended restrictions on its use. In mid-1995, physicians were administering hydroxyurea only to adults, but NIH officials said a two-year study would soon begin to establish appropriate doses for adolescents and younger children.

Controlling bleeding. A genetically engineered form of thrombopoietin, a substance that promotes blood clotting, may soon be available, according to a January 1995 report. Thrombopoietin regulates the production of blood cells called platelets. When a blood vessel is injured, platelets normally form a sticky clump and plug the leaking vessel. In patients who have a very low platelet count, however, life-threatening bleeding can occur—even without an injury to a blood vessel.

In June 1994, researchers at five laboratories announced they had identified thrombopoietin as the protein responsible for platelet production in bone marrow. Researchers then isolated the gene for thrombopoietin. Biologists in Seattle, Washington, reported they had injected mice with a form of thrombopoietin they had produced in a laboratory using the techniques of genetic engineering. After one week, the mice registered a fourfold increase in the number of platelets in their blood. Experts were hopeful that the research would soon lead to a treatment for people with low platelet counts.

Abnormal clotting. A defective gene is responsible for an abnormal tendency to form blood clots, according to findings reported in 1994. Inappropriate clotting, known as thrombosis, plays an important role in heart disease and stroke. Although scientists have known that a tendency to form clots runs in families, they did not know the specific cause of the problem.

Clotting is a complex process in which substances called clotting factors are activated in the blood and combine to form a clot. Once the clotting process is initiated, other substances normally block any further formation of clots. One of the key substances in halting the clotting process is protein C, which destroys an important clotting factor known as clotting factor V. In 1993, Swedish biochemists found that patients with a familial tendency to form blood clots are resistant to the effects of protein C.

In August 1994, researchers at the University of Leiden in the Netherlands found that resistance to protein C was caused by an abnormality in the gene responsible for the production of factor V. In September, British geneticists reported finding an abnormal factor V gene in about 3.5 percent of the 144 healthy people they tested. These findings suggest that resistance to protein C may be a major contributing cause in all families with a tendency to form abnormal blood clots.　　• G. David Roodman

In the section A Healthy You, see DRAWING FROM YOUR OWN BLOOD BANK. In WORLD BOOK, see BLOOD.

Tall elderly men are twice as likely to fracture a hip as shorter men the same age. That finding was reported in November 1994 by researchers at the National Heart, Lung, and Blood Institute in Bethesda, Maryland.

The investigators studied health data compiled since 1986 on about 50,000 male health professionals 40 to 75 years of age. They found that the only factors significantly related to the incidence of hip fracture in the men were advanced age and tallness. For men 70 years of age and older, the risk of hip fracture was almost 4½ times higher than for men aged 40 to 44 years.

The most surprising finding, however, was that among men the same age, those 6 feet (1.8 meters) or taller were slightly more than twice as likely to suffer a hip fracture as men who were less than 5 feet 9 inches (1.75 meters) tall. The researchers said further studies would be required to explain that difference.

Nutrition and osteoporosis. Doctors have long warned women that failure to obtain proper nutrition can lead to *osteoporosis,* the weakening of bones due to loss of minerals. Further evidence that inadequate nutrition is a risk factor for osteoporosis was reported in January 1995 by investigators at the University of Alcalá de Henares in Madrid, Spain.

The researchers studied 60 women between the ages of 59 and 88 who had suffered a hip or spine fracture and compared them with 60 women of similar ages who had not experienced such injuries. They also compared the nutritional status of the women in both groups, using the level of three biochemical substances in the blood as indicators of either adequate or inadequate nutrition.

The blood of the women who had suffered fractures was found to have lower amounts of the biochemicals, indicating poorer nutrition. The most marked nutritional deficiencies were found in women 75 years and older with hip fractures. These results support the view that elderly women—at least those who have not eaten a good diet—should take nutritional supplements. Supplements, along

with mild physical exercise such as walking, help combat osteoporosis and reduce the risk of hip fracture.

Detecting kids' bone infections. Ultrasound—high-frequency sound— can be an effective tool for diagnosing and managing a type of bone infection called acute osteomyelitis in young children. That finding was reported in November 1994 by researchers at Women's and Children's Hospital in Adelaide, Australia.

Children are more susceptible than adults to acute osteomyelitis, a condition that most often affects arm or leg bones. Discovering the infection early

Gray hair, brittle bones? Premature gray hair, researchers at Boston University reported in late 1994, may be a risk factor for osteoporosis, the weakening of bones caused by a gradual loss of minerals. They found that early graying was associated with a fourfold increase in osteoporosis risk.

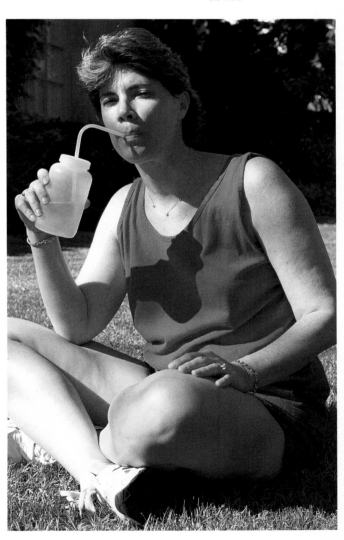

Books of Health and Medicine

Swimming may help strengthen bones

Doctors have long advised patients that only weight-bearing exercises such as walking and aerobics build bone mass. But researchers at Hebrew University in Jerusalem, Israel, reported in late 1994 that swimming may be at least as effective. The scientists studied 64 women over age 50 who swam or did calisthenics and found that the swimmers gained more bone mass than the women who worked out on land.

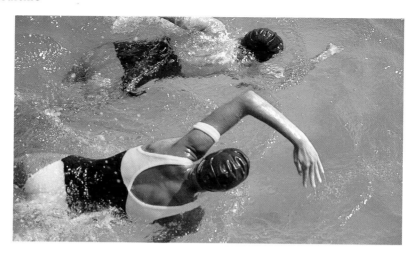

in its course is critical because at that stage it can usually be cured with antibiotics. If not diagnosed early, the infection may spread into a neighboring joint or become a chronic infection requiring multiple operations to cure. But bone infections can be difficult to detect at an early stage because of a lack of symptoms and because they are not visible on X rays.

The Australian investigators diagnosed 38 cases of osteomyelitis with ultrasound. They found that the earliest sign of the infection, clearly visible in the ultrasound images, was swelling of the deep soft tissues next to the affected bone. All the patients were diagnosed early enough to be

cured with antibiotics, and ultrasound enabled the investigators to evaluate the drug treatment and watch the infections subside.

Anesthesia for setting bones. A child with a broken bone may need general anesthesia to allow a doctor to set the bone. Surgeons at Children's Mercy Hospital in Kansas City, Missouri, reported in March 1995 that an intravenous solution of a narcotic and an antianxiety drug was a safe and effective way of sedating children. The physicians used the method with 104 children and had no problems.   • John J. Gartland

In WORLD BOOK, see BONE.

Books of Health and Medicine

The following books on health and medicine were written for the general reader. All were published in 1994 or 1995.

Aging. *Choosing Medical Care in Old Age: What Kind, How Much, When to Stop* by Muriel R. Gillick. Gillick, a gerontologist, uses insights gleaned from her work with elderly patients to explain how the goals of medical care change depending on whether a patient is robust, frail, demented, or dying. (Harvard, 1994. 213 pp. $19.95.)

Arthritis. *Arthritis: Take Care of Yourself Health Guide for Understanding Your Arthritis,* 4th ed., by James F.

Fries. Fries describes eight major categories of arthritis and discusses arthritis prevention, diagnosis, pain management, and surgery. (Addison-Wesley, 1995. 320 pp. $14.)

Cancer. *After Cancer: A Guide to Your New Life* by Wendy S. Harpham, a Dallas physician and cancer survivor. Written in a question-and-answer format, Harpham's book covers the medical aspects of recovery and follow-up as well as practical issues relating to work, school, parenting, exercise, and diet. (Norton, 1994. 364 pp. $23.)

Caregiving. *At Home with Terminal Illness* by Michael Appleton, director of a Los Angeles hospice service, and Todd Henschell. A "family guide to hospice in the home," the book contains advice for caregivers in an A-to-Z format. (Prentice Hall, 1995. 103 pp. $14.)

Giving Comfort: What You Can Do When Someone You Love is Ill by Linda B. Milstein. Milstein provides simple, practical recommendations for comforting the sick—including tips on brightening the surroundings and enhancing physical comfort. (Penguin, 1994. 132 pp. $6.95.)

Helping Yourself Help Others: A Book for Caregivers by Rosalynn Carter with Susan K. Golant. The former First Lady writes from personal experience about the blessings and frustrations of caring for the sick. (Times Books, 1994. 278 pp. $20.)

Drugs. *Thueson's Guide to Over-the-Counter Drugs: A Symptom-by-Symptom Handbook of the Best Nonprescription Drugs* by pharmacologist David O. Thueson. Thueson's handbook is organized so that readers can find out which drugs are used for various ailments and then make comparisons among the medications. (New Harbinger Publications, 1995. 234 pp. $13.95.)

General reference. *Consumer's Medical Desk Reference: Information Your Doctor Can't or Won't Tell You—Everything You Need to Know for the Best in Health Care* by Charles B. Inlander and the staff of the People's Medical Society. This comprehensive volume includes topics such as medical procedures, medications, insurance, government health resources, and consumer protection. (Hyperion, 1995. 656 pp. $24.95.)

The Human Body. Editor Charles B. Clayman compiled over 1,000 color images for this illustrated guide to the body's structure and function. More than 150 medical disorders are also covered, and the illustrations are accompanied by easy-to-understand text. (Dorling Kindersley, 1995. 240 pp. $29.95.)

Heart. *American Heart Association's Your Heart: An Owner's Manual* by the staff of the American Heart Association. This guidebook describes the

normal heart and its proper "service and maintenance." A "troubleshooting" section highlights symptoms of heart problems. (Prentice Hall, 1995. 368 pp. $27.95.)

Immune system. *How Your Immune System Works.* Baltimore physician Jeff Baggish focuses on the healthy human immune system, explaining its functions using simple language enhanced by illustrations. (Ziff-Davis, 1994. 153 pp. $19.95.)

Medical education. *Harvard Med: The Story Behind America's Premier Medical School and the Making of America's Doctors.* Written by John Langone, a medical journalist and Harvard fellow, this unauthorized examination of Harvard Medical School in Boston describes the curriculum and atmosphere of the elite institution. (Crown, 1995. 383 pp. $25.)

Learning How the Heart Beats: The Making of a Pediatrician by Claire McCarthy, a physician at an inner-city clinic in Boston. McCarthy presents 23 stories of real-life medical dramas on hospital wards. (Viking, 1995. 247 pp. $21.95.)

Medicine and society. *Cancer Wars: How Politics Shapes What We Know and Don't Know about Cancer.* Science historian Robert N. Proctor explains how social biases, economic interests, and politics have influenced cancer research. (Basic Books, 1994. 288 pp. $25.)

Defying the Gods: Inside the New Frontiers of Organ Transplants. Author Scott McCartney uses the stories of four transplant patients to describe the history of organ transplantation, the science behind the procedures, and the surrounding ethical issues. (Macmillan, 1994. 298 pp. $22.)

Equal Partners: A Physician's Call for a New Spirit of Medicine. One week after graduating from Harvard Medical School, author Jody Heymann became a patient in a neurological intensive care unit. In *Equal Partners*, she discusses her experiences as a patient and how they changed her ideas about the practice of medicine. (Little, Brown and Company, 1995. 257 pp. $22.95.)

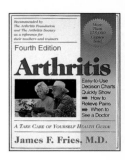

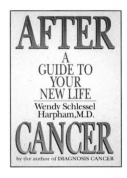

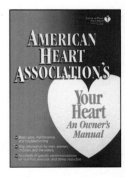

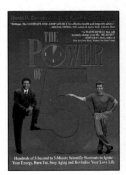

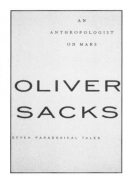

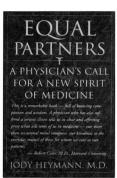

Seeking Fair Treatment: From the AIDS Epidemic to National Health Care Reform. Norman Daniels, a professor of philosophy and expert on health care reform, argues that the plight of AIDS patients highlights the inefficiencies, inequities, and social injustices of the U.S. health care system. (Oxford, 1995. 204 pp. $25.)

Memoirs. *In Love with Daylight* by Wilfrid Sheed. Sheed's "memoir of recovery" is a humorous account of the writer's struggles with polio, depression, addictions, and cancer. (Simon and Schuster, 1995. 252 pp. $23.)

Taking Care of Our Own: A Year in the Life of a Small Hospital. Author Susan Garrett describes her experiences as a manager in a hospital in Maine. (Dutton, 1994. 177 pp. $19.95.)

Wrongful Death: A Medical Tragedy by Sandra Gilbert. Gilbert, whose husband died shortly after what was purported to be a "successful operation," writes of her family's suffering. (Norton, 1995. 364 pp. $22.50.)

Neurology. *An Anthropologist on Mars: Seven Paradoxical Tales.* This critically acclaimed book by neurologist Oliver W. Sacks profiles patients and acquaintances such as a surgeon whose Tourette syndrome tics disappear when he steps into the operating room and an autistic scientist with

an intuitive understanding of animals. (Knopf, 1995. 327 pp. $24.)

Pain control. *Freedom from Chronic Pain.* Norman Marcus and Jean S. Arbeiter teach readers physical and mental techniques designed to end chronic pain. (Simon and Schuster, 1995. 236 pp. $11.)

Self-help. *The Power of 5.* Psychiatrist Harold H. Bloomfield and Robert K. Cooper offer hundreds of "five-second to five-minute techniques" for boosting energy, losing weight, and feeling more youthful. (Rodale, 1995. 524 pp. $24.95.)

Sports medicine. *The Sports Medicine Bible: Prevent, Detect, and Treat Your Sports Injuries Through the Latest Medical Techniques.* Lyle J. Micheli, former president of the American College of Sports Medicine, and Mark Jenkins describe sports injuries involving the foot, wrist, shoulder, knee, and other body parts. (Harper-Perennial, 1995. 339 pp. $20.)

Women's health. *The Good News About Women's Hormones: Complete Information and Proven Solutions for the Most Common Hormonal Problems.* Geoffrey P. Redmond, a specialist in hormone disorders, explains the tests and treatments for hormone imbalances. (Warner, 1995. 510 pp. $12.99.)   • Margaret E. Moore

Brain and Nervous System

Evidence of functional differences between the brains of males and females was reported in February 1995 by researchers at the Yale University School of Medicine in New Haven, Connecticut. Neuroscientists had known for years that brains of males and females are different in some ways. For example, certain structures in the brain are larger in men, while others are larger in women. Still, there was little evidence that the brains of the two sexes differed in the way they function.

The research team, directed by pediatrician and neurologist Bennett A. Shaywitz, used a scanning technique called functional magnetic resonance imaging (fMRI) to study the

brains of 19 men and 19 women as the subjects carried out tasks related to language processing. fMRI revealed areas of the brain in which there was increased blood flow and thus heightened mental activity.

The men and women, all of them right-handed, were asked to read nonsense words and decide whether or not they rhymed. The scientists noted that when men performed these reading tasks, an area in the left side of the brain next to a major speech center showed increased blood flow. This finding was expected, because in right-handed individuals the left half of the brain controls both spoken and written language.

The results with the women were

quite different, however. When the women performed the identical language task, the same area in the left side of the brain showed increased blood flow, but so did the corresponding area in the right half of the brain. This finding showed that the women's brains were processing the information differently.

But does this difference—and perhaps other variations between male and female mental functioning—represent fundamentally divergent ways of thinking? That is, do men and women reach different conclusions when processing the same information? Further research will be required to answer that question.

Insight into dyslexia. Findings that point to an anatomical basis for the language disorder known as dyslexia were reported in August 1994 by brain researcher Albert Galaburda and his colleagues at Beth Israel Hospital in Boston. Neuroscientists had long suspected that dyslexia results from a malfunction in areas of the brain that process the sounds of speech. But they had been unable to identify any anatomical abnormalities in the brain that might be responsible for such malfunctioning.

Dyslexic individuals, though usually of normal intelligence, have difficulty with reading and writing and sometimes also with speech. Because language skills are so central to the process of learning, dyslexics typically have a great deal of difficulty in school and are often incorrectly labeled as retarded.

Galaburda and his associates studied the brains of deceased dyslexics and compared them with the brains of deceased individuals who had possessed normal language abilities. They found that the dyslexics' brains contained considerably fewer *neurons* (nerve cells) in a portion of the brain called the medial geniculate nucleus (MGN), an area involved in the processing of sounds and speech. Two groups of neurons in the MGN, called small neurons and large neurons, receive auditory signals from the ear and encode them. The neurons then transmit the coded signals to thought centers in the brain, where they are interpreted.

It was the large neurons that were deficient in number in the dyslexic brains examined by Galaburda's team. These cells are important in the processing of short sounds, such as consonants, and of the transitions between consonants and vowels—such as the change from "T" in the word "Tom" to the slower "ah" sound. This kind of sound processing, called spatial processing, is impaired in persons with dyslexia.

The findings of Galaburda and his associates may lead to new ways of helping dyslexic children acquire language skills. For example, speech sounds can be altered by computer, so that short sounds are stretched

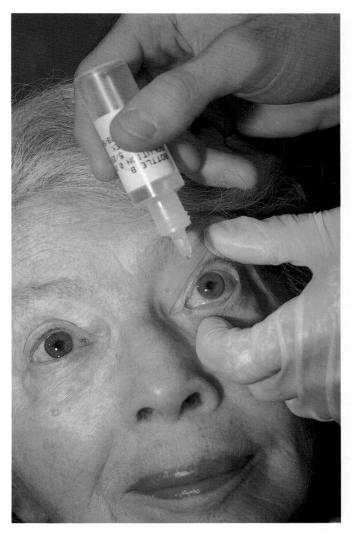

Eye test for Alzheimer's
Drops of the drug tropicamide, routinely used by eye doctors to dilate patients' eyes for examination, are applied to a woman's eyes as a diagnostic test for Alzheimer's disease. A group of U.S. researchers reported in November 1994 that the eyes of people with Alzheimer's dilate three times as much in response to the drug as the eyes of normal individuals.

Brain and Nervous System

Differences between the male and female brain
Images of a male (left) and a female brain made while the individuals were performing a language task show a higher level of activity in the female brain. The finding, reported by researchers at Yale University in February 1995, is the first evidence that males and females use their brains differently for at least some kinds of mental processing.

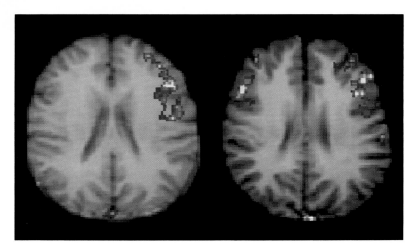

out, making them more intelligible. The ultimate treatment, however, will come when scientists understand what causes the changes in the MGN in the first place. It may then be possible to prevent such abnormalities or to correct them.

Resilient adult brains? Evidence that the adult brain possesses considerable potential for regeneration was reported in December 1994 by neuroscientist Steven A. Goldman and his associates at the Cornell University Medical College in New York City. It had been the accepted wisdom among neuroscientists that the adult human brain has little ability to regenerate after losing neurons to injury or disease. This is in contrast to the brains of infants and small children, which contain large numbers of neurons able to multiply and replace dead neurons.

Goldman and his colleagues studied tissues removed from the brains of patients undergoing surgical treatment for epilepsy. They placed the specimens in laboratory culture dishes for one to four weeks and then examined the tissues for the presence of new nerve cells.

The investigators noted the growth of immature cells called nerve cell precursors, which have the capacity to develop into fully functioning neurons. Significantly, they saw the precursor cells in tissues from parts of the brain called the subependymal zones. These are the regions in which

nerve cell precursors are found in the infant brain during its development.

The researchers' observations indicate that the adult brain has the potential to form new neurons that might replace ones destroyed by injuries, strokes, or degenerative neurological disorders such as Alzheimer's disease and Parkinson's disease.

What scientists must now discover is why neuron precursors in the adult brain do not multiply spontaneously to replace dead nerve cells. There are at least two possible explanations. One is that the adult brain produces substances that inhibit the growth of new neurons. Another is that the adult brain is deficient in the growth factors that are needed to stimulate the development of neurons.

Good news on tissue transplants. The first proof that human fetal nerve tissue survives transplantation into the brain and helps curb the symptoms of Parkinson's disease was reported in April 1995 by neurologist Jeffrey H. Kordower and his associates at Rush-Presbyterian-St. Luke's Medical Center in Chicago and several other institutions.

Parkinson's disease is a degenerative disorder of the brain characterized by the death of neurons that produce a vital chemical called dopamine. Dopamine relays nerve signals to neurons elsewhere in the brain, but especially to an area called the striatum, which is essential for controlling body movements. When dopamine-producing neurons die, the concentration of dopamine in the striatum decreases, and the individual develops tremors, muscle stiffness, and loss of balance.

Since the 1980's, researchers have tried to treat Parkinson's disease in some patients by transplanting fetal nerve cells into the brain. The results of these treatments have been mixed. In some cases, the patients did very well, but others experienced only a temporary improvement. In cases where the patient received minimal benefit from the procedure, the transplanted cells may have been identified as foreign tissue by the patient's immune system and destroyed.

Kordower and his colleagues studied a 59-year-old man with Parkinson's disease who had received two injections of fetal dopamine-producing cells into the striatum of his brain. The man was also given drugs to suppress his immune system and prevent a rejection reaction against the new tissue. The patient improved markedly as a result of this combined treatment.

After 18 months, the man died from a cause unrelated to his treatment for Parkinson's disease. An autopsy of his brain showed the striatum contained dense clusters of dopamine-releasing neurons that looked healthy and were fully integrated into the surrounding tissues of the striatum. Further studies will be required to learn whether transplanted fetal cells can survive and flourish over a period of many years.

New light on MS. Findings shedding light on a puzzling aspect of the nervous system disease multiple sclerosis (MS) were announced in May 1995 by neuroscientists Kai Wucherpfennig and Jack L. Strominger of Harvard University in Cambridge, Massachusetts. MS is an inflammatory disease of the *central nervous system* (brain and spinal cord). The disease, which usually begins in early adulthood, is believed to occur when the immune system mistakenly attacks myelin, a fatty material that insulates nerve fibers. As myelin is destroyed, nerve impulses short-circuit.

MS attacks can occur at any time and can affect any part of the central nervous system. In some people with MS, attacks subside completely for months or years; in others, one attack follows the other, with little recovery and increasing disability. One of the major unanswered questions about MS is what causes these recurrent and increasingly disabling attacks.

Scientists have known for years that an MS patient's risk of suffering an attack increases after the person has had an infection. That observation indicated that there was a link between infections and attacks of MS, but the immunologic mechanism involved was a mystery.

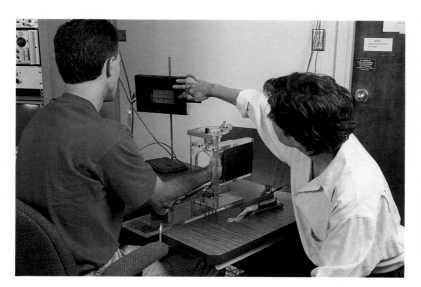

Test for Parkinson's
A test developed at the University of Arizona in Tucson could make it possible to diagnose Parkinson's disease—a brain disorder that causes a loss of muscle control—in its earliest stages. Part of the test involves measuring coordination as a person tries to match hand motions to flashing lights. The test may enable doctors to begin treating Parkinson's patients soon enough to slow and maybe even stop the course of the disease.

Wucherpfennig and Strominger's research may lead to an understanding of how attacks occur. They found that certain immune system cells called lymphocytes from persons with MS are activated by proteins from common viruses and bacteria.

The scientists isolated lymphocytes that responded to a protein in myelin called myelin basic protein. They compared the structure of myelin basic protein with that of thousands of proteins associated with infectious agents such as viruses and bacteria. They were looking for proteins that were similar enough to myelin basic protein to stimulate lymphocytes into mounting an immune reaction.

The researchers found several hundred proteins from the infectious agents that were similar to myelin basic protein. They then tested each of the proteins on antimyelin lymphocytes. Of all the proteins tested, only a handful stimulated the antimyelin lymphocytes, but that was enough to prove conclusively that proteins from viruses and bacteria have the capacity to provoke the kind of immune reaction seen in MS. This discovery takes us one step closer to finding a cure for MS.   • Gary Birnbaum

In the section A Healthy You, see HEADACHE: A COMPLEX PAIN WITH ORIGINS IN THE BRAIN. In WORLD BOOK, see BRAIN; NERVOUS SYSTEM.

Cancer

Mindful of the evidence that reproductive hormones play a role in breast cancer, physicians have worried about the possibility of increasing breast cancer risk by using these hormones to ease the effects of menopause, when a woman's natural production of estrogen drops. Two studies published in 1995 came to opposite conclusions about whether such hormone replacement therapy (HRT) does, in fact, raise breast cancer risk.

Many women take estrogen supplements for a few years to relieve hot flashes and other symptoms of menopause. Some continue to use estrogen much longer because it can lower the risk of heart disease and *osteoporosis* (a bone-thinning disorder that can lead to disabling fractures). Because estrogen increases the risk of uterine cancer, many women on estrogen therapy also take the hormone progestin, which reduces this cancer risk. Still, regimens that include progestin are relatively new, so little information exists yet on their long-term effects.

In June 1995, a team of scientists from Harvard Medical School and Harvard School of Public Health in Boston reported the results of a study of more than 69,000 nurses who had reached menopause. The women were enrolled in the Nurses' Health Study, an ongoing research effort to track the long-term health of 121,700 women.

The researchers found that women who took estrogen—either alone or with progestin—for more than five years had a 46 percent greater risk of developing invasive breast cancer than those who had never used HRT. Older women (aged 60 to 64) who had taken estrogen for five years or longer had the highest risk, 71 percent more than that of nonusers. Still, for long-term users who stopped HRT, risk appeared to return to normal within two years.

Just one month later, however, a second study made it clear that the effect of HRT on breast cancer risk is far from settled. Researchers at the University of Washington in Seattle studied more than 1,000 women 50 to 64 years old—537 who had breast cancer and 492 who had no history of the disease. This study found no evidence that women who took estrogen, alone or combined with progestin, experienced an increased risk of breast cancer.

Both the Harvard and University of Washington teams said more research is needed on the potential risks and benefits of hormones in older women. Experts also cautioned that women should discuss their medical histories with their physicians before deciding whether to undergo HRT.

Regular exercise can significantly reduce a woman's risk of developing breast cancer by age 40, according to a study of more than 1,000 women. If confirmed, health experts said, the finding of such a protective effect is particularly encouraging, because unlike other factors increasing breast cancer risk—such as early onset of menstruation, late menopause, or having a mother or sister with the disease—physical activity is something women generally can control.

The study, reported in September 1994 by researchers at the University of Southern California School of Medicine in Los Angeles, involved 545 newly diagnosed breast cancer patients age 40 or younger. The researchers matched each of these patients with a woman without cancer who lived in the same neighborhood and was the same age and race. All 1,090 of the women were asked about their lifetime exercise habits and other potentially relevant factors, such as use of oral contraceptives, body size, family history of breast cancer, and number of pregnancies.

Even after accounting for these factors, the researchers found that the more women exercised, the less their risk of developing breast cancer by age 40. Those who had exercised an average of four or more hours a week since they started menstruating were nearly 60 percent less likely to get breast cancer than inactive women.

Although the most active women had the greatest reduction in risk, the researchers noted that women who exercised as little as one to three hours a week could reduce their risk by about 30 percent over sedentary women. The findings also showed that exercise just in the 10 years after the onset of menstruation was beneficial, but the researchers added that the protective effect was most pronounced when they looked at life-long exercise patterns.

The study did not attempt to determine how exercise protects against breast cancer. The researchers noted, however, that exercise alters a woman's production of estrogen and progesterone, reproductive hormones known to influence the development and growth of breast cancer.

Prostate cancer screening. Medical researchers debated in 1994 and 1995 whether the benefits of a blood test used to screen men for signs of

Don't take chances with a mammogram

A mammogram may save a woman's life by revealing early breast cancer—but only if the test is done correctly. The Department of Health and Human Services suggests that women follow these guidelines:

- Use only centers certified by the Food and Drug Administration. If the center can't show its certification, leave.
- Schedule the appointment for the time of your menstrual cycle when your breasts are least tender.
- Be prepared to provide information on past or current breast problems, breast disease in your family, previous mammograms, and timing of your menstrual cycle.
- On the day of the test, wear a two-piece outfit. Don't wear deodorant, lotion, or powder. They can show up on the picture.
- Find out whom you should call if you don't receive results. If you don't get results within 10 days, call and demand the information.
- If the test suggests anything unusual, talk to your doctor right away.

More detailed advice appears in the brochure "Things to Know about Quality Mammograms." To request a copy, write AHCPR Publications Clearinghouse, P.O. Box 8547, Silver Spring, MD 20907, or call 1-800-358-9295 weekdays.

prostate cancer outweigh the test's drawbacks. The test measures prostate-specific antigen (PSA), a protein produced by the prostate gland. An elevated PSA level may indicate cancer but can also be a sign of benign prostatic hyperplasia, a noncancerous condition common in older men.

In a September 1994 report, researchers from the University of Toronto, Canada, calculated the risks and benefits of widespread prostate cancer screening and predicted that it would "result in net harm rather than net health improvement." They argued that many men who have a positive PSA test and are then treated would never have experienced problems from the disease, that many of those who undergo treatment experience incontinence or impotence, and that screening and treatment only slightly extend an individual's life.

Critics said the study had several limitations, including the fact that it was based on a one-time screening effort. An editorial that appeared in the same journal as the report cautioned that while the study "suggests that a one-time screening effort is not worthwhile, it provides no information about the impact of more frequent screening policies like those used for breast cancer or cervical cancer." Others noted that because many men with prostate cancer die of it, the test provides a useful way of detecting the cancer while it is still curable.

To help settle the related question of whether early diagnosis and treatment of prostate cancer significantly improve survival, the U.S. Department of Veterans Affairs and the National Cancer Institute announced plans to launch a large study called the Prostate Intervention Versus Observation Trial, or PIVOT, in fall 1995. Prostate cancer usually grows so slowly that most men with the disease eventually die of a completely unrelated cause. Because of this, plus the chance of complications or death from surgical removal of the prostate, some physicians recommend a strategy called "watchful waiting" or "expectant management." This strategy entails deferring surgery or other treatments—perhaps permanently—unless the

tumor causes symptoms or spreads beyond the prostate.

Although current data suggest that both surgery and watchful waiting may be equally effective, the evidence is far from conclusive. Because of this, researchers hope that PIVOT will confirm either that the two strategies are equally helpful or that one is clearly more likely to improve survival.

Alcohol, diet, and colon cancer.
People who combine alcohol with a poor diet substantially raise their risk of colon cancer, according to a study of nearly 48,000 male health professionals aged 40 to 75. Researchers from Harvard Medical School and Harvard School of Public Health reported in February 1995 that men who had more than two drinks daily and ate few fruits, vegetables, fish, and low-fat foods had a risk of colon cancer more than three times that of men who drank less and ate smarter.

Experts say there is good reason to suspect that the combination of poor diet and high alcohol intake helps foster colon cancer. Animal studies suggest that disruption of a biochemical process called DNA methylation may promote cancer. DNA methylation requires folic acid and methionine—substances found in fruits, vegetables, and protein. Moreover, alcohol blocks the process. The researchers therefore suspected that individuals who ingest too little folic

Dyeing without fear
Although experts have long worried that hair dyes may pose a risk of cancer, an October 1994 report suggests that most salon clients can change their locks without harm. Harvard University researchers who tracked the health of 99,000 women over a period of 14 years found no increased cancer risk from hair dye. However, some uncertainty remained regarding long-term use of black hair dye.

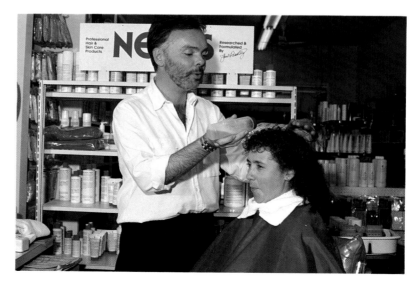

acid and methionine and too much alcohol would be particularly prone to developing the disease.

The researchers used a detailed questionnaire to evaluate the men's dietary intake for one year. None of the men had colon cancer at the beginning of the study. Within six years, 205 had developed the disease.

The investigators then compared the diets of those with colon cancer with those who were cancer-free. Although they found that men who took more than two drinks daily and ate poorly more than tripled their colon cancer risk, they also noted that a healthful diet seemed to offer some protection against the effects of heavy drinking. The drinkers who ate better foods had about the same risk of colon cancer as men who drank little or no alcohol.

The researchers also said that their study does not support taking pills containing methionine as a supplement, because excess methionine can increase blood levels of a chemical linked to heart disease. But they added that vitamin supplements containing folic acid are worth considering, especially for groups who tend to get too little folic acid (such as older people and people who drink regularly), though such supplements "should not be used as a substitute for a diet abundant in fruits and vegetables."

Immunizing against cancer. Scientists successfully immunized a woman with a rare blood cancer against her own cancer cells by transferring immunity to the cells through a bone marrow transplant from her healthy brother, researchers from the National Cancer Institute in Bethesda, Maryland, reported in April 1995. At the time of the report, the woman, who suffered from multiple myeloma, a blood cancer that strikes about 13,000 Americans each year, had been in remission for two years after the novel procedure.

The researchers first purified a protein from the patient's cancerous cells, coupled it to another protein, and combined it with an immunity-boosting substance to create a kind of vaccine. The woman's brother was then given two doses of this mixture to induce his body to mount a re-

Cutting off a tumor's supply lines

To grow, cancerous tumors need a steady supply of blood, which brings nutrients and carries off wastes. For years, researchers have sought ways of cutting off a tumor's blood supply and starving the tumor.

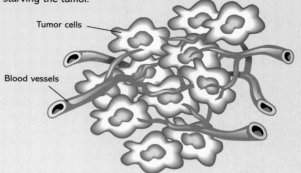

Tumor cells

Blood vessels

A pair of proteins shows promise in tricking new blood vessels in cancerous tumors into self-destructing, researchers at the Scripps Research Institute in La Jolla, California, reported in December 1994. Starved of blood, the tumors in laboratory animals shrank. But tests on human subjects were years away, the researchers cautioned.

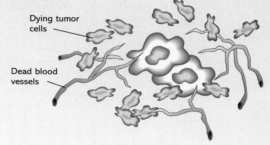

Dying tumor cells

Dead blood vessels

sponse against the cancer cell protein.

Meanwhile, the woman received anticancer drugs to reduce the number of cancerous cells in her body. She then received a bone marrow transplant from her brother, a process that involves replacing the patient's bone marrow (the body's blood-cell factory) with that of a healthy donor.

Within two months, laboratory tests showed that the woman's white blood cells—derived from the transplanted marrow—were "activated" to fight her cancer protein. If the procedure works as hoped, these cells will detect and destroy any stray cancer cells in her body. • Joan Stephenson

In the section On the Medical Frontier, see ARE WE WINNING THE WAR ON CANCER? In WORLD BOOK, see CANCER.

Child Development

Managing the sleep problems of toddlers can help them behave better by day, according to a report in October 1994 from a group of investigators at McGill University in Montreal, Canada. The researchers—Klaus Minde, André Faucon, and Suki Falkner—specialize in the problems of very young children. They reported on using techniques of behavioral psychology in as many as six training sessions with parents, so that the parents could work on improving their toddlers' disturbed sleep patterns.

Treating sleep problems. Children in the study were considered sleep-impaired if they awoke three or more times on at least four nights in a week, awoke for more than 20 minutes per night, were taken into their parents' bed, refused for more than 30 minutes to go to sleep at bedtime, or required a parent's presence to fall asleep. The poor sleepers, a group of 28 children, were compared to a group of 30 children of similar ages and with a similar sex ratio who did not have sleep problems.

The researchers determined the severity of a child's sleep problems by using a scoring system developed in 1981 by English child psychologist Naomi Richman. Using a scale of 1 to 24, Richman considered scores of 8 and above an indication of moderate-to-severe sleep disturbances. The scores were recorded in sleep diaries.

The parents of each of the 28 poor sleepers in the study kept a sleep diary for two weeks. The children designated by the researchers as sleep-disturbed scored 9 or more on the Richman scale. Each child in the normal group received a score of less than 6.

The researchers used two different behavioral approaches with the children. In two-parent families, they tried having the father take over all bedtime responsibilities. This approach was chosen to eliminate the possibility that the mother's anxiety was contributing to the sleep problem. The father's duties included arranging for specific and consistent bedtime routines, keeping the child in bed once put there, responding to all nighttime awakenings, and repeatedly soothing a crying child at regular intervals until the child fell asleep.

In families in which there was either a single parent or one parent who was unwilling to work on the child's sleep disturbance, a "shaping" technique was employed. In this technique, the parent would move from lying down with the child, to sitting up on the bed, to sitting in a chair at the side of the bed, to moving the chair away from the child's side, and eventually to leaving the room.

After initiating the parents in these behavioral techniques and providing psychotherapy sessions, the researchers checked on the toddlers

Taming toddler tantrums

Temper tantrums are a normal part of life for 1- to 3-year-olds, who can be easily frustrated by their inability to communicate, physical limitations, and the confusion of learning many new things at once. Fortunately, tantrums usually abate by age 4. These tips from the American Academy of Pediatrics can help parents survive in the meantime.

- Minimize frustration by keeping expectations reasonable and rules consistent.
- When you say "no" to a demand, offer an acceptable alternative.
- Take care of physical problems that may contribute to tantrums, such as hunger, fatigue, illness, or discomfort.
- Ignore mild attention-getting tactics like whining or door slamming.
- For violent tantrums, remove the child to another room and stay with the child until the tantrum is over.
- Keep calm. Shouting or spanking will only make matters worse.
- Don't give in, particularly when safety is a question. And don't offer rewards for stopping a tantrum. That may encourage more.
- Consult a physician if tantrums are frequent, severe, or destructive; if the child has frequent headaches, stomachaches, or nightmares; if the child does not seem happy and healthy most of the time; or if tantrums don't taper off during the child's fourth year.

Source: American Academy of Pediatrics.

after three months and again after six months. They found that both treatment programs decreased the toddlers' sleep problems by more than a third in the first three months and by a slightly higher percentage at the six-month mark.

The researchers used two standard tests to rate the children's progress—the Child Behavioral Checklist, developed by Stephanie McConaugh and Thomas Achenback in 1988, and the infant version of the Behavioral Checklist developed by Naomi Richman in 1977. From these tests, the researchers determined that the daytime organizational, attentional, and social skills of the sleep-disturbed children improved significantly after their parents attended the counseling sessions. The children exhibited less uncontrollable emotion, less irritability, and less negative behavior, as well as better interactions with their caregivers. Thus, intervention in their sleep problems helped these toddlers' overall behavior.

Two sets of rankings in this otherwise optimistic study concerned the researchers. Both before and after the behavior modification sessions, the researchers observed and scored the interactions of the mothers and toddlers during free play. The mothers' interactions did not change appreciably after counseling.

Of even greater concern was the fact that from observations of the mothers' feeding of their toddlers, the researchers could still differentiate the sleep-disturbed children from the normal toddlers. It appeared that the sleep-disturbed toddlers had changed more readily than had their mothers.

This study suggested that when one aspect of a toddler's life improves, his or her general behavior may improve as well. But the study also indicated that something more than highly focused attention on a specific parent-child problem is needed if parents are to change their behavioral patterns as parents. Unless a more general approach is taken, mothers and fathers may not alter these patterns easily.

Smallest babies at risk. The first report appeared in September 1994 on the long-term development of ba-

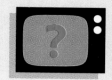

Small screen, big impact

By the time today's children reach age 70, they will have spent 7 to 10 years watching television. The American Academy of Pediatrics has some suggestions on how parents can take charge of their children's TV viewing.

- Limit viewing to one to two hours daily.
- Don't put a TV set in the child's room, where you can't supervise viewing.
- Don't "channel-surf." Choose what to watch before turning the TV on.
- Watch TV with your children. Ask them why they like their favorite shows.
- Talk about what TV characters do. Ask your children if they can think of more realistic ways to solve problems.
- Use shows you find bad to start discussions about ways TV can create misperceptions.
- Encourage children to watch high-quality shows—and talk about why.
- Ban programs you strongly oppose—and talk about why.
- Avoid commercials. Explain that they're someone's attempt to make money.
- Find constructive alternatives to TV.
- Become active in determining local programming.

bies born too tiny to survive without assistance from advanced technology. Pediatric researcher Maureen Hack and her colleagues at Case Western Reserve University Medical School in Cleveland, Ohio, looked at what happens to these children once they enter school.

Hack followed 68 children who had weighed less than 1.5 pounds (0.7 kilogram) at birth and compared them with 65 children who had weighed from 1.5 to 3 pounds (1.4 kilograms) and 61 children who had been born at full term. Hack's team found that the tiniest babies were the most likely to suffer from disabilities and learning problems when they reached school. At school age, as many as 21 percent of these children

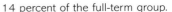

scored below 70 on IQ tests, whereas only 8 percent of the group with higher birthweights had such low IQ's and none of the full-term babies did. Nine percent of those who had been tiniest at birth had cerebral palsy—brain damage that results in a lack of muscle control—compared with 6 percent of the larger group and none of the full-term babies.

Very poor vision troubled 25 percent of children in the tiniest group, compared with 5 percent of children in the larger group and 2 percent of the full-term group. Forty percent of the tiniest group required special education classes, compared with 25 percent of the larger group and

14 percent of the full-term group.

This study brought the long-term risks of premature birth to the attention of doctors and child development specialists and highlighted the importance of preventing such births. Earlier and better prenatal care for pregnant women and assistance with quitting smoking can increase the chances that a baby will be born at or near term and at normal weight. However, these actions do not prevent extreme prematurity, the causes of which remain unclear.

The study raised another question. The cost of keeping alive a baby who weighs about 1.5 pounds can run from $100,000 to $150,000. However, little money is available for helping these babies and their families as they grow older. Hack's research team showed that the problems of these very premature babies continue long after birth. Future research is needed to determine what can be done to help them at later stages.

Retaining childhood memories. From how early can a college student capture his or her first memory? Psychologist Mary K. Mullen gave questionnaires designed to answer this question to 768 students, most of them at Harvard University in Cambridge, Massachusetts. She reported her findings in May 1995.

Mullen found unexpected differences by gender and race. The most striking difference occurred between Asians and Caucasians. While Caucasian respondents on average recalled their earliest memory at just over age 3, Asian students' earliest memories dated back to age 3½ to 4½. Mullen also found that women and first-born children could recall first memories from earlier ages than could men or children born later.

Mullen conducted a similar survey among 41 Korean students and their spouses, who had grown up in Korea. The questionnaire was in Korean because Mullen wanted to tap memories that might have been inaccessible in an adopted language. The average age from which this group's earliest memories stemmed was 4 years 7½ months—more than a year and a half later than the first memories of Caucasians.

Home alone

Children should not be left home alone until age 7, and even then only once in a while and for no more than an hour or two, child welfare experts say. By age 10, they may stay alone occasionally for up to three hours, and for longer periods by age 12—assuming they have no overriding emotional or medical problems and are comfortable with the situation. When children must be home alone, parents should post phone numbers for where they plan to be, along with numbers for a neighbor and emergency services, and make sure the child knows how and when to use them.

Also write down the child's own address and phone number—it's easy for a child to panic and forget these when calling for help. Children who come home to an empty house should learn the following rules:

- Do not talk to strangers.
- Keep your key out of sight.
- Do not go in if something about your home looks different.
- Lock the door after you come into the house.
- Call a parent when you get home.
- If someone telephones, never say you are home alone.

Source: Fairfax County (Va.) Department of Human Development and North Arundel Hospital, Glen Burnie, Maryland.

One interesting finding in Mullen's report was the effect that moving had on children's memories. A person who had changed homes before the age of 4 related earlier memories than someone who had stayed put as a child. Houses were special markers that helped people recall how early in their lives memorable events had taken place.

Status of research funding. In February 1995, at about the same time many children received their first-semester report cards, the American Academy of Child and Adolescent Psychiatry (AACAP) sent out its own report card. The AACAP graded the United States government midway through a five-year plan to boost research funding for mental disorders of the young.

The AACAP's Report Card on the National Plan for Research on Child and Adolescent Mental Disorders gave high marks to the National Institute for Mental Health (NIMH) for improving the funding for research on services for children, biomedical research, training and career development of researchers, and patient-based (clinical) research, especially in regard to preventing mental illnesses.

But NIMH received poorer grades for other actions or inactions during the first half of its five-year plan. Research on children carried out within NIMH declined by 9 percent and

faced the possibility of greater cuts. Public education about childhood mental conditions had been given short shrift. The proportion of NIMH's research money that was devoted to childhood and adolescent disorders— about 20 percent—had not risen since 1987, even though total funding for research had increased.

NIMH had a long way to go before it could receive a straight-A report card, the AACAP found. More than 26 percent of Americans are under age 18, yet only 20 percent of mental health research money is spent on them. Almost 8 million American children and adolescents suffer from mental illnesses. Many of these conditions are serious, and many of them last a lifetime.

NIMH realized that it was not fully meeting the goals the U.S. Congress asked it to set up in 1990. After merging with the National Institutes of Health (NIH) in 1990, NIMH received directions from the NIH's central leadership, which favored biological research over clinical research. NIMH, however, responded to the AACAP Report Card. The chief of the child and adolescent disorders branch of the NIMH, Peter Jensen, commented, "We are similarly concerned."
● Lenore Terr

In the section A Healthy Family, see How Children Learn to Talk and Talking to Your Child About Sex. In World Book, see Child.

Childbirth
See Pregnancy and Childbirth

Contraception
See Birth Control

Dentistry

Parents should make sure that young children use only a small amount of fluoride toothpaste and avoid swallowing it, the American Dental Association (ADA) said in February 1995. The ADA, which is based in Chicago, said that children whose permanent teeth have not yet appeared should use a pea-sized dab of toothpaste.

Most children in the United States ingest beneficial amounts of cavity-fighting fluoride from community water supplies and food, and from the traces of mouth rinses and toothpaste that enter their bodies with normal use. As a result, half the children entering first grade have never had a cavity, and tooth decay has declined among older children.

But young children, who tend to swallow small amounts of toothpaste at each brushing, may end up getting too much. This may put them at risk for a mild form of dental fluorosis—a cosmetic defect that can develop in a young child's teeth while they are still forming, before they erupt through the gum. Mild cases of dental fluorosis involve small white specks in the teeth and often can be detected only by a dentist or dental hygienist. Very severe cases, due to ingestion of larger amounts of fluoride, can cause pitting of the teeth. These cases are rare in the United States.

The ADA recommended that parents monitor their children's toothbrushing habits periodically to ensure

Dentistry

The number of cavities filled in the United States has declined steadily since 1959, according to figures released by the American Dental Association (ADA) in October 1994. The ADA attributed the decline to fluoride treatments in dentists' offices, the addition of fluoride to public drinking water supplies, and more frequent checkups.

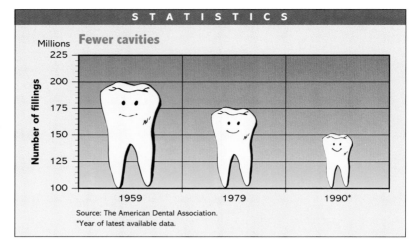

S T A T I S T I C S

Fewer cavities

Millions

Number of fillings

Source: The American Dental Association.
*Year of latest available data.

they use fluoride toothpaste properly. Children under age 6 also should avoid using fluoridated mouth rinse, since they may swallow that as well, the ADA said.

Basketball players' injuries. Basketball players are far more likely than football players to suffer injuries to the teeth, mouth, and jaw, according to a study reported in April 1995. One reason, the study's authors say, is that basketball players rarely wear mouth protectors like the mouth guards routinely worn by football players.

Researchers from the Illinois Department of Public Health studied injury reports on 820 high school football players and 120 basketball players over the course of a school year. They found only one oral injury among the football players, compared with 14 among the basketball players, despite their much smaller number. Moreover, oral injuries accounted for 34 percent of all injuries in basketball, but less than one-tenth of 1 percent in football.

The researchers concluded that school officials should encourage basketball players to use mouth guards during practice sessions and games. They also suggested that such sports as soccer and field hockey might call for similar study.

Teeth out of tune

Playing brass, string, or woodwind instruments may exert damaging pressure on the teeth or jaw, say University of Michigan researchers. Still, problems such as tooth movement, bite misalignment, and jaw joint dysfunction are usually preventable with proper dental care. And if a child already has a bite problem, a dentist may advise parents on a musical instrument to help correct it.

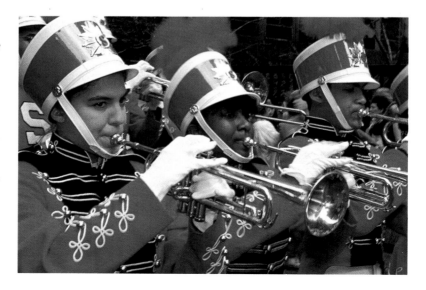

Laser therapy protects teeth. Zapping the teeth with short pulses of low-energy laser light dramatically increases resistance to cavities, scientists reported in February 1995. The technique works by melting and fusing a tooth's outer enamel coating, in somewhat the same way that heat is used to strengthen glass or steel, according to John Featherstone, chairman of the Department of Oral Sciences at the University of Rochester in New York.

Tooth enamel consists of two minerals. One, calcium carbonate, dissolves easily in acids—such as those produced by the bacteria responsible for tooth decay. The other, calcium phosphate, is resistant to such acids.

Experimenting on extracted human teeth, Featherstone and his associates applied laser light to heat the outermost surface of tooth enamel to about 1,800 °F (1,000 °C) for a fraction of a second. The heat momentarily melted the enamel, eliminating some of the decay-prone calcium carbonate. When the enamel fused, or solidified, it was 75 times more resistant to acid attack.

Lasers already are being used experimentally to remove tooth decay. But the new research indicates that lasers may help prevent such decay in the first place.   • Michael Woods

In World Book, see Dentistry.

Diabetes

Women have more than twice the risk of dying of diabetes as of breast cancer, according to statistics released in June 1995 by the Centers for Disease Control and Prevention (CDC) in Atlanta, Georgia. Data based on national surveys conducted in the mid-1980's showed that 47,000 women aged 25 years and older die of breast cancer each year, compared with 109,000 deaths of diabetes among women. According to the CDC, the risk is particularly high for women aged 65 and over: Three times as many women in this group die of diabetes as of breast cancer.

The report prompted the American Diabetes Association (ADA) to recommend regular screening for diabetes, particularly in women who are over age 45, overweight, and physically inactive. These are the women most at risk for diabetes.

New drug. On Dec. 29, 1994, the United States Food and Drug Administration approved metformin (sold as Glucophage) for treating Type II (noninsulin-dependent) diabetes. Metformin has been used in Europe and Canada to treat Type II diabetes since 1959.

In Type II diabetes, the body fails to use the hormone insulin properly. Insulin is normally secreted by the pancreas when levels of *glucose* (sugar) rise in the blood, as they do after a meal. Insulin helps glucose enter the body's cells, where it is converted into energy. In people with Type II diabetes, glucose can build up in the blood, leading to such serious consequences as diabetic coma.

Metformin can be used alone or in combination with sulfonylureas, the only other class of oral drugs approved in the United States for Type II diabetes. Unlike sulfonylureas, which stimulate the production of insulin, metformin helps the body use insulin more efficiently. The ADA said that metformin is the least likely of the drugs used for treating Type II diabetes to cause hypoglycemia, a condition in which blood sugar drops dangerously low. Hypoglycemia can lead to weakness, confusion, and profuse sweating. If not treated quickly, loss of consciousness may follow.

Prevention potential. Troglitazone, a new drug under development for treating diabetes, could also become the first medication to prevent the disease in at-risk individuals, according to a November 1994 report. Researchers at the University of California at San Diego studied the drug's effects in 15 obese people who did not have diabetes but who had been diagnosed with insulin resistance, a condition in which glucose builds up in the bloodstream. Insulin resistance often precedes Type II diabetes.

The scientists reported that they administered troglitazone to a group of six men and three women over 12 weeks. Another group of six men were given a *placebo* (inactive substance). During the period, neither group took steps that might have improved their condition, such as exercising more or losing weight.

At the end of the study, those taking troglitazone were significantly less resistant to insulin and showed an improvement in glucose levels. Those in the placebo group experienced no change in insulin resistance. In mid-1995, the drug was undergoing further study to determine if these results would hold up in a larger group.

Risks for diabetes. Even a modest weight gain significantly increases a woman's risk of developing diabetes, according to a study reported in April 1995 by researchers at the Harvard School of Public Health and Brigham and Women's Hospital, both in Boston. The study involved 114,281 female nurses who were aged 30 to 55 in 1976, when the study began, and who did not then have diabetes.

In follow-up evaluations until 1990, researchers found that weight increases of 11 to 17 pounds (5 to 7.7 kilograms) after age 18 doubled the women's chances of developing Type II diabetes. In contrast, weight losses of 11 pounds or more lowered the risk by 50 percent or better.

In a separate study, investigators at the Harvard School of Public Health reported in March 1995 that smoking elevates the risk of diabetes in men.

The researchers followed 41,810 male health professionals (ages 40 to 75) for six years, beginning in 1986. None had diabetes at the start of the study. The study found that men who smoked 25 or more cigarettes a day had nearly twice the risk of developing Type II diabetes as the nonsmokers. After quitting, the smokers still had a higher risk than men who had never smoked.

Diabetes linked to cancer. In May 1995, researchers from the National Institute of Diabetes and Digestive and Kidney Diseases in Bethesda, Maryland, said that "at present diabetes is perhaps the only common risk factor other than smoking to have a clear, positive association with pancreatic cancer." The researchers had evaluated 20 studies published between 1975 and 1994, of which 18 found that pancreatic cancer was more common in people with diabetes than in those who did not have the disease.

Genetic ties. Scientists in late 1994 identified two genes that increase the likelihood of developing Type I (insulin-dependent) diabetes. In this form of the disease, the body either produces no insulin or produces inadequate amounts, requiring patients to receive daily doses of insulin.

British scientists reported in July 1994 that they had identified 18 re-

Genes identified
Canadian geneticist Leigh Field examines a scan indicating the location of two genes that make a person susceptible to Type I (insulin-dependent) diabetes. A team of researchers from the University of Calgary led by Field reported in October 1994 that they had discovered the genes from their study of 250 families with two or more diabetic children.

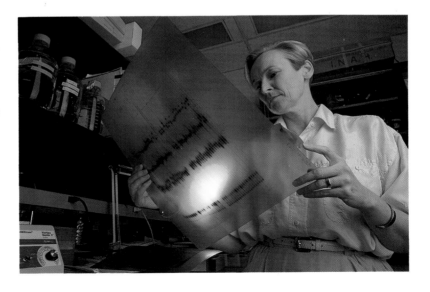

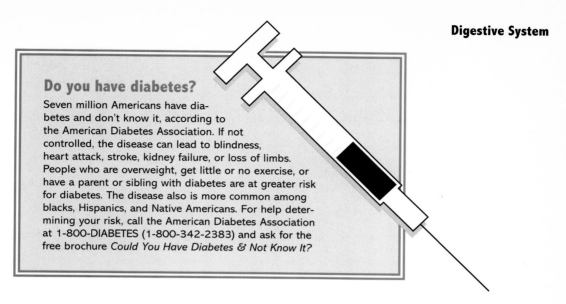

Do you have diabetes?

Seven million Americans have diabetes and don't know it, according to the American Diabetes Association. If not controlled, the disease can lead to blindness, heart attack, stroke, kidney failure, or loss of limbs. People who are overweight, get little or no exercise, or have a parent or sibling with diabetes are at greater risk for diabetes. The disease also is more common among blacks, Hispanics, and Native Americans. For help determining your risk, call the American Diabetes Association at 1-800-DIABETES (1-800-342-2383) and ask for the free brochure *Could You Have Diabetes & Not Know It?*

gions on three chromosomes associated with Type I diabetes. Instead of attempting a laborious gene-by-gene search, the researchers had used an advanced technique that analyzes all 46 human chromosomes at once. In September, they reported that a study of almost 300 families with one or more diabetic members had indicated that regions on chromosomes 6 and 11 were linked with the disease. They also found evidence for a third gene site on chromosome 18. In October 1994, a team of Canadian researchers reported locating two genes for the disease through genetic screening of 250 families with two or more diabetic children.

Vitamin E research. An animal study reported in November 1994 concluded that vitamin E may play a role in minimizing injury that diabetes can cause to blood vessels. Researchers at centers in Boston and Fukuoka, Japan, injected a form of vitamin E into laboratory rats that had a type of diabetes similar to the human disease. Vitamin E interfered with biochemical processes triggered by high blood glucose levels. These processes are believed to play a role in blood vessel injuries that contribute to such complications of diabetes as stroke and kidney failure.   • Richard Trubo

See also EYE AND VISION. In WORLD BOOK, see DIABETES.

Digestive System

Researchers in March 1995 reported successfully treating a disorder of the esophagus with very small doses of the *toxin* (poison) that causes a serious form of food poisoning known as botulism. The disease, achalasia, disrupts the movement of food into the stomach as muscles in the esophagus fail to relax during swallowing.

Drug treatment for achalasia. Researchers do not know what causes achalasia, but they believe it involves damage to nerves that coordinate the functioning of the muscles in the walls of the esophagus or that it results from an imbalance in the chemicals called neurotransmitters that transmit messages between nerve

cells. As the disorder progresses, normal contractions that move food through the esophagus may cease, and food and fluids may remain in the esophagus for many hours after a meal. If this material spills into the lungs, recurrent bouts of pneumonia may occur.

Currently, there is no drug treatment for achalasia. Traditional therapies have relied on surgery or a special balloon to enlarge the esophagus. Physicians inflate the balloon after placing it inside the esophagus. As the balloon expands, it weakens muscle fibers at the base of the esophagus, widening the esophagus and allowing food to pass more easily into the stomach.

The major drawback of this treatment is the risk of perforation of the esophagus, which occurs in about 5 percent of patients. Immediate surgery is then required to remove the balloon and repair the esophagus. The technique effectively opens the esophagus in 60 to 70 percent of achalasia patients but sometimes must be repeated once or twice to achieve the desired results.

If balloon treatment fails, physicians perform surgery to weaken the lower muscles of the esophagus and prevent them from contracting. Surgery is successful in 90 percent of cases, but it can cause unwanted side effects. The inability to contract prevents muscles in the lower esophagus from performing their normal action of blocking a backward flow of acidic stomach contents into the esophagus. This condition, called gastroesophageal reflux, can cause a severe burning sensation in the chest and inflammation of the esophagus.

These potential complications make a drug treatment for achalasia highly desirable. Researchers at the Johns Hopkins Medical Institutions in Baltimore suspected that botulinum toxin given in small, nontoxic amounts would block the release of acetylcholine—a neurotransmitter that regulates muscle contraction. The results of a previous small study of achalasia patients had led researchers to suspect that an imbalance of acetylcho-line might be causing muscles in the esophagus to tighten unnaturally. The Johns Hopkins researchers sought to determine whether the toxin could relax the esophagus muscles.

The researchers injected 21 achalasia patients with either the botulinum toxin or a *placebo* (inactive substance). The researchers evaluated the patients' symptoms after a week by measuring how wide their esophagus was able to open and how well it emptied after meals. The patients who had received the placebo were then treated with the toxin. After six months, the researchers evaluated the patients again.

After the first week, symptoms decreased significantly in patients treated with botulinum toxin but very little in the placebo group. The width of the esophagus in patients treated with botulinum increased by an average of 204 percent compared with a 14 percent decrease in the placebo group. Retention of food in the esophagus also decreased by 21 percent in the treated group but increased by 22 percent in the placebo group. After six months, two-thirds of the patients treated with the toxin continued to experience an improvement in their symptoms, and no side effects had occurred.

New drug for Crohn's disease. The drug budesonide can effectively treat an inflammation of the small intestine

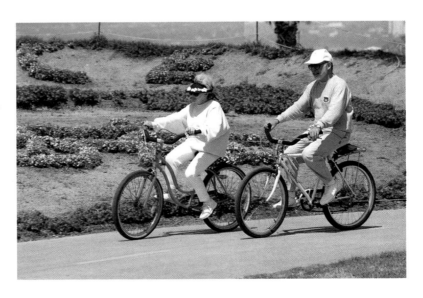

Preventing intestinal bleeding in the elderly
Researchers reported in September 1994 that exercise three times a week can lower the risk of severe intestinal bleeding in persons over age 68 by 30 percent. Such bleeding affects thousands of people over age 65 each year in North America and can be fatal.

High fiber, low risk

A recent study suggests that a diet high in fiber can help head off diverticulosis, a potentially dangerous condition in which the colon develops pouches. Researchers from the Harvard School of Public Health in Boston tracked 47,888 men for four years and found that the men who ate the least fiber (no more than 13 grams daily) were almost twice as likely to develop the disease as the men who ate the most (32 grams or more daily). Nutritionists have some suggestions for introducing more fiber into your diet:

- Favor whole-grain breads, pastas, and cereals.
- Use high-fiber vegetables, such as broccoli, cauliflower, potatoes, sweet potatoes, and peas—alone or in other dishes.
- Snack on such fruit as oranges, apples, pears, bananas, strawberries, and raisins.
- Eat more legumes—beans, lentils, and split peas.

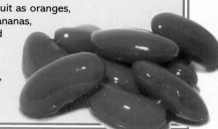

known as Crohn's disease without the severe side effects that standard treatments for the disease can cause. That was the conclusion of research reported in September 1994 by gastroenterologist Gordon R. Greenberg and his colleagues in the Canadian Inflammatory Bowel Disease Study Group.

Crohn's disease most often strikes people in their 20's and 30's and causes abdominal pain, fever, diarrhea, rectal bleeding, and weight loss. The cause of Crohn's disease is unknown, but researchers believe that *antibodies* (immune system molecules) may mistake tissue of the intestine for foreign tissue and mount an attack against it.

Research has shown that drugs called corticosteroids, which reduce the activity of the immune system, can effectively treat Crohn's disease. But many of these drugs also can cause severe side effects. The corticosteroid prednisone, for example, is highly effective in controlling attacks, but long-term use carries the risk of weight gain, especially in the trunk; acne; and *osteoporosis*, a thinning of the bones that increases the likelihood of bone fractures.

Greenberg's group gave the corticosteroid budesonide in three different doses to three groups of patients, each consisting of 60 to 65 people. A fourth group received a placebo. The liver rapidly breaks down budesonide, which lessens the likelihood of severe side effects.

The researchers observed significant improvement in the patients treated with the two higher dosages compared with the placebo group. Fifty-one percent of patients receiving 9 milligrams (mg) and 43 percent of patients receiving 15 mg experienced a remission in symptoms after eight weeks, compared with 20 percent of the placebo group.

Alternative to prednisone. Some Crohn's disease patients develop chronic symptoms when taken off prednisone, the standard treatment for the disease, or when given a lower dosage of the drug. Methotrexate, an anti-inflammatory drug used to treat rheumatoid arthritis and the skin disease psoriasis, may be effective in these patients, according to a study reported in February 1995 by gastroenterologist Brian G. Feagan of the University of Calgary in Canada and his colleagues.

Feagan's team administered methotrexate or a placebo to 141 people who were taking prednisone and had tried unsuccessfully to withdraw from the drug at least once. The dosage of prednisone they received was gradually reduced during the study period. After 16 weeks, 39 percent of the patients treated with methotrexate were in remission, compared with 19 percent of the patients in the placebo group.   • James L. Franklin

In the section A Healthy You, see TREATING HEMORRHOIDS. In WORLD BOOK, see DIGESTIVE SYSTEM.

Drug Abuse
See Alcohol and Drug Abuse

Drugs

A new class of medication for treating hypertension was approved in April 1995. Hypertension is a disorder that typically involves the *constriction* (narrowing) of small blood vessels called arterioles. This constriction increases the pressure blood exerts on arteriole walls as it flows through the vessels. The condition requires the heart to work harder to pump blood through the body, and over time, it can lead to heart disease, *stroke* (an interruption of the blood supply to the brain), and other serious medical problems. According to the American Heart Association, about 50 million Americans suffer from hypertension.

The United States Food and Drug Administration (FDA) approved for marketing losartan potassium (sold as Cozaar), the first antihypertensive medication known as an angiotensin II receptor antagonist. The drug works by blocking the action of angiotensin II in blood vessels. Angiotensin II is a chemical produced by the body that causes blood vessels to constrict, thereby elevating blood pressure.

Another class of antihypertensive drugs known as angiotensin-converting enzyme (ACE) inhibitors works by decreasing the production of angiotensin II. But a number of patients who regularly take these drugs develop a persistent cough as a side effect. In clinical studies, regular use of Cozaar did not cause coughing.

A new alcoholism drug. In December 1994, the FDA approved a drug designed to treat alcoholism by manipulating chemicals in the brain. The drug, naltrexone hydrochloride (sold as Revia), became only the second drug on the market for treating alcohol addiction. Revia has been sold in the United States since 1984 for the treatment of heroin dependence.

Disulfiram (sold as Antabuse) had been the only medication marketed to treat alcoholism. This drug causes people taking it to become nauseous if they drink alcohol.

Naltrexone was approved based on two federally funded 12-week studies of its effects on alcohol-dependent men who were trying to stop drinking. The studies were conducted at Yale University in New Haven, Connecticut, and the University of Pennsylvania in Philadelphia.

Of the 167 study participants, 23 percent of those who took naltrexone returned to drinking, compared with 54 percent of those who received a *placebo* (inactive substance). In addition, those taking naltrexone who relapsed had fewer drinks than those who relapsed in the placebo group.

Naltrexone acts by blocking *receptors* (proteins on cell surfaces) that bind to chemicals in the brain called opioids. Opioids help relieve pain and promote feelings of well-being. Drinking alcohol causes the release of opioids, but by blocking their use by the

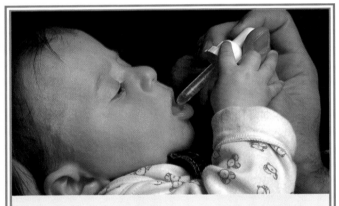

A dose of sugar?

It isn't easy to get a bitter-tasting antibiotic down the throat of a cranky infant or toddler. Pediatricians offer several tips to help the medicine go down.

- Ask your doctor or pharmacist if the medicine can be chilled. This may reduce the bad taste. Or let a toddler suck on an ice pop first.

- Use a calibrated dropper or a tubular medicine spoon. Infants who refuse these may be willing to suck the medicine through a hand-held nipple.

- Have someone else hold an infant to control squirming.

- Deposit the medicine deep in the back of the cheek to bypass the taste buds. To avoid a gag reflex, don't touch the back of the tongue.

- If the medicine can be taken with food, try mixing it with a small amount of fruit or another strong, sweet substance—but be sure the child takes all the mixture.

- Offer a bottle or cup of your child's favorite beverage immediately afterward. (Milk or a milk-based formula can counteract some medicines, so ask your doctor first.)

brain, naltrexone reduces the pleasurable effects of drinking.

Physicians say that naltrexone is not a cure for alcoholism and that it should be used in combination with traditional treatments. Such treatments include individual and group counseling.

Alcohol abuse and dependence affect about 15.3 million adults in the United States, according to the National Institute on Alcohol Abuse and Alcoholism (NIAAA) in Rockville, Maryland. Approximately 5 percent of all U.S. deaths each year can be attributed in some way to alcohol abuse, according to the NIAAA.

New pain treatment. A new drug became available in March 1995 for the treatment of pain. Tramadol hydrochloride (sold as Ultram) was approved by the FDA for treating moderate to moderately severe pain.

According to the results of an October 1994 poll commissioned by the American Medical Association, nearly one in five American adults suffers from pain that has lasted at least six months. Respondents who experienced arthritis pain, lower back pain, or migraine headache pain reported that they were often unable to sleep, they were less effective at work, and their relationships with friends and family suffered because of their pain.

Ultram appears to relieve pain in two ways. One way involves binding

to receptors to block the transmission of pain signals in the brain. The other way involves prolonging the action of certain pain-modifying chemicals in the brain.

Ultram does not reduce inflammation, as do aspirin and related nonsteroidal anti-inflammatory pain relievers. But studies show that Ultram also is less likely to cause the side effects sometimes associated with long-term use of anti-inflammatory drugs, including *ulcers* (sores) in the lining of the stomach and kidney damage. But ultram can cause dizziness, nausea, and constipation in some patients.

An old drug with a new use. A drug used since the 1970's to treat cancer has shown promise in the treatment of sickle cell anemia. The National Heart, Lung, and Blood Institute in Bethesda, Maryland, announced the results of clinical tests of the drug on Jan. 30, 1995.

In the United States, sickle cell anemia affects about 72,000 African Americans. The disease occurs when red blood cells lack normal hemoglobin, the substance in blood that carries oxygen. These blood cells develop a sickle shape as a result. Sickled cells can become trapped in small blood vessels, thereby depriving body tissues of oxygen and bringing on painful attacks. These attacks can last several days and, in many cases, they eventually damage body organs.

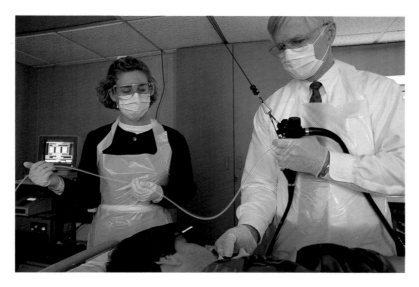

Light-activated drug
An optical fiber guides light from a laser (shown in red) down the throat of a cancer patient at the Knoxville Cancer Center in Tennessee. In late 1994, doctors there and elsewhere experimented with a new treatment in which a patient's tumor is coated with a drug that is activated only by certain wavelengths of light. The light triggers chemical reactions that attack the tumor and small blood vessels that feed it.

Cracking the prescription code

If you can't read a written prescription, don't blame it just on poor handwriting. Doctors and pharmacists use a code to relay information. Usually the name of the drug comes first, then its strength—often in milligrams (mg) or grams (g). Next is the amount the pharmacist should put in the bottle—a number sign (#) and the quantity for pills, or ounces (oz.) or milliliters (ml.) for liquids. Then come dosage instructions, couched in abbreviations for such Latin words as *ante* (before), *cum* (with), and *die* (day), as shown in the accompanying table. Finally, doctors who want to specify a certain brand of medicine may check a box on the prescription form or write "do not substitute" or "D.A.W." (dispense as written). Otherwise, the pharmacist may substitute a generic equivalent.

Some common prescription abbreviations

a.c.	before meals	man.	in the morning
agit. a. us.	shake before using	p.c.	after meals
b.i.d.	twice a day	p.r.n.	as needed
c.	with	q.h.	every hour
gtt.	drops	q.2h.	every 2 hours
h.	an hour	q.i.d.	four times a day
hor. som. or H.S.	at bedtime	t.d. or t.i.d.	three times a day
		semel in d.	one a day

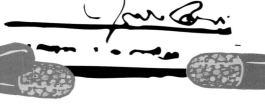

In tests, hydroxyurea (sold as Hydrea) reduced by 50 percent the frequency of sickle cell attacks and subsequent hospital admissions. Patients who took the drug also required half as many blood transfusions as those who received a placebo. Hydrea's effectiveness was so compelling that health officials stopped the study earlier than planned.

New use for ibuprofen. The anti-inflammatory pain reliever ibuprofen may slow the progression of cystic fibrosis in children. That was the result of a study reported in March 1995 by researchers from Case Western Reserve University School of Medicine in Cleveland.

Cystic fibrosis is an inherited disease that afflicts more than 30,000 children and young adults in the United States. A genetic defect in people with the disease causes thick mucus to accumulate in the respiratory passages. The mucus build-up causes breathing difficulties and increases the likelihood of infections and inflammation that eventually damage the lungs and lead to death.

The researchers administered ibuprofen or a placebo to 85 study participants for four years. During the study, the patients taking ibuprofen experienced 60 percent less deterioration of the lungs than did those who received the placebo. Patients under age 13 who took ibuprofen experienced even less lung deterioration—88 percent less, according to the researchers.

Researchers said a reduction in inflammation as a result of taking the drug probably helped limit lung damage. Attempts to treat cystic fibrosis with stronger anti-inflammatory drugs had shown promise, but the drugs had caused serious side effects.

Two popular drugs for treating stomach and intestinal ailments, which had been available only with a prescription, received nonprescription status from the FDA in 1995. The drugs, famotidine (sold as Pepcid AC) and cimetidine (sold as Tagamet), belong to a class of drugs known as histamine H_2-receptor antagonists. Pepcid AC was approved in April, and Tagamet in June. Physicians have treated ulcers and other gastrointestinal problems with these drugs since cimetidine came on the market in the late 1970's.

H_2-receptor antagonists block the secretion of acid by cells in the stomach. Pepcid AC and Tagamet offer an alternative to antacids for the estimated 95 million Americans who experience heartburn and acid indigestion. The most commonly used antacids include calcium carbonate, magnesium hydroxide, and aluminum hydroxide. They neutralize stomach acid after it has already been produced.

Ibuprofen approved for children. A study released in March 1995 concluded that ibuprofen can safely bring down fevers in children. The study, conducted by researchers at Boston University's School of Public Health, was the first large-scale look at ibuprofen's potential for causing side effects in children. On the basis of the study's findings, the FDA on June 20, 1995, approved the nonprescription sale of ibuprofen for treating fever and pain in children between the ages of 2 and 11.

The FDA had approved ibuprofen for reducing fevers in children under age 12 in 1989. But the drug could be obtained only by prescription because of the lack of information on its side effects in children. Acetaminophen (Tylenol), which was available over the counter, has been the drug most widely used to bring down children's fevers.

Between 1991 and 1993, the Boston researchers gave either ibuprofen or acetaminophen to 83,915 children aged 6 months to 12 years to reduce fevers. The researchers reported that the children developed no serious side effects as a result of either treatment. But 4 of the 56,000 children taking ibuprofen experienced temporary bleeding in the intestinal tract. None of the children in the acetaminophen group did.　　• Daniel A. Hussar

In the section Medical and Safety Alerts, see KEEPING THE WONDER IN WONDER DRUGS. IN WORLD BOOK, see DRUGS.

Deaf people who receive cochlear implants, small electronic devices implanted in the inner ear to improve hearing, experience both psychological and economic benefits from the implants. That finding was reported in April 1995 by investigators at the University of California at San Diego and San Diego State University.

Cochlear implants provide some auditory sensations but do not restore normal hearing. Nonetheless, they have proven effective in improving deaf people's ability to speak intelligibly, understand other people's words, and read lips.

The California researchers assessed the progress of nine patients between the ages of 18 and 60 who had recently received cochlear implants. During the three-year study, the individuals showed increased confidence to take jobs or go to school in preparation for work. The patients also experienced a steady upward growth in personal income.

Communicating with deaf patients. Most physicians believe it is a good idea to enlist the aid of a sign language interpreter when treating deaf patients. But, as investigators at the University of Illinois at Chicago reported in January 1995, it appears

Food allergies a cause of ear infections?

Food allergies may be the cause of many middle-ear infections, allergist Talal M. Nsouli and his colleagues at Georgetown University in Washington, D.C., reported in September 1994. Nsouli's research team tested 104 children with recurring ear infections for food allergies and found that 81 of them were allergic to a food they commonly ate—most often milk or wheat. When the children stopped eating the foods to which they were allergic for a four-month period, 70 of them experienced a significant improvement in their ear troubles. When those children resumed eating the offending foods, 66 developed new ear infections. Nsouli explained that a food allergy may cause the middle ear to swell, thereby preventing fluids from draining from the ear. Bacteria can build up in the fluids, leading to an ear infection.

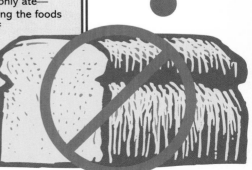

The world can be hard on our ears

Ear specialists warn that as many as 20 million Americans are routinely exposed to noise levels that could permanently damage their hearing. That number includes many fire fighters, police officers, military personnel, construction and factory workers, farmers, truckdrivers, and musicians. People regularly engaged in certain leisure activities, such as operating snowmobiles or power tools or listening to loud music, may also be putting their hearing at risk. Sound levels are expressed in units called decibels. A single short exposure to an extremely loud noise, such as a shotgun blast (140 decibels), can cause hearing loss by damaging tiny hairs in the inner ear. Hours of exposure to noise over about 85 decibels—the level of a power lawnmower—can produce the same effect. Doctors advise those who are around loud noise on a regular basis to protect their ears with ear plugs.

Some common sounds	Decibel level
Normal conversation	50 to 60
Busy traffic	70
Vacuum cleaner	75
Shop tools	80 to 95
Snowmobile	105
Rock concert	110 to 140
Jet plane takeoff	130
Civil defense siren	140

Source: National Institute on Deafness and Other Communication Disorders.

Surgical tubes for ear infections.

Eighty percent of small children will have at least one ear infection by the age of 2, John Niparko, director of ear surgery at Johns Hopkins Hospital in Baltimore reported in January 1995. He said the surgical implantation of a tube to drain fluid buildup in the middle ear is becoming the preferred treatment for controlling recurrent ear infections in children.

Normally, fluid produced in the ear drains through the Eustachian tube, a tiny channel that connects the middle ear to the back of the throat. Fluid accumulation in the middle ear is common in children because their Eustachian tubes tend to be shorter, narrower, and more horizontal than those of adults.

The placement of tubes in the middle ear to control this problem is a quick and simple outpatient procedure. The surgeon makes a tiny incision in the eardrum, draining the accumulated fluid behind it, and then inserts a tiny ventilation tube in the incision. The tube enables air to reach the middle ear and prevents further buildup of fluid.

The procedure—believed to be the most common childhood operation now performed—is used on more than 1 million children each year when antibiotics have failed to stop recurrent infections. After 6 to 24 months, the tubes loosen and fall out. By then, the Eustachian tubes have usually developed to the point where they are not so prone to infection.

Despite the procedure's effectiveness, it has been somewhat controversial because many doctors think most middle-ear infections will clear up on their own. In 1994, an advisory panel of the Agency for Health Care Policy and Research, a federal agency that develops guidelines for medical procedures, issued a recommendation that children with persistent fluid buildup in the ears should first be treated with "watchful waiting," which can include antibiotics. The panel said fluid buildup should not be treated until it has lasted at least three months.   • Julie Foreman

In the section On the Medical Frontier, see COCHLEAR IMPLANTS: DELIVERING SOUND TO THE DEAF. In WORLD BOOK, see DEAFNESS; EAR.

that only a minority of doctors actually use interpreters.

The researchers surveyed 73 physicians at the university's College of Medicine about their prior contacts with deaf patients and their methods of communicating with those patients. The survey found that 63 percent of the physicians said that signing should be the initial method of communication with deaf patients who sign, but only 22 percent of the doctors had used interpreters as their primary means of communication.

Writing was the most common way of communicating, reported by 34 percent of the doctors. After that, in declining order, were sign language interpreters, translation by friends and relatives, lip reading, and gestures.

Research reported in 1994 and 1995 highlighted several health risks associated with the everyday environment. Studies reported finding potentially harmful bacteria in some meats and in drinking water. Other studies reinforced long-standing concerns about the risks of air pollution and certain chemicals in the environment.

E. coli in salami. A potentially lethal strain of the *Escherichia coli* bacterium can survive in salami, according to investigators from the Centers for Disease Control and Prevention (CDC) in Atlanta, Georgia. CDC officials reported in March 1995 that *E. coli* had been responsible for an outbreak of diarrhea in 23 people in California and Washington in November and December 1994. The same bacterium in undercooked hamburgers killed several children in the United States and sickened thousands of children and adults in 1992 and 1993. The 1994 outbreak was the first one known to result from *E. coli* contamination of so-called fermented meats, a category that also includes pepperoni and summer sausage.

The latest outbreak of *E. coli* poisoning was traced to dry-cured salami bought from deli counters. Some scientists had known for at least two years that the bacteria could survive the processing of meats, but *E. coli's* presence did not become an issue

until the outbreak in November and December.

The bacteria are a problem only in meats that have not been *pasteurized* (heated to kill bacteria). Yet manufacturers do not routinely label such meats to indicate whether they have undergone pasteurization.

Particulates and health. Breathing particulates—tiny airborne bits of dust, soot, smoke, and acid aerosols from automobile exhausts and industrial emissions—increases the risk of death by 15 to 17 percent in the most polluted U.S. cities. This was the March 1995 conclusion of the largest study ever conducted on air quality and health. Even in cities that met federal clean-air standards, the risk of death was 3 to 8 percent higher than in the cleanest cities, the study found. Researchers from Harvard University in Cambridge, Massachusetts, and Brigham Young University in Provo, Utah, conducted the study.

The researchers studied more than 550,000 adults in 151 cities over the period 1982 through 1989. They observed an increased risk of early death in the polluted cities, whether they considered all causes of death or deaths from heart and lung diseases alone.

The researchers also looked at the effects of smoking, and they concluded that the increased risks from par-

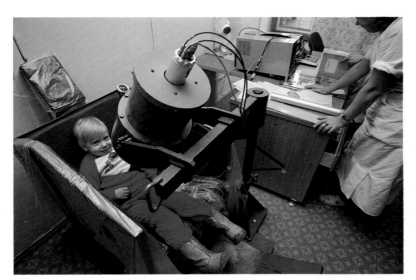

Chernobyl legacy
Medical researchers in late 1994 reported a fivefold increase in thyroid cancer among children who lived in the vicinity of the Chernobyl nuclear reactor in Ukraine in 1986, when an accident at the site spewed large amounts of radioactive material into the environment. Radiation from the reactor contaminated food and water supplies in neighboring Belarus, where this child was monitored for radiation exposure.

Environmental Health

Gulf War syndrome
Some 37,000 American veterans of the Persian Gulf War (1991) have experienced persistent dizziness, rashes, and fatigue since returning home, though no cause has ever been found for their symptoms. In May 1995, President Bill Clinton appointed a panel to look into the ailment, widely known as Gulf War syndrome.

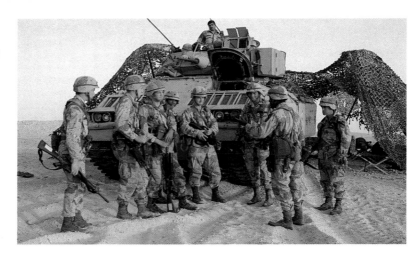

ticulate pollution were the same for smokers as for nonsmokers. They noted, however, that the increased risk from air pollution was small in comparison with the added risk from smoking. Smoking might reduce life span by about 10 years, compared with a 1-year reduction from particulate air pollution, according to Harvard epidemiologist and study participant Douglas W. Dockery.

The finding that smoking carries greater health risks than polluted air contradicts the conclusions of a study conducted by researchers at the University of California at Los Angeles (UCLA) and the American Lung Association. That study was reported in 1994.

Beginning in the early 1970's, the team monitored residents of Long Beach and Glendora—heavily polluted cities in the Los Angeles area—and compared them with residents of the much cleaner community of Lancaster, 75 miles (120 kilometers) north of Los Angeles. Results showed that nonsmoking men from the most polluted area had nearly as steep an annual decline in lung function as smokers living in the cleanest area.

Nonsmoking men living in Long Beach experienced a decline in lung function equal to 71 percent of the decline among men living in Lancaster who smoked one pack of cigarettes per day. Nonsmoking women living in Glendora had a 44 percent higher annual reduction in lung function than nonsmoking women in Lan-

caster, whereas nonsmoking women in Long Beach had a 58 percent higher decline. Smoking men who lived in the two polluted communities had the greatest decline of all.

Pollutants and fertility in men. A study by French medical researchers, reported in February 1995, added to a growing body of evidence that sperm counts are declining, possibly because of exposure to environmental pollutants. The team studied 1,351 preserved sperm samples taken between 1973 and 1992 from donors to a sperm bank in Paris. They found that the concentration of sperm in the men was 32.5 percent lower in 1992 than in 1973. The sperm donated in 1992 were also of significantly poorer quality in terms of vigor and normal shape than the 1973 sperm samples from men of the same age group.

The researchers speculated that the decline in sperm counts and sperm quality might result from exposure to certain pesticides and other environmental chemicals that disrupt normal male sexual development. Previous studies in the early 1990's had also shown declines in human sperm levels, but most of these studies had one or more defects that made experts skeptical of the findings. The previous research had claimed that the chemical structure of certain pollutants disrupts male sexual development by mimicking the female sex hormone estrogen.

Ulcers and drinking water. Gastro-enterologists reached agreement in the early 1990's that a bacterium called *Helicobacter pylori* causes most *ulcers* (painful irritations of the stomach or small intestine). Experts believe that the bacteria disturb the lining of the stomach, allowing digestive acids to attack the stomach wall.

Researchers are uncertain about how the bacteria spread, though many of them suspect that the bacteria may spread from person to person through contact with infected feces. But evidence reported in May 1995 indicated that *H. pylori* may exist in water, which would make it more widespread than previously thought.

The researchers, led by veterinarian David B. Schauer of the Massachusetts Institute of Technology in Cambridge, employed a highly sensitive technique called polymerase chain reaction to detect the presence of *H. pylori* bacteria in the water supply of Narino, Colombia, a town in which infection with the bacteria is common. The researchers were unsure, however, whether the strain of *H. pylori* in the water was the one that most commonly infected the townspeople.

• **Thomas H. Maugh II**

In the section Medical and Safety Alerts, see POISON ON THE MENU. In WORLD BOOK, see ENVIRONMENTAL POLLUTION.

Vigorous exercise, but not light or moderate exercise, helps increase the life span of men, according to a study reported in April 1995 by researchers at the Harvard School of Public Health in Boston and Stanford University in California.

The researchers studied 17,321 middle-aged, male Harvard graduates who were free of cardiovascular disease, cancer, and chronic lung disease. Each participant had completed questionnaires in the 1960's that asked how many hours he spent each week climbing flights of stairs, walking city blocks, and participating in sports. It also asked what types of sports or recreational activities he engaged in. This information gave researchers an assessment of each participant's level of physical activity.

Using these data, the researchers estimated how much energy each participant expended in such vigorous activity as brisk walking, jogging, swimming, and playing tennis and in such light or moderate activity as golf, bowling, and walking at a casual pace. The study continued until 1988, by which time 3,728 of the men had died.

In analyzing the data, researchers took into account a number of factors that could hasten death, including

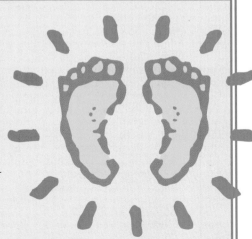

Keeping feet fit

Exercise may be good for the body, but it can be hard on the feet. The American Podiatric Medical Association offers a series of free brochures on foot health for specific activities—walking, running, aerobics, fitness, baseball, basketball, cycling, golf, tennis, and winter sports—as well as one on sports and children's feet. To request a copy of any of these, call 800-366-8227.

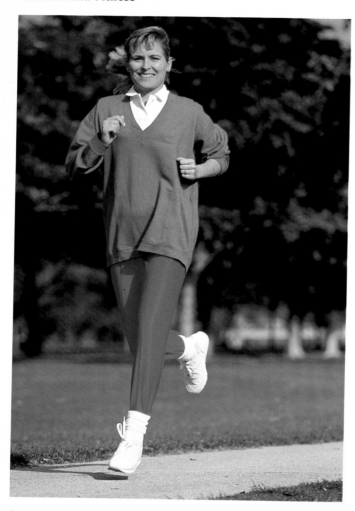

span, according to a study reported in April 1995 by researchers at the Cooper Institute for Aerobics Research in Dallas. Unlike previous studies, which have shown that a lack of physical fitness can shorten life span, this study examined the effect of changes in fitness and how they relate to life span.

The researchers studied 9,777 men who ranged in age from 20 to 82 years. In each of two examinations over a period of about five years, the researchers assessed each participant's level of physical fitness by his performance on a treadmill endurance test. The men were then categorized as fit or unfit at each examination. The researchers followed the men for another five years to determine whether changes in fitness affected their life span.

Men who were rated physically unfit at both examinations had the highest death rate, and men who were rated fit at both examinations had the lowest. The unfit men who improved their level of fitness between the first and second examination had on average a death rate 44 percent lower than men who were rated unfit at both examinations. Because the improvement in physical fitness was related to an increase in physical activity, the researchers recommended that physicians encourage unfit men to start a physical activity program.

Exercise may reduce breast cancer risk

Regular exercise may reduce the risk of breast cancer for women under 40 by as much as 60 percent, according to a study at the University of Southern California's North Cancer Center. Authors of the study note that the more frequent the exercise, the lower the risk of cancer. However, even two to three hours of moderate exercise a week may be beneficial.

obesity, smoking, hypertension, diabetes, and a family history of early death. When the researchers examined the participants' energy expenditure, they found that only energy expended in vigorous exercise was associated with increased longevity.

How intense physical activity needs to be to provide health benefits has been a source of controversy, in part because few studies have compared vigorous and nonvigorous activity. The researchers cautioned that their findings applied only to early death and said that light or moderate exercise can still provide health benefits.

Longer life with improved fitness.

Physically unfit men who become physically fit can increase their life

The benefits of strength training.

Intensive strength training helps reduce the risk of fractures associated with *osteoporosis* (thinning of bone tissue) in women 50 to 70 years old, according to a study reported in December 1994 by researchers at Tufts University in Medford, Massachusetts, and at Pennsylvania State University in University Park. The risk factors for fractures include bone fragility, muscle weakness, and poor balance.

Researchers recruited 40 postmenopausal women and randomly assigned them to either a strength-training group or a control group that did not take part in strength training. Women assigned to the strength-training group participated in high-intensity strength training two days per week for one year. The exercises included in the training—hip extension, knee extension, lateral pull-down, back extension, and abdominal flexion—worked the major muscle groups attached to the bones that most commonly fracture as a result of osteoporosis.

The researchers found that among the women who participated in the strength training, bone density increased in both the lower spine and the hip, which indicates increased bone strength. They also noted that bone density decreased in these sites among the control women. Similarly, total body bone density was preserved in the strength-trained women, but it tended to decrease in the control women. Muscle mass and

strength also increased and balance improved among the strength-trained women, whereas each of these potentially protective factors decreased among the control group.

Reducing falls among seniors. Exercise may help prevent falls among older people, according to a study sponsored by the National Institute on Aging and the National Institute for Nursing Research. The study was reported in May 1995.

Falls are common among older people and constitute a potentially serious threat to their health. Poor balance, reduced strength, slow reaction time, and lack of flexibility all

Keep to a comfortable lace

The standard "crisscross" way of lacing athletic shoes may work for most people, but those with specific foot problems should customize their lacing style, says orthopedic surgeon Carol Frey of the University of Southern California. She recommends the following lacing patterns for special needs:

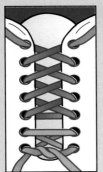 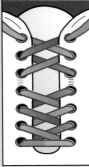 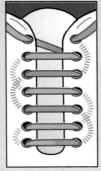 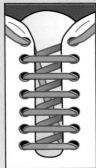 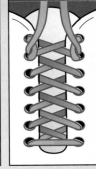

1. **Narrow heel and wider forefoot:** Use two laces, one in the front and another further back, and adjust separately.

2. **Painful spot:** To avoid pressure over a bump, protruding bone, or other sensitive area, leave a space in the lacing at that spot.

3. **High arches:** Lace in parallel lines to avoid pressure from laces crossing over the top of the foot.

4. **Toe problems:** Lace one end using a spiral, and let the other end run straight from the front to the back. Pull that lace to raise the toe area, providing extra room for hammertoes, corns, or other toe troubles.

5. **Loose heel:** To keep the heel firmly in place, use the top two eyelets to form a loop of lacing on each side. Thread each end through the opposite loop; then tie.

contribute to the higher risk of falls among senior citizens. To determine whether short-term exercise programs could reduce frailty and the risk of falls, researchers compiled data from seven independent clinical trials. Each trial included an exercise regimen lasting from 10 to 36 weeks for study participants, who were 60 to 75 years old. Participants in the studies were followed for two to four years to establish whether the exercise programs had a long-term impact on preventing falls and fall-related injuries.

The character, duration, frequency, and intensity of the exercise programs varied across the studies. But each training program included at least one of the following elements: endurance, flexibility, balance, or resistance training.

The researchers found that seniors who participated in a general exercise program experienced 10 percent fewer falls during the follow-up period and those who also had balance training experienced 17 percent fewer falls. The researchers said that additional research was needed to determine whether exercise programs for seniors can reduce fall-related injuries.   • David S. Siscovick

In the section A Healthy You, see HOW MUCH EXERCISE IS ENOUGH? In WORLD BOOK, see PHYSICAL FITNESS.

Eye and Vision

The full results of a study that found an eye surgery procedure ineffective and potentially harmful were reported in February 1995. The National Eye Institute, one of the National Institutes of Health, had already recommended in October 1994 that the procedure be halted and had alerted physicians to its potential harm. The study was conducted at 25 clinics across the United States.

The study involved patients who underwent optic nerve decompression surgery (ONDS) for treatment of a disease of the optic nerve called nonarteritic anterior ischemic optic neuropathy (NAION). NAION causes sudden, painless loss of vision in one eye. It is brought on by swelling of the optic disc, a region at the back of the eye that connects the retina with the optic nerve, which leads to the brain. An estimated 1,500 to 6,000 cases of NAION are diagnosed in the United States each year. Early studies had indicated that ONDS could reduce swelling and improve vision. But many doctors remained skeptical about its effectiveness.

For this reason, the federal government launched a large clinical trial of ONDS in 1992. Researchers recruited 244 patients with NAION and randomly assigned 119 of them to un-

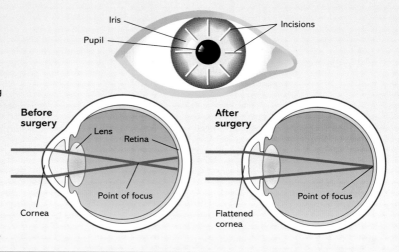

Correcting near-sightedness surgically

Radial keratotomy (RK) is a surgical procedure to correct near-sightedness, which occurs when light rays focus before reaching the light-sensitive retina. Incisions are made in the cornea to flatten it, moving the point of focus back to the retina. A National Eye Institute study of 374 patients, reported in 1995, found RK effective but said 43 percent of the patients needed reading glasses afterward.

Iris — Incisions
Pupil —

Before surgery
Lens
Retina
Point of focus
Cornea

After surgery
Point of focus
Flattened cornea

dergo surgery and 125 to receive close monitoring only. After six months, the researchers found that the patients who were monitored had a higher rate of vision improvement than the patients who had the surgery. Moreover, 23.9 percent of the surgical patients had actually lost some vision, whereas vision worsened in only 12.4 percent of the monitored group. The scientists said this finding suggests that many patients improve on their own.

Correcting vision with lasers. In October 1994, an advisory panel to the U.S. Food and Drug Administration (FDA) recommended that the FDA approve the use of lasers to correct *myopia* (near-sightedness). The panel also recommended that FDA approval depend on the manufacturer's ability to show the FDA that 75 percent of the people undergoing the procedure would no longer need corrective lenses and that the surgery would worsen vision in only a tiny percentage of patients.

People with myopia have difficulty seeing objects at a distance because light rays that enter their eyes focus before reaching the light-sensitive cells of the retina. In the laser procedure, called photorefractive keratectomy (PRK), a surgeon sculpts the transparent cornea covering the pupil with a computer-guided laser. By removing a thin layer of corneal cells, the surgery moves the point of focus back to the retina.

A number of studies have reported success in using PRK on patients with mild myopia. But in April 1995, researchers at the University at Melbourne in Australia reported preliminary findings of PRK's effectiveness in treating extreme myopia. Vision tests six months after surgery found a 90 percent improvement in myopia in the majority of patients. One side effect of the therapy was a loss of corneal transparency. The scientists said this "corneal haze" had started to clear in the majority of patients by a year after surgery but that more data were needed to confirm the findings.

Reducing diabetic blindness. About half of the adults with diabetes in the United States are not having recom-

A blight of sore eyes

Children know it as "pinkeye" because the white of the eye turns red. Doctors call this common condition conjunctivitis—meaning an inflammation of the *conjunctiva*, the membrane that lines the eyelids and the white of the eye. In addition to redness, symptoms include burning, itching, or watering of the eye, which may also produce a sticky pus. Cold compresses, soothing eyedrops, and time can help relieve eyes inflamed from allergies, sleeplessness, or irritants like smoke or chlorinated pool water. Many cases, though, result from infection. Viral infections often pass on their own within a few days, and antibiotic drops or ointments will usually clear up bacterial conjunctivitis. Because stubborn cases may lead to eye damage, it's wise to consult a doctor whenever pinkeye occurs. Meanwhile, remember that eye infections can spread through secretions, so wash an infected child's hands—and yours—frequently.

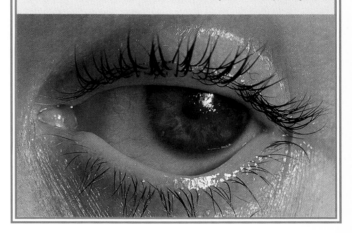

mended eye examinations to detect and treat diabetic retinopathy, according to an October 1994 report from the Centers for Disease Control and Prevention (CDC) in Atlanta, Georgia. Damage to the retina known as retinopathy occurs when tiny blood vessels in the retina leak fluid. It is a common complication of unregulated diabetes, and it can lead to blindness. Regular eye examinations, in which the pupil is dilated to permit examination of the retina, can detect diabetic retinopathy at an early, treatable stage, reducing the risk of blindness.

The CDC researchers reviewed questionnaires included in the 1989 National Health Interview Survey sent to more than 84,000 people in the United States. About 2,400 had been returned by people diagnosed with diabetes. Only 49 percent of these respondents—1,179 people—said they received an eye examination each year. The older the person was, the more likely that he or she had an annual eye examination, and people who said they attended diabetes education classes also were more likely to have had an examination.

The study prompted the American Diabetes Association to repeat its recommendation that people with insulin-dependent (Type II) diabetes have a dilated eye examination annually, starting five years after the diagnosis of diabetes. The association also recommended that people diagnosed with noninsulin-dependent (Type I) diabetes have a dilated eye examination immediately and every year thereafter.

Vegetables and vision. Eating dark green, leafy vegetables may decrease the risk of blindness from an age-related degeneration of the retina known as macular degeneration. In November 1994, researchers from the Massachusetts Eye and Ear Infirmary in Boston and other institutions reported results of a study to determine whether certain molecules in foods, called carotenoids, might slow the progression of the disease. Carotenoids are a family of yellow, orange, and red pigments. The best known carotenoid is beta-carotene.

Food
See Nutrition and Food

Macular degeneration is the most common cause of blindness in people over age 65. It is caused by fluid leaking into the center of the retina, an area called the macula where vision is sharpest. The leakage is often followed by hemorrhaging, scarring, and permanent loss of central vision, though peripheral vision usually remains unimpaired. There is no known means of prevention, and treatment for the disorder is effective for only a fraction of patients.

The researchers studied 356 men and women aged 55 to 80 who had been diagnosed with advanced macular degeneration within one year prior to enrolling in the study. The patients were surveyed extensively about their diet, and from the surveys, the researchers calculated the amounts of vitamins and other nutrients each person consumed each day.

The researchers found that the people with the highest intake of carotenoids had a 43 percent lower risk of macular degeneration than those with the lowest intake. The carotenoids most responsible for lowering risk—lutein and zeaxanthin—were found primarily in dark green, leafy vegetables, such as spinach and broccoli. The two substances also form the yellow pigment in the macula. The researchers emphasized that further studies were needed to confirm the findings.   • Julie Foreman
In WORLD BOOK, see EYE.

Genetic Medicine

The identification of a gene that increases the risk of breast and ovarian cancer was reported in October 1994 by a team of biologists and physicians in the United States and Canada. The finding may lead to a test that would identify women who carry the gene.

Cancer is a disease in which cell division, the normal process that produces new cells in the body, runs out out of control. Put simply, cancerous cells do not know when to stop multiplying. Although all cancers are genetic in the sense that the cellular damage and loss of control involves genes, not all cancers are hereditary. Only about 5 percent of breast cancers, for example, may be caused by

an inherited faulty gene. Hereditary forms of breast cancer, however, probably account for about 25 percent of breast cancer cases that occur before age 30.

In 1990, geneticists mapped a hereditary breast cancer gene called BRCA1 to chromosome 17 by studying families that had a history of breast cancer. (Human genes are contained in 23 pairs of chromosomes, tiny threadlike structures in the cell nucleus.) That discovery touched off a worldwide race to isolate the gene. The U.S. and Canadian researchers, led by geneticist Mark H. Skolnick of the University of Utah Medical Center in Salt Lake City, succeeded at that task.

The investigators said as many as 1 in 200 women may carry the BRCA1 gene. The gene, they said, may "account for 45 percent of families with increased incidence of breast cancer and at least 80 percent of families with increased incidence of both early-onset breast cancer and ovarian cancer." A second gene associated with breast cancer, labeled BRCA2, is located on chromosome 13. This gene may be responsible for as much early-onset breast cancer as BRCA1, but scientists do not think that it is involved in ovarian cancer.

The BRCA1 gene probably *codes for* (contains encoded information for producing) a type of protein that biologists call a tumor suppressor, which helps regulate cell division. If the gene is altered by any of several types of *mutations* (molecular changes), the gene's protein will be improperly formed and unable to carry out its role.

A woman who inherits one copy of the altered BRCA1 gene has inherited a predisposition to breast cancer. If dietary factors, smoking, exposure to radiation, or other environmental influences cause a mutation in the second, functional copy of the gene, the tumor-suppressing function of that gene, too, will be lost. Cancer is then likely to develop.

The isolation of BRCA1 has raised optimism about the possibility of developing a test to identify women who carry the gene. That prospect, however, poses certain scientific and ethical difficulties. Who, for instance, will ensure the quality of the testing, and who will provide education and counseling for those women whose test results contain bad news? Furthermore, should employers or insurance companies have access to the test results? To address these issues, the Office of Human Genome Research at the National Institutes of Health in Bethesda, Maryland, has funded some 30 special projects to investigate the implications of widespread testing for breast and ovarian cancer.

A rare but important gene. Yet another gene involved in breast cancer came to light as a result of the search for the gene associated with a rare genetic disorder called ataxia telangiectasia (AT). An international team of scientists at Tel Aviv University in Israel reported in June 1995 that it had isolated the gene. Although AT afflicts no more than 1 in 40,000 people around the world, the AT gene could yield important insights into the nature of cancer.

The AT gene produces a variety of symptoms, including a lack of coordination, caused by deterioration of the cerebellum, the part of the brain primarily responsible for balance and coordinating movement. Affected individuals usually do not live beyond

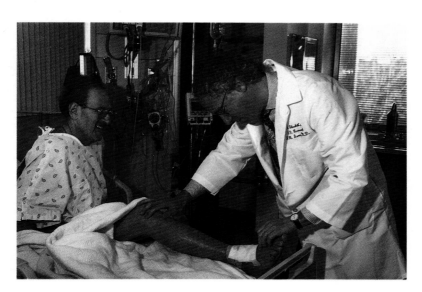

New genes to save a leg

Physician Jeffrey Isner checks the leg of his patient Michael Ruo at St. Elizabeth's Hospital in Brighton, Massachusetts, in December 1994. Ruo had faced amputation of the leg because of blockages that had reduced blood flow to a trickle. Genes that direct the production of new blood vessels were introduced into the leg to improve circulation. It may someday be possible to use the technique to bypass blockages in the heart.

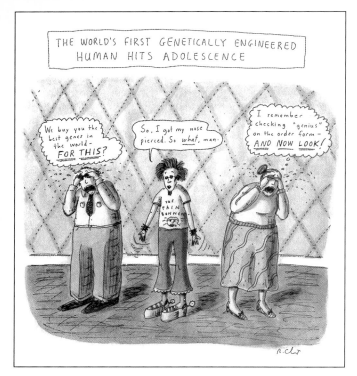

tists believe, one of the key proteins controlling cell division.

If that proves to be the case, the AT gene may be one of the most important discoveries in genetics in recent years. An understanding of the gene and its protein may lead to a better understanding of cellular reproduction and the onset of cancer. In addition, the isolation of the AT gene offers the prospect of improved cancer screening in the general population, though that is still some time in the future.

Genes and obesity. The isolation of a gene associated with excess weight gain was reported in December 1994 by geneticist Jeffrey M. Friedman and his colleagues at Rockefeller University in New York City. Friedman's team built on work done nearly 50 years ago, when U.S. geneticists discovered a genetic defect that causes some mice to become extremely obese.

The Rockefeller University group pursued the gene responsible for this disorder—called *ob,* for *obese*—for eight years, finally tracking it to mouse chromosome 6. The researchers theorized that the gene is a mutated version of a gene that normally keeps body weight within certain set limits. They said the normal gene probably codes for a protein that tells the mouse's brain when the mouse's stomach is full. Further research revealed that the gene does indeed contain a mutation.

Friedman's team then examined DNA from other species, including human DNA, for a corresponding gene. They found similar genetic sequences in the human DNA and many of the other DNA samples.

The isolation of the *ob* gene and the resulting insights into the related protein raise the possibility of new treatments for obesity. A genetically engineered version of the protein, for example, might be given to an obese patient to replace the defective protein, thereby reintroducing the chemical signals that regulate food intake.

Researchers caution strongly, however, against assuming that with the isolation of *ob,* we have found "the cause" of obesity. Like most human traits, body weight results from a complex interaction of genetic and

their late teens or early twenties. AT is inherited as a recessive trait, which means that a person must inherit two copies of the AT gene, one from each parent, to develop the disorder.

Earlier findings about the AT gene led the research team to a potentially groundbreaking discovery. Previous evidence had indicated that women with one copy of the defective AT gene have perhaps a five-times higher risk of breast cancer than the general population. Moreover, when cells that contain one mutated AT gene are grown in the laboratory and exposed to X rays, they accumulate more damage to their DNA (deoxyribonucleic acid, the molecule genes are made of) than do cells with two normal copies of the gene. This inability to repair DNA damage may lead to the development of cancer.

Analysis of the AT gene by the researchers in Israel indicated that it codes for a protein that is central to cell growth and development. In particular, this protein minimizes any damage that occurs to a cell's DNA and stops cell division until such damage is repaired. It is, the scien-

environmental factors. Much more research is necessary before scientists fully understand the intricacies of weight control.

Genes and sex determination. Research reported in December 1994 goes a long way toward answering a fundamental biological question: "How did a newborn first become a male or female?" Not surprisingly, the new findings reveal a complex series of genetic and biochemical steps leading to the determination of sex. The research project was directed by geneticist Michael A. Weiss of the University of Chicago and also included scientists at Harvard Medical School and Massachusetts General Hospital, both in Boston.

Biologists have long known that the embryos of all mammals, at an early formative stage, start to develop female reproductive organs. This occurs even if the embryo's cells have the male-determining Y chromosome. (The two sex-determining chromosomes are designated X and Y. Female embryos have two X chromosomes in each cell; male embryos have one X and one Y.)

At some point in the development of male embryos, a gene on the Y chromosome—designated SRY—switches on and begins the molecular and biochemical processes that produce a male offspring.

Weiss and his colleagues investigat-ed how SRY works. The gene, they concluded, is probably a regulatory gene that influences the expression of a second gene, called MIS. The MIS gene evidently causes the female structures in the fetus to recede. SRY also influences the production of testosterone, a hormone that stimulates the development of male reproductive organs in the XY embryo.

In earlier research, the team had analyzed the structure of the two genes taken from the cells of people with disrupted sexual development to explore the normal molecular steps in fetal development. These clinical studies supported the scientists' theories about the two genes. They learned, for example, that mutations in the MIS gene result in the persistence of female reproductive structures and that mutations in the SRY gene can result in sex reversal, producing XX males and XY females.

Biologists are hopeful that this new work will lead to additional insights into the genetic and cellular events that regulate sexual development. Such knowledge might lead to improved treatments for reproductive disorders and, perhaps, to improved understanding of the cellular switches that go awry and result in cancer.

• Joseph D. McInerney

See also DIABETES. In the section On the Medical Frontier, see ARE WE WINNING THE WAR ON CANCER? In WORLD BOOK, see CELL; GENETICS.

Some abnormal thyroid conditions result from faulty genes that cause a delicate hormonal interaction to go awry, according to two studies published in January 1995. The thyroid is a gland that wraps around the front of the windpipe. Hormones produced by the thyroid control the rate at which the body's cells convert oxygen and nutrients into energy. The thyroid's production of hormones is regulated by a hormone called thyroid-stimulating hormone (TSH), which is secreted by the pituitary, a gland at the base of the brain.

A precise feedback mechanism operates between the thyroid and pituitary glands. If the thyroid produces too much thyroid hormone, a condition called hyperthyroidism, the pituitary stops secreting TSH. If the thyroid produces too little thyroid hormone, a condition called hypothyroidism develops and the pituitary releases excessive amounts of TSH. Doctors diagnose hyperthyroidism and hypothyroidism by checking TSH levels in the blood.

TSH molecules stimulate the thyroid gland by acting as "keys" to TSH receptors, "keyholes" in thyroid cell surfaces. The 1995 studies showed that defective TSH receptors could upset thyroid hormone regulation. In a study conducted at the University of Chicago, three siblings who had inherited a *mutated* (altered) gene from both parents were found to have defective TSH receptors. Although the children had normal thyroid function, they had abnormally high blood levels of TSH. Elevated TSH alone could have led doctors to conclude mistakenly that the children had hypothyroidism and to prescribe thyroid hormone supplements inappropriately.

The second study was reported by researchers who were led by Peter Kopp of Northwestern University in Chicago. They described a case of hyperthyroidism in a child who had a mutation in the same gene. The mutation left the TSH receptor permanently "turned on" so that the thyroid produced excessive amounts of thyroid hormone. Doctors surgically removed the thyroid gland to cure her.

Fountain of youth. A hormone responsible for growth may slow the aging process, according to research reported in late 1994 by investigators from the University of Virginia in Charlottesville and Merck Research Laboratories in Rahway, New Jersey. Growth hormone (GH) is released by the pituitary gland and is regulated by other hormones. Growth-hormone-releasing hormone (GHRH) stimulates GH release, and somatostatin blocks GH release. Both of these are released by the hypothalamus, a structure at the base of the brain.

During the aging process, GH levels decrease. This decline is accompanied by a decrease in bone mass and muscle mass, a decreased ability to exercise, and an increase in fat deposits. It is not known if the loss of GH is directly involved in all these aspects of aging, but research has shown that body fat decreases and lean body mass increases in people who receive GH injections.

The Virginia and New Jersey researchers developed a chemical they called L-692-429, which raised GH levels in the blood. It seems that the drug stimulated the release of GHRH and blocked the effects of somatostatin. If further studies prove it safe and effective, L-692-429 may become a "fountain of youth."

Conflicting findings on HRT. Two studies reported in June and July 1995 reached different conclusions on the risks of hormone replacement therapy (HRT) taken by women after menopause. The June study, led by researchers at Harvard Medical School in Boston, found a 30 to 40 percent increase in breast cancer cases among women who received HRT for five or more years. The July study, led by epidemiologist Janet L. Stanford at the University of Washington in Seattle, found no difference in hormone use between a group of women who developed breast cancer and a group who did not.

Previous studies have shown that HRT has substantial benefits in lowering the risks of heart disease and os-

Alcohol raises female testosterone levels

After a couple of alcoholic beverages, a woman's normally low level of the male hormone testosterone increases, according to a group of Finnish and Japanese researchers who published their findings in September 1994. The study generated interest because testosterone is thought to stimulate sexual desire in both men and women.

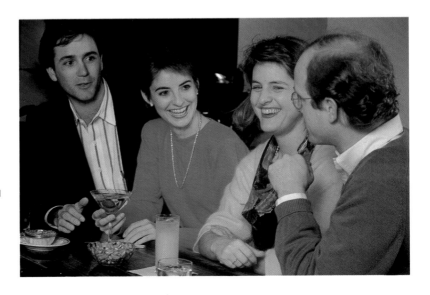

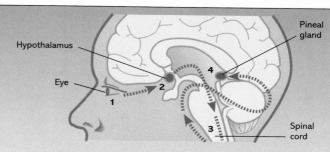

A natural sleep aid?

The brain hormone melatonin, which helps control sleep cycles, may someday provide a safe treatment for such problems as jet lag and insomnia. A March 1995 study reported by researchers at the Massachusetts Institute of Technology in Cambridge, Massachusetts, found that small doses of melatonin worked like a sleeping pill in 20 healthy volunteers. Researchers are now studying ways to use synthetic versions of the hormone to treat sleep disorders.

Daylight entering through the eye (1) helps set the brain's internal clock, a cluster of nerve cells located in the hypothalamus (2). When night comes, the clock sends out a signal that travels a roundabout path down the spinal cord (3) and back up to the brain, eventually reaching the pineal gland (4). In response, this tiny gland produces the hormone melatonin, which encourages sleep.

teoporosis (loss of bone density) in postmenopausal women. The two 1995 studies led researchers to emphasize that each woman should discuss with her doctor specific risks associated with long-term HRT before reaching a decision.

Obesity and hormones. The discovery of a gene that may contribute to obesity was announced in December 1994 by researchers at Rockefeller University in New York City. Obesity is defined as weighing at least 20 percent more than recommended body weight. (See WEIGHT CONTROL.)

The researchers used specially bred obese mice to isolate the gene.

They theorize that the gene normally controls appetite by causing fat cells to secrete a hormone into the blood. This hormone sends signals to the brain that produce a sensation of fullness. If the gene malfunctions, however, the mice do not feel full and go on eating. A nearly identical gene has been found in human beings.

By August 1995, three research teams, including the Rockefeller group, had confirmed the presence of the hormone, named leptin. When obese mice were given leptin, they lost weight rapidly, giving researchers hope that a treatment for obesity may be near.　　　　• Andre J. Van Herle

In WORLD BOOK, see GLAND; HORMONE.

Efforts to reform the nation's health care system were resurrected in 1995, after months of heated debate and a bruising battle in Congress left the fate of the health care system unresolved in 1994. In November 1994, the Republicans gained control of both the U.S. House of Representatives and the U.S. Senate, and their determination to balance the federal budget left even well-established federal and state health care programs at risk of significant cutbacks.

The fight for health care reform. The plan for universal health insurance coverage, cost controls, and major reconfiguring of health care delivery and financing—first proposed by

President Bill Clinton in September 1993—continued to face wave after wave of opposition during the summer of 1994. Even Democratic support for the President's proposal waned, and legislators tried to put together a bill that was acceptable to both Republicans and Democrats.

On Aug. 2, 1994, Senator George J. Mitchell (D., Me.), then Senate majority leader, proposed a bill that was considered a compromise between the wide-ranging Clinton plan and the limited Republican proposals. Mitchell's plan set a goal of insurance coverage for 95 percent of U.S. citizens by the year 2000. In mid-1994, an estimated 15 to 20 percent of U.S. citizens had no insurance.

Health Care Issues

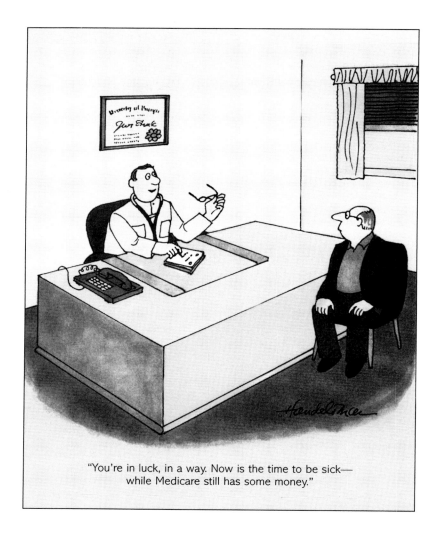

"You're in luck, in a way. Now is the time to be sick—
while Medicare still has some money."

The Mitchell plan also stipulated that if the goal was not achieved, a backup plan would take effect. Financing for the Mitchell plan would come from cuts in spending on Medicare (the government health insurance for retirees), elimination of most of Medicaid (government-funded health care for the poor and some other groups), and tax increases.

The Mitchell bill was widely seen as a last gasp effort in the losing battle to reform health care in the United States. And just as the Clinton proposal drew broad opposition from Republicans, insurance companies, labor interests, and others, so did the Mitchell bill.

In late August, a group of moderate senators, led by John H. Chafee

(R., R.I.) and John Breaux (D., La.), tried to formulate a less sweeping and more bipartisan bill. But their efforts were also defeated as employers, labor, and other interest groups criticized it.

As time went on, it looked less and less likely that both sides of Congress would reach a consensus on a plan for health care reform. Finally, on September 26, Senator Mitchell admitted failure and declared health care reform dead for the year.

Robert J. Dole (R., Kans.), who was then Senate minority leader, had been a major opponent of the Democratic proposals. He stated that the Clinton plan failed because it was too big, too complex, too costly, and too bureaucratic. Democrats, on the other hand, blamed Republicans and special-interest lobbies for the defeat of health care reform in 1994.

New Congress tackles health care. The mid-term election of 1994, held on November 8, completely changed the health policy landscape. For the first time since the 1950's, Republicans were in control of both houses of Congress. Many new members of Congress were conservative and pledged to reduce the federal budget deficit, no matter what the cost—a pledge that threatened the funding of federal health care programs.

However, in July 1995, Senator Nancy Landon Kassebaum (R., Kans.), the new chair of the Senate Labor and Human Resources Committee, introduced a reform proposal to Congress that appealed to many. The bill, which was cosponsored by Senator Edward M. Kennedy (D., Mass.), would supposedly make it easier for people to keep insurance coverage if they became ill or changed jobs.

The bill would prohibit insurers from denying coverage to workers whose health was poor. It would also allow workers leaving a company and starting their own business to keep their group health insurance from their former company as long as they met all payments. The bill had the support of the majority of Kassebaum's committee, and the committee approved it on Aug. 2, 1995.

Health insurance lobbyists said that it would lead to higher premiums.

Mantle gets liver transplant. The continuing shortage of donor organs and the issue of how scarce organs are distributed made news in June 1995 with reports that baseball Hall of Fame outfielder Mickey Mantle was in need of a liver transplant. Mantle, who had been hospitalized on May 28 for stomach pains, was suffering from liver cancer, the liver disease hepatitis, and cirrhosis—a disease often associated with heavy drinking, to which Mantle admitted.

Although many patients must wait weeks or months for organs, Mantle received a liver within days of his diagnosis. Several newspapers voiced suspicions that he had been allowed to receive a transplant ahead of others because of his celebrity status. His surgeons insisted that this was not the case. Other questions about the appropriateness of Mantle's transplant were raised a few weeks later, when it was revealed that his cancer had spread. Mantle died on August 13, nine weeks after the transplant.

Physician-assisted suicide was on the election agenda in Oregon in 1994. Voters approved a referendum called Measure 16 that allows physicians to prescribe to their dying patients medications with which the patients could end their lives.

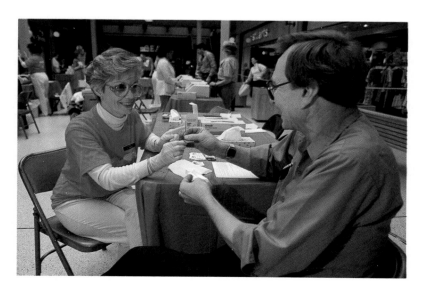

Get a second opinion! Some instant cholesterol tests, such as those often performed in shopping malls, can be inaccurate by as much as 50 percent, according to government investigators. Health officials say that even clinical laboratory results can vary and advise patients not to rely on only one blood test to determine cholesterol level.

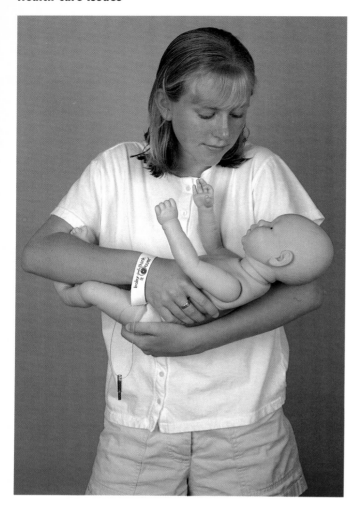

Life with baby

High schools and health clinics around the country are using lifelike dolls to encourage young people to hold off on parenthood. The dolls, called Baby Think It Over, are programmed to cry at different times, both day and night. The only way to get the doll to stop crying is to hold a key in its back for 5 to 35 minutes, about the length of time it takes to feed an infant.

Measure 16, also known as the Death with Dignity Act, stipulated that patients covered by the act would need to have less than six months left to live and would be required to make the request three times, the last time in writing. The patient would also have to obtain from a second physician an opinion stating that the patient's condition was terminal. The doctor prescribing the lethal dose of medication would have to inform the patient of any treatment options available and would have to wait 15 days from the first oral request before fulfilling the request for the prescription.

Voter approval of the bill set off a bitter controversy between right-to-die advocates and those who oppose assisted suicide. On Dec. 27, 1994, a federal judge issued a preliminary injunction, preventing the law from going into effect. And on Aug. 7, 1995, the judge ruled the measure unconstitutional. Supporters of assisted suicide filed an immediate appeal.

The Kevorkian case. In December 1994, the Michigan Supreme Court ruled that there is no constitutional right to suicide and that those who aid patients in taking their own lives can be prosecuted for common-law felony. Conviction for the felony carries a five-year prison term.

Despite this ruling, retired physician Jack Kevorkian, who has received widespread publicity for assisting in the suicides of terminally ill people, was present for two suicides in May 1995, one in June, and one in August. These deaths brought the total number of suicides in which he has been involved to 25. The June death occurred in his "obitorium," a building he had rented to provide a place in which patients could commit suicide.

The owner of the building where the June death occurred gave Kevorkian one month to close his operation. The prosecutor's office in Oakland County indicated that it would probably file charges in the case. Kevorkian already faced two counts of murder for his past involvement in the deaths of terminally ill persons.

Surgeon general battle. On Dec. 9, 1994, President Clinton fired Surgeon General Jocelyn Elders after she stated publicly that there was an argument for teaching children about masturbation as a means of combating the spread of AIDS. It was the latest of several remarks she had made that the President and others felt were too controversial to be coming from someone in her position.

Clinton subsequently nominated Henry Foster for the post. Foster, an obstetrician-gynecologist from Tennessee, was known for his much-praised plan to reduce teen pregnancies by building job skills, self-esteem, and responsibility in young women. However, his confirmation became controversial after reports surfaced that he had performed legal abortions as a physician. Just how many abortions he had performed was also called into question. The White House first reported that he had performed fewer than a dozen abortions, but eventually, after Foster said he had reviewed his records, the total was revised to 39.

During his May confirmation hearings before the Senate Labor and Human Resources Committee, Foster impressed many senators, and the committee approved his nomination.

However, Senator Phil Gramm (R., Tex.), an announced candidate for the 1996 Republican presidential nomination, promised that he would filibuster to block the nomination if it came to the Senate floor. Majority Leader Dole, another Republican presidential hopeful, announced that there would not be a direct vote on the Foster nomination. Instead, there would be a vote to see if there were enough votes to break a filibuster. The vote, taken on June 22, 1995, indicated that a filibuster would succeed, so the nomination never came to a vote. Clinton angrily denounced the maneuver and did not submit another nomination.

Proposition 187. In November, 1994, California voters approved a controversial state ballot referendum called Proposition 187, which was aimed at curbing illegal immigration. The initiative would have denied nonemergency health care and a number of other social services to undocumented aliens. It would also have required health care providers to report to the immigration authorities anyone suspected of being an illegal immigrant. On December 14, a federal district judge in Los Angeles ruled that the initiative conflicted with federal law on health and social services and banned California from carrying out most provisions of the measure.

Medicare budget crisis. Efforts to limit spending on Medicare gained new urgency in April 1995, when the trustees of the part of Medicare that pays for hospital services reported on April 3 that its trust fund could run out of money by the year 2002. The fund, which is financed by payroll taxes, accounts for about two-thirds of all Medicare spending.

Looming budget cuts. The House and the Senate began outlining plans to balance the budget in early 1995. Part of the plan included significant cuts in Medicare and Medicaid.

The Republican budget plan called for Medicaid to become a block grant, through which state governors would receive a lump-sum payment from the federal government. The plan would include fewer restrictions than the federal government had previously placed on use of the funds. Many governors like the block-grant idea, though some expressed concern that the grants might contain less federal money than would have been spent on Medicaid otherwise.

By late June, the House and the Senate had agreed to take $270 billion from Medicare over seven years and $180 billion from Medicaid over the same period. President Clinton agreed that some cuts in Medicaid and Medicare were necessary to balance the budget, but he proposed cutting only $127 billion from Medicare and $54 billion from Medicaid.

The actual reductions would be determined later. However, Clinton hinted strongly that he would veto any proposal that included what he considered "unacceptable" cuts.

Growth in managed care. Managed care programs continued to grow in popularity in 1994 and 1995. The most common form of managed care is the health maintenance organization (HMO). At the end of 1994, an estimated 51.4 million Americans belonged to HMO's. A patient in an HMO uses only hospitals and other services that participate in the plan and sees only physicians who work for or have contracts with the plan. Many physicians have been unhappy with HMO's because the plans often demand discounts from physicians or else refuse to contract with them. HMO's have also been accused of making it difficult for patients to use specialists and certain hospitals.

In March 1995, Speaker of the House of Representatives Newt Gingrich (R., Ga.) called for congressional hearings on HMO's to explore accusations that some plans' concern for profit negatively affected the quality of patient care. • Emily Friedman

Hearing
See Ear and Hearing

Although research has made clear that people with high blood cholesterol levels are more likely to develop heart disease, it has been less certain whether lowering high blood cholesterol levels actually helps people live longer. A study reported in November 1994 provided strong evidence that drug treatment to lower cholesterol may indeed reduce heart attacks and death in people who already have heart disease.

The study, which was conducted in several Scandinavian countries, involved 4,444 patients with both heart disease and high blood cholesterol. About half received the cholesterol-lowering drug Simvastatin for five to six years; the rest received no treatment. Cholesterol levels dropped an average of 25 percent in the treated patients and stayed constant in the untreated group.

Compared with the untreated patients, people in the treated group proved 42 percent less likely to die of heart disease. They were also 37 percent less likely to have a nonfatal heart attack, 37 percent less likely to undergo major heart surgery (coronary bypass or angioplasty), and 30 percent less likely to have a stroke. Similar patterns emerged when the scientists looked just at women and people aged 60 or older.

Simvastatin is one of several drugs that prevent the liver from manufac-turing cholesterol from dietary fat. It has been shown to have stronger effects on blood cholesterol than other drugs and diet therapy. Although this study looked specifically at Simvastatin, some physicians believe that related drugs would bring similar results. The study suggests that while the expense of lifelong drug treatments may not be justified in a young person with high cholesterol but no heart disease, it might well be worth the cost in patients known to have heart disease.

High cholesterol in older people.
Physicians frequently recommend that people with high levels of blood cholesterol undergo therapy to lower those levels, in hopes of preventing *atherosclerosis,* a condition in which fatty deposits form inside the arteries and hamper blood flow. But because atherosclerosis starts during adolescence and builds gradually throughout adulthood, physicians have questioned whether there is much benefit in aggressively testing for and treating high blood cholesterol in very old individuals—who have had a lifetime in which cholesterol could do its damage. A study reported in November 1994 indicates that in certain cases, such treatment might indeed be unproductive.

Researchers at Yale University School of Medicine in New Haven,

Cholesterol and old age
High blood cholesterol can be a sign of impending heart disease in most adults. But among people over age 70 who do not have heart problems, blood cholesterol levels appear unrelated to heart risk, Yale University researchers said in November 1994. They theorize that people who live that long with high cholesterol are relatively resistant to its effects.

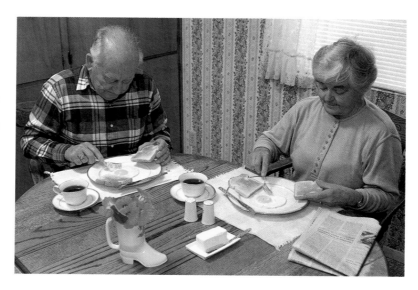

Connecticut, followed 997 people over age 70 to see if their blood cholesterol levels bore any relation to their likelihood of dying or entering the hospital because of heart conditions. One-third of the women and 16 percent of the men had cholesterol levels of at least 240 milligrams per deciliter, a level generally recognized as risky.

Over the course of four years, however, these high blood cholesterol levels were not associated with higher rates of death or heart attack, after adjustment for other risk factors. Even when the researchers compared the group with the least blood cholesterol to the group with the most, they found no significant difference in risk.

The researchers concluded that blood cholesterol levels may not be as important a risk factor in older people as they are in younger people. The researchers suggested that those people with high cholesterol levels who reach their late 70's without dying of heart disease may be relatively resistant to cholesterol's effects.

Chelation therapy, a treatment to remove undesirable substances from the body, has long been used to treat such problems as lead poisoning or excessive iron deposits. The treatment involves infusing agents called chelators into the bloodstream; these agents seek out and *bind* (chemically attach) to the targeted substances.

Because one chelator, ethylene diamine tetracetic acid (EDTA), also binds to calcium, some clinicians have begun using EDTA to try to extract calcium from diseased arteries. But a study reported in September 1994 by physicians from the University of Otago Medical School in Dunedin, New Zealand, cast doubt on the effectiveness of this procedure for that purpose.

Studies of atherosclerotic arteries removed from cadavers show that the fatty deposits in these blood vessels contain variable amounts of calcium, which produces the characteristic "hardening" of the arteries that occurs in atherosclerosis. Theoretically, removing this calcium might break up the deposits and, in turn, lessen the risk of heart attack, stroke, and limb loss due to atherosclerosis.

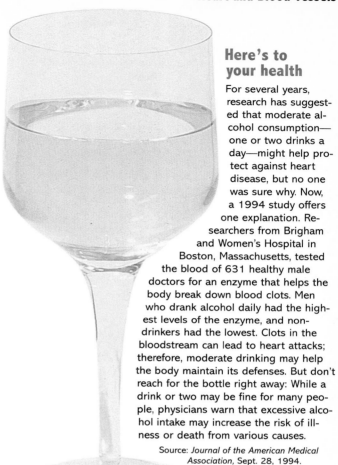

Here's to your health

For several years, research has suggested that moderate alcohol consumption—one or two drinks a day—might help protect against heart disease, but no one was sure why. Now, a 1994 study offers one explanation. Researchers from Brigham and Women's Hospital in Boston, Massachusetts, tested the blood of 631 healthy male doctors for an enzyme that helps the body break down blood clots. Men who drank alcohol daily had the highest levels of the enzyme, and nondrinkers had the lowest. Clots in the bloodstream can lead to heart attacks; therefore, moderate drinking may help the body maintain its defenses. But don't reach for the bottle right away: While a drink or two may be fine for many people, physicians warn that excessive alcohol intake may increase the risk of illness or death from various causes.

Source: *Journal of the American Medical Association*, Sept. 28, 1994.

Although this is an attractive theory, it has not been proven. Still, chelation therapy clinics have sprung up around the United States, and many patients with atherosclerosis spend a considerable amount of money on chelation treatment—despite the lack of solid data supporting its use.

The New Zealand team examined the effects of chelation therapy on atherosclerosis of the arteries in the legs. The doctors tested walking ability and other factors in 32 patients with leg pain caused by atherosclerosis. Then 15 of the patients received 10 weeks of chelation therapy with EDTA. The patients were reassessed at the end of the treatment period and again three months later.

The treated patients showed significant improvement in treadmill walking distances—but so did the untreated patients (60 percent in the chelation group and 59 percent in the untreated group). The investigators concluded that while chelation therapy may seem to bring improvements in patients with atherosclerosis of the large arteries of the legs, those improvements are just as likely to happen without treatment.

Anxiety and sudden death. Some people may literally be scared to death, according to a study published in November 1994. A team of Boston scientists conducting a long-term study for the U.S. Veterans Administration tracked the health of 2,280 men from the Boston area from 1961 to 1993. At the start of the project, the patients filled out a questionnaire that included questions about nervousness, fear of strangers, and other signs of anxiety. The researchers used the patients' responses to rank the men on a scale of zero (least anxious) to five (most anxious).

During the next 32 years, 131 of the men died of heart disease, 26 of them suddenly. Compared to men with an anxiety score of zero, men reporting a score of two or more had almost twice the risk of dying of heart disease and more than four times the risk of dying suddenly of heart disease—even after the researchers adjusted for several other

factors. The investigators concluded that there is an association between anxiety and death from heart disease, particularly sudden death.

The researchers theorized that intense psychological stress may trigger episodes of irregular heartbeat that can cause death. Interestingly, anxiety and panic disorders are more common in women, yet there is very little information about the risk of sudden death among women with anxiety disorders. The same research team was conducting a new study in 1995 to see if anxiety poses a similar risk to women.

Heart help from a vitamin. Lack of the vitamin folic acid could contribute to the development of heart attacks and strokes in American men, a Canadian researcher announced in July 1995. If confirmed, the finding would mean that taking vitamin supplements might ward off many of these attacks.

Judith Hall, a geneticist at the University of British Columbia in Vancouver, Canada, based her estimate on the results of several dozen studies showing the vitamin's protective effect. Folic acid is found in green leafy vegetables such as spinach and lettuce, fruits such as apples and oranges, and most multivitamin pills. Because the vitamin has already been shown to help prevent certain birth defects, the U.S. government is considering requiring its addition to some

Worried to death?
Anxiety may literally cause some people to drop dead. In a Harvard University study reported in November 1994, men prone to anxiety proved four times more likely to have sudden, fatal heart attacks than other men. The researchers say that in anxiety-prone people, stress may trigger episodes of irregular heartbeat that can cause sudden death.

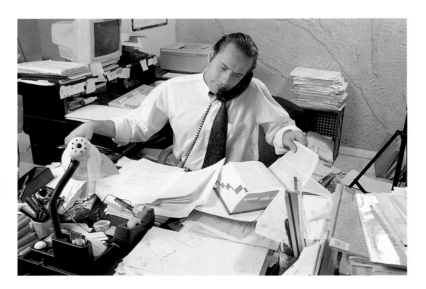

commonly consumed grain products.

Studies have shown that folic acid reduces blood levels of homocysteine, a natural substance essential to the body's functioning. High levels of homocysteine have been linked to increased risk of heart attack and stroke. Now, scientists say, it is necessary to scientifically test the theory that using folic acid to lower high homocysteine levels will lessen heart disease.

In the meantime, medical experts caution that taking folic acid will not counteract the heart-endangering effects of a diet high in fat and cholesterol. But, they add, eating more fruits and vegetables is a good step toward heart health in any case.

Avoiding valve surgery. Nifedipine, a widely used heart drug, may delay or eliminate the need for heart valve surgery, researchers at the University of Padua, Italy, and the University of Southern California, Los Angeles, reported in September 1994. Nifedipine, one of a class of drugs known as calcium channel blockers, has been used since 1982 to treat high blood pressure and *angina* (chest pain related to heart disease).

The researchers tested the drug on 143 patients with a condition called severe aortic regurgitation, in which blood leaks backward through the heart's aortic valve. Normally blood flows from the left ventricle—the heart's main pumping chamber— through the valve to the aorta, the artery that carries blood to the rest of the body. The backward flow, or regurgitation, forces the left ventricle to work harder, enlarging it and eventually interfering with its ability to pump. When this happens, the patient generally needs surgery to replace the valve.

Nifedipine works by relaxing blood vessels. In patients with aortic regurgitation, the drug increases the blood's forward flow and reduces the amount of regurgitation, resulting in a short-term improvement in left ventricular function.

The patients in the study all had aortic regurgitation, but their left ventricles were still pumping properly and none had experienced symptoms yet. Half the patients began taking

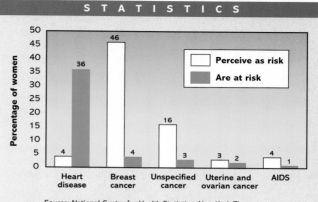

STATISTICS				

Percentage of women

- Perceive as risk
- Are at risk

	Heart disease	Breast cancer	Unspecified cancer	Uterine and ovarian cancer	AIDS
Perceive as risk	4	46	16	3	4
Are at risk	36	4	3	2	1

Source: National Center for Health Statistics; *New York Times*.

Women and heart disease: No small threat

Although heart disease will strike 36 percent of American women, only 4 percent recognize it as a serious health threat, according to the National Center for Health Statistics. But almost half of American women consider breast cancer a threat to their health, though only 4 percent will develop it. The American Heart Association offers these facts about American women and heart disease:

- Heart attack is the top killer of women.
- Of the 485,000 people who die of heart attack each year, nearly 49 percent are women. About 20,800 of those women are under age 65.
- More than twice as many women die of heart attack annually than breast cancer and lung cancer combined.
- Nearly twice as many women die of all cardiovascular diseases annually than of all forms of cancer combined.

nifedipine, and the rest took digoxin, another common heart medication. Over the course of six years, 34 percent of the digoxin patients eventually needed valve surgery, compared with only 15 percent of those receiving nifedipine. None of the patients taking nifedipine required surgery for the first two years of treatment.

When the nifedipine patients did have surgery, their heart's ability to pump blood returned to normal. This finding, the researchers noted, allayed the concern that in delaying the need for surgery, nifedipine might have masked the development of irreversible damage. • Michael H. Crawford

In the section Medical and Safety Alerts, see HYPERTENSION: A TICKING TIME BOMB. In WORLD BOOK, see HEART.

Infectious Diseases

Public health authorities in the United States warned Americans of a new, potentially fatal tick-borne disease in 1995. The new disease, called human granulocytic Ehrlichiosis, or HGE, had stricken dozens of people in wooded areas of New York, Minnesota, Wisconsin, and a few other states by mid-1995, causing four deaths.

Infectious disease experts believe that HGE is spread by the *Ehrlichia* bacterium, which is found in some ticks that live primarily on deer. *Ehrlichia* is related to the bacterium that causes Rocky Mountain spotted fever, another tick-borne disease, according to health officials. Scientists discovered the *Ehrlichia* bacterium in the 1930's, but they thought it infected only dogs and horses.

Symptoms of the disease appear 2 to 15 days after a bite and can include a high fever, severe headache, chills, lethargy, mental confusion, and sweating. However, health officials say that HGE has no telltale signs, such as the bull's-eye rash around the site of a tick bite that appears in most cases of Lyme disease, another tick-borne disorder.

Many HGE infections are mild, but 5 to 10 percent of cases can be life-threatening, according to health officials. The antibiotic doxycycline can cure the infection if it is taken in time, according to medical experts.

Ebola virus strikes Zaire. An outbreak of hemorrhagic fever caused by the Ebola virus, one of the deadliest known microbes, began in April 1995 in the African nation of Zaire. The outbreak killed 244 of the 315 people known to have been infected, according to the World Health Organization (WHO), a United Nations agency based in Geneva, Switzerland.

Ebola hemorrhagic fever involves high fever and severe bleeding from the eyes, nose, and other body openings. The disease usually strikes pigs, monkeys, and other animals. But it occasionally infects human populations. There is no vaccine or cure, and the fatality rate can reach 90 percent. WHO said the outbreak began April 10 in Kikwit, a city about 300 miles (480 kilometers) east of Kinshasa, Zaire's capital.

Health experts said there was little risk of an Ebola outbreak in the United States or in other industrialized countries. Unlike such highly contagious diseases as influenza and tuberculosis, Ebola hemorrhagic fever cannot be transmitted by coughs or sneezes. It requires close contact with an infected person's blood or other body fluids—usually after the person is bleeding and obviously ill.

Chickenpox vaccine approved. The United States Food and Drug Administration (FDA) on March 17, 1995,

Ebola takes a toll

Members of the International Red Cross prepare to lower the body of a nun who died of Ebola hemorrhagic fever into her grave. The outbreak of Ebola— one of the deadliest microbes known—began in Zaire in April 1995. It had killed 244 people by August 24, when the World Health Organization declared that the outbreak was officially over.

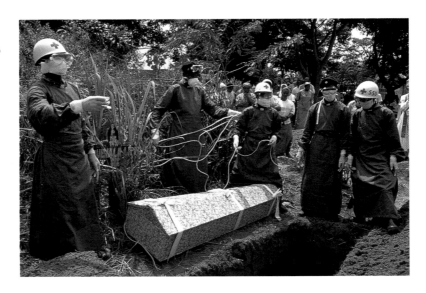

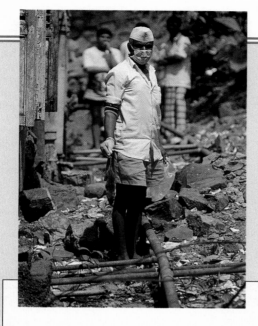

Plague strikes India

A worker in India removes a dead rat, *left*, in an effort to stem an outbreak of pneumonic plague that struck the city of Surat in September 1994, killing more than 50 people and sickening thousands more. Plague is a highly infectious disease caused by the bacterium *Yersinia pestis*. The disease spreads to human beings through contact with infected rats and fleas that feed on these rats. Pneumonic plague, one of three forms of the disease, also can spread in the coughs and sneezes of an infected person.

Plague bacteria	Rat	Flea	
	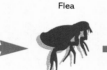		

The plague-causing bacteria typically move from host to host in the gut of fleas that live on animal blood.

Rats and other rodents are common hosts for the plague bacterium. If the rodents should die off, their fleas may bite other animals or human beings.

Fleas that carry the plague bacteria can transmit them to human beings through bites. A person with pneumonic plague can transmit the bacteria in sneezes or coughs.

approved a vaccine for chickenpox, or varicella, a highly contagious viral disease that strikes about 3.3 million children in the United States each year. The disease causes fever, headache, loss of appetite, and a rash consisting of hundreds of itchy lesions. Each year about 9,000 children with chickenpox must be hospitalized, and about 100 children die of the disease.

The FDA said the vaccine, sold under the trade name Varivax, is 70 to 90 percent effective in preventing the disease. Clinical trials on about 11,000 volunteers showed that those vaccinated either do not develop chickenpox or develop a mild form.

The American Academy of Pediatrics (AAP), a professional organization of pediatricians, on May 1 recommended that the new vaccine be administered to all children, adolescents, and young adults who have not been infected with chickenpox.

Beating diarrhea-causing bacteria. A new vaccine can help prevent severe diarrhea caused by rotaviruses. The National Institute of Allergy and Infectious Diseases (NIAID) reported the results of studies on the new vaccine in April 1995. NIAID, which developed the vaccine, is one Δ321 of the National Institutes of Health in Bethesda, Maryland.

Rotaviruses are a group of viruses with a wheellike appearance. They are the leading cause of severe diarrhea in young children.

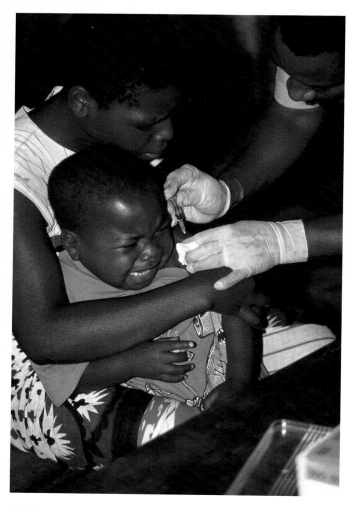

(inactive substance). Researchers then monitored the children for two years, comparing the number of diarrhea cases in each group. One vaccine was 82 percent effective in protecting against severe diarrhea and 49 percent effective in preventing milder cases. The other vaccine's effectiveness ranged from 73 percent for severe cases to 31 percent for mild cases. NIAID researchers said the vaccines have the potential to reduce the extent of serious illness from rotavirus infections.

Protecting adults from tetanus. Many adults in the United States are not properly immunized against tetanus, a rare but serious disease transmitted through cuts and other breaks in the skin. Researchers from the National Institutes of Health (NIH) and the CDC reached this conclusion in a study reported in March 1995.

Common bacteria that exist in ordinary soil cause tetanus. A minor wound from a splinter or thorn can provide an opening for the bacteria to enter the body, where it produces a poison that causes muscle stiffness and contractions of the jaw muscles, which make it hard for victims to open their mouth.

Researchers from the NIH and the CDC studied tetanus immunity among 10,618 people. They found that about 88 percent of children aged 6 to 11 were fully protected against tetanus, because children get tetanus vaccine shots as part of their routine childhood immunizations.

The study found lower levels of immunity to tetanus among people over age 40. Immunity gradually fades as *antibodies* (disease-fighting cells of the immune system) lose their effectiveness against the disease. Only 50 percent of men and women aged 60 to 69 were fully protected against tetanus. By age 70, immunity levels dropped below 30 percent. Physicians recommend that adults receive a tetanus booster shot every 10 years to maintain their immunity.

• **Michael Woods**

In the section Medical and Safety Alerts, see KEEPING THE WONDER IN WONDER DRUGS; and GERM WARFARE: BATTLING THE STREP A "BUG." In WORLD BOOK, see VIRUS.

Malaria vaccine test

A doctor injects a child in Tanzania with an experimental vaccine against malaria. Biochemist Manuel Patarroyo of Colombia, who developed the vaccine, reported In October 1994 that tests had shown it reduced the risk of contracting the disease by 31 percent in Tanzanian children. Malaria kills about 2 million people each year, according to the World Health Organization.

Diarrhea is usually a symptom of an intestinal disorder and not a disease itself. Yet diarrhea can lead to dehydration and death. About 1 million cases of rotaviral diarrhea occur in U.S. children under the age of 5 each year, with about 65,000 cases severe enough to require hospitalization. The condition takes a greater toll in developing countries, where 18 million cases and 870,000 deaths occur each year.

In the study, researchers at 31 U.S. medical centers tested two vaccines against rotavirus on 898 healthy infants aged 4 weeks to 26 weeks. Some infants received the vaccines, which researchers administered orally in several doses at two-week intervals, and others received a *placebo*

Patients with kidney failure are waiting an increasingly long time for a transplant because of an inadequate supply of donor kidneys. One potential solution to this shortage is xeno-transplantation—transplantation from one species into another. In May 1995, researchers at Duke University Medical Center in Durham, North Carolina, announced progress toward that goal. They succeeded in prolonging the survival of pig organs transplanted into baboons.

The main obstacle to xenotransplantation is rejection by the immune system—a response in which the immune system identifies the transplanted organ as foreign and attacks it. In this response, *antibodies* (immune system proteins) bind to the surface of cells lining the blood vessels within the transplanted organ, triggering inflammation and subsequent destruction of tissue. The body's own blood vessels are protected from antibodies by other proteins called complement regulatory proteins.

The researchers prolonged the survival of the transplanted pig organs by inserting a human gene that directs the production of complement regulatory proteins into the red blood cells of the pig. The pig blood cells could then produce the human complement regulatory proteins and carry them to the cells lining the blood vessels of the pig organ. The researchers used the human gene because of its similarity to the baboon gene. The scientists hope eventually to transplant genetically engineered animal organs into human beings.

The organs transplanted from the genetically engineered pigs survived longer than organs from pigs without the human gene, but they did not survive indefinitely. Either additional complement regulatory proteins are required on the cells lining the blood vessels or other immune system mechanisms must be blocked to prolong organ survival further.

Kidney disease gene identified. In April 1995, a research group at Johns Hopkins University in Baltimore reported that they had completed identifying a gene that causes most cases of autosomal dominant polycystic kid-

ney disease (ADPKD). One of the most common inherited diseases, ADPKD causes the gradual development of many cysts within the kidney, which leads to a progressive loss of kidney function and eventually to kidney failure. About 10 percent of all people who require long-term dialysis or kidney transplants have ADPKD. Research is now underway to find out how this abnormal gene causes the development of renal cysts.

Dialysis membranes affect survival rate. The survival rate of patients afflicted with sudden and severe kidney

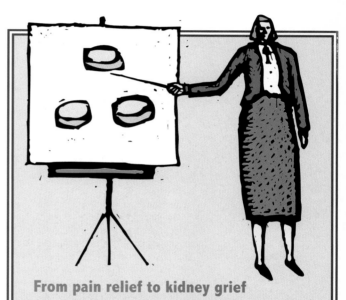

From pain relief to kidney grief

One in 10 cases of kidney failure in the United States—about 5,000 each year—may stem from frequent, long-term use of the common pain reliever acetaminophen (sold as Tylenol and other brands). Researchers at the Johns Hopkins School of Public Health in Baltimore, Maryland, compared the use of pain relievers by a group of healthy people and by 716 patients who developed kidney failure. They found that the risk of kidney failure was 40 percent higher among people who took acetaminophen twice a week or more for at least a year, compared with those who used it less. Those who took the drug at least once a day for a year had twice the risk compared with occasional users. Experts emphasized, however, that such complications are exceedingly rare. Used in moderation, acetaminophen appears to be a safe remedy for headache, pain, or fever.

Source: *New England Journal of Medicine,* Dec. 12, 1994.

failure who undergo hemodialysis is affected by the type of membrane used. That finding was reported by researchers at Ludwig-Maximilians University in Munich, Germany, in August 1994 and by researchers at Vanderbilt University in Nashville, Tennessee, in November 1994.

Over 100,000 people in the United States receive hemodialysis three times weekly because of kidney failure. During hemodialysis, blood is pumped out of the patient's body and through a filter that removes wastes. The blood is then pumped back into the body. In the filter, the patient's blood runs through thousands of miniature tubes bathed in a dialysis solution. The walls of these tubes can be constructed from different materials, and some materials provoke an inflammatory response when blood passes through them. Certain dialysis membrane materials, however, produce only a minimal reaction and are therefore considered biocompatible.

Both research groups found a higher survival rate among patients who had hemodialysis using a biocompatible filter rather than a filter that could induce an inflammatory reaction. A study to investigate whether long-term dialysis patients would experience similar improvement was underway in 1995   • Jeffrey R. Thompson

In WORLD BOOK, see KIDNEY.

Medical Ethics

Guidelines for research on human embryos were approved by an advisory panel at the National Institutes of Health (NIH) in December 1994, ending a 13-year ban on government funding of embryo research. Supporters of the panel's recommendations believe such research could provide information on the nature of genetic diseases, infertility, and other medical problems. Critics of embryo research argue that it is an unacceptable manipulation of human life.

The panel limited the research to certain studies and specified that embryos used in research must be less than 14 days old—the time at which the first trace of a nervous system appears. The panel also decided that embryos produced in private fertility clinics through a technique called in vitro fertilization could be used in research. In this technique, a woman's eggs are fertilized in a laboratory dish and then implanted in the uterus, where they may develop into fetuses. This process often produces extra embryos, and the panel decided that these embryos could be used in research. In its most controversial decision, the panel also approved the creation of embryos specifically for certain types of research.

The Administration of President Bill Clinton agreed with many of the panel's recommendations but rejected the creation of embryos specifically for research. The NIH has not yet finalized rules for embryo research.

A case of life and death. U.S. courts came to inconsistent conclusions in 1995 on the issue of whether terminally ill patients should be given life-prolonging treatment. This issue was the centerpiece of two legal battles that pitted the family members of patients against physicians and hospital administrators.

In one case, the Supreme Court of the United States let stand in early 1995 a ruling that denied a Virginia hospital permission to discontinue emergency treatment of a child born missing most of her brain, a condition known as anencephaly. At her mother's insistence, the child, known nationwide as "Baby K," had been kept alive in a pediatric nursing home for more than two years, with admissions to the hospital whenever she developed breathing problems. The hospital had sought a court order to discontinue treatment of Baby K.

Many medical experts felt that treating Baby K was merely prolonging the inevitable death of a child who was unconscious and unable to think, hear, or see. Some physicians were also concerned that a court decision in favor of continued treatment would force professionals to provide medical care that they considered ineffective.

After reviewing the case, the courts had discovered several laws that protected the continued emergency treatment of Baby K. However, despite continued treatment, Baby K died of cardiac arrest in April 1995.

In another decision, a Massachusetts court ruled in April 1995 that a hospital and its doctors can halt life-prolonging treatment that they feel is futile. The decision stemmed from a case in which doctors refused the request of Joan Gilgunn to revive her elderly mother, Catherine F. Gilgunn, should her heart stop. Mrs. Gilgunn was in a coma and had irreversible brain damage. She died in August 1994 after her doctors issued a "do not resuscitate" order. Her daughter sued, but a jury found the doctor was not negligent in his treatment.

The medical meaning of death.
The Council on Ethical and Judicial Affairs of the American Medical Association concluded in May 1995 that although anencephalic newborns are alive under the current medical definitions of death, it is ethically permissible, at the parents' request, to consider them potential organ donors, because they neither have nor ever will experience consciousness. The council's statement prompted debate over the medical definition of death.

HIV screening of newborns. The Centers for Disease Control and Prevention (CDC) in Atlanta, Georgia, announced in May 1995 that it was suspending a controversial program to screen newborns anonymously for the presence of antibodies to the AIDS-causing HIV (human immunodeficiency virus). The program has been the subject of a debate over the ethics of collecting HIV-related data in a way that does not identify and inform those infected with HIV.

The CDC has conducted anonymous HIV screening in various populations in an attempt to determine the course of the AIDS epidemic. This testing uses blood drawn from unidentified people so that consent is not needed. By testing newborns, who carry their mother's antibodies, the CDC was able to track the course of HIV in childbearing women.

Many pediatricians have recommended that the CDC "unblind" the screening, which would link names with results. That way, a doctor could start treating an infected mother's child—who may have gotten the virus

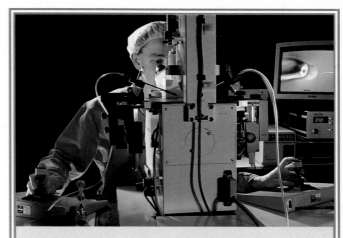

The debate over gene alteration

A technique reported in November 1994 enables scientists to alter genes in sperm. Because it alters germ cells from which mature sperm develop, the altered gene would be passed on to all future generations. Although the experiment was performed on mice, and human applications remain far off, medical ethicists called for debate to begin now on the implications of inheritable gene modification.

- Arguments in favor: Alteration of genes could eliminate inherited disorders, and parents should have the right to improve their children's health. Scientific knowledge that could come from such research should be supported.

- Arguments against: The technique could obliterate potentially beneficial genes or create new, potentially devastating genetic diseases. Mistakes would be irreversible. Parents inevitably will want to enhance the genetic makeup of their offspring.

from the mother during pregnancy or birth or through breast milk—to prevent the onset of illness. But opponents argue that unblinding the test forces mandatory screening of mothers without their consent. Also, all babies born to HIV-infected mothers test positive in the first months of life, but only about 25 percent are infected. Thus, unblinding the test would not truly identify infected babies.

In July 1995, the CDC recommended that pregnant women consider HIV testing and that HIV-infected pregnant women begin treatment with the drug zidovudine (AZT). Treatment with AZT can reduce the risk that HIV-infected women will transmit HIV to their babies by as much as 66 percent. • Carol Levine
See also HEALTH CARE ISSUES.

Mental Health

Mental Health

In late 1994, the United States Food and Drug Administration approved the drug naltrexone, sold under the trade name Revia, for the treatment of alcoholism. Medical professionals greeted the news with enthusiasm, because alcoholism is a debilitating disease for which there has been very little medical treatment.

A new use for an old drug. For many years, naltrexone has been used in treating narcotics addiction. Naltrexone counters the effects of opioids, compounds in narcotics that produce feelings of well-being and reduce sensitivity to pain. It has also been used in hospital emergency rooms to counteract overdoses of such narcotics as heroin, morphine, and demerol. Naltrexone renders the opioids powerless and, if injected in time, can save the life of someone poisoned by illicit drugs. Studies have found that naltrexone is relatively safe and carries few side effects.

Physicians began to use naltrexone experimentally in the 1980's to treat war veterans who suffered from post-traumatic stress disorder. The drug has had some success in countering the harrowing flashbacks and nightmares that the veterans experience. In other experiments, naltrexone has been used to stop self-injurious actions of people with borderline per-

The roots of obsession
Images produced by researchers at Johns Hopkins University in Baltimore show areas of increased brain activity, *top* (red), in people experiencing the uncontrollable, repetitive thoughts associated with obsessive-compulsive disorder (OCD). Another technique shows heightened brain activity during the throes of obsession, *bottom* left (red triangle at top), compared with normal brain activity, *bottom* right. With these tools, researchers hope to gain greater understanding of OCD.

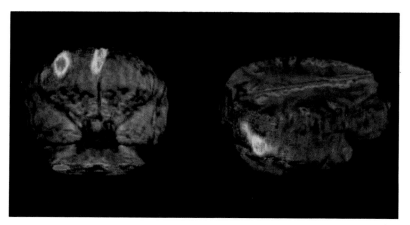

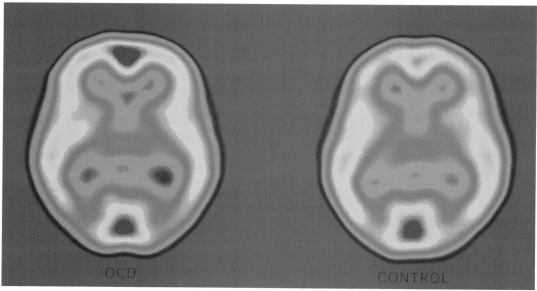

OCD　　　CONTROL

sonality disorder, which is characterized by angry outbursts, mood swings, and an inability to maintain stable relationships. Naltrexone has also been used to counter *hyperactivity* (continual, purposeless motion) and impulsive behavior in children with a developmental disorder known as autism.

But naltrexone has shown even greater promise for curbing a craving for alcohol. In the early 1990's, a number of studies showed that alcoholics who took naltrexone lost their taste for alcohol and were able to stay off alcohol far longer than alcoholics who received a *placebo* (substance with no active ingredients). Animal studies produced similar findings: Addicted animals significantly lowered their alcohol intake when given naltrexone.

Only one other drug, disulfiram (sold under the trade name Antabuse), has been available to treat alcoholism. When Antabuse combines with alcohol in the body, it forms formaldehyde, a poison that causes dizziness, vomiting, and heart palpitations. Although Antabuse makes the user sick upon drinking alcohol, it does not stop the craving for alcohol. For the few people who cannot tolerate naltrexone, however, Antabuse offers a backup choice.

A person recovering from alcoholism typically enters an inpatient treatment program for about 30 days. In that setting, he or she receives psychotherapy and participates in meetings of Alcoholics Anonymous (AA). Effective approaches for combating alcoholism often include group or family therapy and medication when appropriate.

Progress against Alzheimer's disease. In a major scientific breakthrough, researchers announced in February 1995 that they had created a mouse that develops the damage to brain cells which characterizes Alzheimer's disease. This so-called transgenic mouse offers researchers an opportunity for studying how the disease develops and for testing possible treatments. The researchers who created the mouse were from Athena Neurosciences, Incorporated, in South San Francisco, California, and

Eli Lilly & Company, a pharmaceutical firm in Indianapolis.

Alzheimer's involves a gradual deterioration and destruction of brain cells, which greatly impairs memory and other mental abilities. It occurs primarily among people aged 65 and over, and affects some 4 million to 7 million people in the United States, according to the Alzheimer's Disease Association. In looking at the brains of people who died of Alzheimer's disease, researchers have found abundant deposits called plaques, which consist of proteins and degenerated nerve endings.

The transgenic mice were created by inserting a human gene for Alzheimer's disease into mouse embryos. The mice appear fine when young, but by middle age, the parts of their brains involved in learning and memory contain the same sort of plaques that appear in diseased human brains. The mice do not, however, develop another brain abnormality associated with Alzheimer's disease: the presence of tangled fibers within nerve cells. The missing tangles have raised some questions about how useful the mouse model might be to Alzheimer's researchers.

In June 1995, an international group of researchers reported the discovery of a third gene linked with Alzheimer's. The gene causes a rare form of the disease that can strike people as young as 30 years old. Also in 1995, the Metropolitan Life Foundation gave an award to a team of researchers led by Alison Goate of Washington University in St. Louis. Goate and her colleagues found the first genetic link to Alzheimer's disease—a gene responsible for some early-onset cases that occur in people in their 40's and 50's.

Managed care in mental health. In the summer of 1995, the American Medical Association (AMA) gave strong support to a Patient Protection Act that was to go before the United States Congress. The act addressed several issues concerning the rights of patients enrolled in managed care programs, including the rights of mental health patients. A version of the Patient Protection Act had been attached to the health reform act pro-

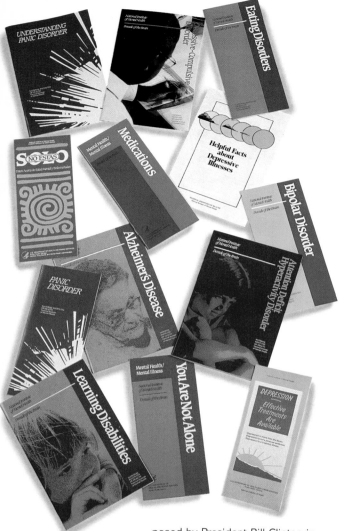

Mental health pamphlets
The National Institute of Mental Health (NIMH) conducts and supports research on many mental illnesses. In addition, the NIMH provides information for consumers. Pamplets that explain a variety of disorders are available free of charge by sending a request in writing to:
NIMH
Office of Public Inquiries
Room 7C-02
5600 Fishers Lane
Rockville, MD 20857

posed by President Bill Clinton in 1994 but later defeated by Congress.

The AMA said the Patient Protection Act was intended to force managed care systems to improve the quality of health care they deliver. It requires plans to disclose to consumers any financial incentives that it offers physicians not to refer patients to specialists or to provide less treatment. The act also requires full disclosure of the plan's provisions to its members. These measures, the AMA said, would enable patients to select plans that better suit their needs—both physical and mental.

The Patient Protection Act also reflects the concerns of many mental health professionals about the level of mental health care that patients can

receive under managed care plans. Managed care insurance plans that offer mental health benefits have burgeoned, and many employers contract with managed care plans that offer these benefits to employees. Although these plans have the advantage of reducing costs and discouraging overtreatment, some mental health experts fear that they have drawbacks for mental health patients.

In a managed care program, the patient selects a primary care physician from a list of general practitioners. Before the patient can see a mental health specialist, he or she must first consult the primary care physician.

In many cases, the primary care physician chooses to treat the patient's condition, usually by prescribing psychoactive medications, instead of providing a referral. Although most generalists understand the importance of psychotherapy, they do not ordinarily have the time or training to provide it. Mental health professionals prefer to combine psychotherapy with medication in treating a problem, rather than rely on drugs alone.

If the patient receives permission from the primary care physician to see a mental health specialist, the patient must accept the specialist to whom he or she is assigned. In many cases, when primary care physicians make a mental health referral, they refer the patient to a professional who charges less than a psychiatrist—a nurse, counselor, or social worker, for example. These therapists do not have the extensive training that psychiatrists have, and they may lack the expertise to handle the patient's problem.

Managed care plans also determine the allowable length of a hospital stay for the treatment of specific mental disorders. Patients often continue their recovery in such facilities as halfway houses, rehabilitation centers, or day-treatment programs, which may be unable to provide the treatment needed.

In spite of these limitations on the care they can receive, employees covered under some managed care plans sign a paper saying that they will not hold the plan liable for medical malpractice. In addition, managed care plans ask patients to assign control of their medical records to the plan. This means that the managed care plan can release patient records to employers in certain circumstances—for example, when the cost of treatment comes into question. Such breaches of confidentiality can be especially intrusive for patients who are receiving psychiatric care. For these reasons, psychiatric patients with the financial means to pay for their treatment may elect to stay out of the managed care system.

Computer addiction. In February 1995, federal agents in North Carolina arrested 31-year-old Kevin Mitnick, a computer hacker who had been on a two-year high-tech crime spree. During the spree, Mitnick allegedly broke into some of the nation's largest computer networks and amassed about 20,000 credit card numbers, though he never used them.

In 1989, Mitnick had been convicted of computer fraud in southern California. Mitnick and his lawyer convinced a judge that Mitnick suffered from computer addiction, an addiction that the lawyer said was as powerful as drinking or gambling to excess. The judge sentenced Mitnick to one year of rehabilitation treatment for the disorder.

Some mental health professionals think that computer addiction may

constitute a significant, but overlooked, problem. The commercial online service CompuServe, in recognition of the problem, has set up a library file entitled "Coping with Computer Addictions."

People who admit to addictive computer usage describe losing all sense of time as they become mesmerized by their online activity. Howard Shaffer, the associate director of the addictions division of Harvard Medical School in Boston, called this kind of computer usage a "relieving experience, like low-level alcohol use."

Some people report spending so many hours at a computer terminal that they begin to ignore family and friends. Some strike up friendships online that are both intimate and anonymous. Online communication provides a relatively safe way to tell all to someone.

Not all experts agree that such behaviors signify addiction. Some think that obsession may be involved. Nat Sandler, an expert on obsessive-compulsive disorder (OCD) from Lexington, Kentucky, has worked with a number of people whose obsession focuses on their computers. OCD is marked by uncontrollable, repetitive thoughts and actions.

• Lenore Terr

In the section A Healthy Family, see WHEN A PARENT DIES. In WORLD BOOK, see MENTAL ILLNESS.

Nervous System
See Brain and Nervous System

New guidelines on school lunch programs have been designed to reduce the fat and sodium in school meals and increase the servings of fruits, vegetables, and grains. The guidelines, published in June 1995 by the United States Department of Agriculture (USDA), called for schools to provide healthier meals by the 1996-1997 school year. One of the requirements of the plan is that schools limit fat content to 30 percent of the total calories in a meal.

Earlier in 1995, the U.S. House of Representatives had voted to eliminate federal nutrition standards and to fund school lunch and breakfast programs through a block grant given to states. But public outcry over the

issue convinced the Senate Agriculture Committee that the federal government should retain responsibility for school meals.

To kick off the new program, the USDA became partners with businesses and health associations in an education campaign to promote nutritious food and encourage children to make healthy food choices.

Benefits of fruits and vegetables. Fruits and vegetables may protect against stroke, according to a study published in April 1995 by researchers from Harvard University in Boston and Boston University. This conclusion was based on a study of 832 men from 45 to 65 years of age who

Nutrition and Food

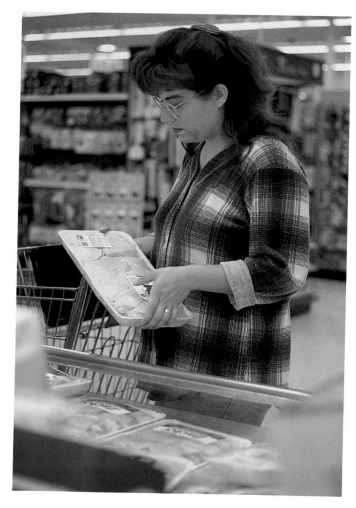

It's really fresh!
Consumers can soon be confident that poultry labeled "fresh" has not been previously frozen. A 1989 rule had allowed chickens and turkeys chilled to 0 °F (−18 °C) to be labeled "fresh." Consumer groups said the labels cheated customers who readily paid higher prices for birds they believed to be fresh. The new rule, to take effect in 1996, allows producers to apply the "fresh" label only to poultry that has never been chilled below 26 °F (−3.3 °C).

duce stroke risk. This may explain why fruits and vegetables, which are a rich source of potassium, have a protective effect. Another theory is that the B vitamin folic acid, which is abundant in leafy green vegetables, may help lower the risk of stroke. Folic acid prevents the build-up of homocysteine, a natural substance that has been linked to increased risk of heart disease and stroke.

The study was limited in a couple of respects, other researchers noted. First, the study included data only on middle-aged men. Second, the study assessed each man's daily fruit and vegetable intake in terms of what the man thought he had eaten over a single 24-hour period. Because diets can vary greatly from day to day, critics pointed out, the estimate of each individual's usual fruit and vegetable intake was hardly precise.

Despite these limitations, the Boston researchers were confident that a more precise assessment of diet would bear out their conclusion. To support this assertion, they pointed to preliminary data from a similar study in women, which also indicated that vegetables have a protective effect against stroke.

were free from heart disease and who were part of a long-term health trial called the Framingham Study.

The researchers assessed the diets of the study participants by recording what each had eaten over a single 24-hour period. They defined one serving of most fruits and vegetables as ½ cup.

By the end of a follow-up period of about 20 years, 97 strokes had occurred among the men. The researchers found that the men's risk of stroke decreased by 22 percent for every three additional daily servings of fruits or vegetables consumed.

Researchers are uncertain how fruits and vegetables affect stroke risk. Previous studies have shown that the mineral potassium may re-

Fish and heart disease. Consuming large amounts of fish does not significantly lower the risk of heart disease. This finding was published in April 1995 by researchers at the Harvard School of Public Health.

The finding came from a study begun in 1986, in which 44,895 men aged 40 to 75 answered questions on their diet and their risk factors, such as smoking, for heart disease. The men were followed for six years.

Among the men free of heart disease at the start of the study, those who increased their weekly number of fish servings from one or two to five or six servings did not significantly lower their risk of suffering a heart attack. On the other hand, the group of men who ate just a little fish—one to three servings per month—did cut their risk of dying of heart disease by 25 percent.

Even though the study challenged the notion that eating a lot of fish protects against heart disease, health experts say that eating some fish is

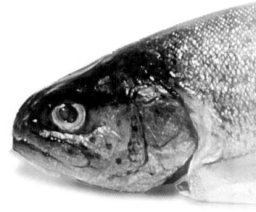

A fishy link to heart health

Research has long hinted that eating lots of seafood can help ward off heart disease—but a 1995 study suggests this is a fish tale. Researchers at the Harvard School of Public Health in Boston tracked the health and eating habits of 44,895 men for six years. They found no difference in heart health between those who consumed fish or fish-oil supplements six or more times a week and those who did so less than once a month. This study is not likely to be the end of the line, however. Scientists still don't know why some countries that rely on seafood-laden cuisine boast low heart disease rates. Nutritionists speculate that high fish consumption may indeed provide benefits, but only in combination with other heart-healthy diet and lifestyle factors.

Source: *New England Journal of Medicine*, April 13, 1995.

still good for one's health because it contains a variety of important nutrients. In addition, people who eat fish tend to eat less red meat, which is rich in heart-damaging saturated fats.

Selenium and cancer. The mineral selenium may not protect against cancer as was thought, according to a study published in April 1995 by researchers at the Harvard School of Public Health. The mineral had gained widespread attention after animal studies showed that, in high doses, it has a protective effect against cancer.

Selenium, which is found in seafood, Brazil nuts, and other foods, is an antioxidant, a compound capable of blocking the destructive effects of molecules called free radicals. In the human body, free radicals can cause damage to cells, including the genetic damage that may lead to cancer. Scientists believe that selenium may also help the body's immune system hunt down and fight cancer cells.

The new study was designed to examine further the protective effects of selenium, particularly the relationship between selenium levels and cancer incidence among women. The study measured selenium levels in toenail clippings, because dietary selenium is deposited in nails and the deposits were thought to reflect levels of the mineral in the women's bodies.

Vegetables improve the view

Carrots have long been touted as good for vision. Now a study suggests that green leafy vegetables can benefit the eyes—specifically by protecting against age-related macular degeneration, a decay of the retina that is the chief cause of blindness in people over 65. Researchers at the Massachusetts Eye and Ear Infirmary in Boston, Massachusetts, compared the diets of 356 men and women with advanced macular degeneration and a similar group of people with different eye diseases. They found that people whose diets included the most carotenoids—chemical compounds that give vegetables their color—had 43 percent less risk of advanced macular degeneration than those who ate the least. The most helpful carotenoids were lutein and zeaxanthin, yellow pigments plentiful in such vegetables as spinach and collard greens. Both of these pigments are also found in the retina.

Source: *Journal of the American Medical Association*, Nov. 9, 1994.

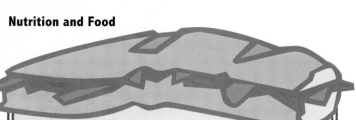

One fat sandwich, coming up

Beware: That healthy-looking tuna salad sandwich may have three times the fat of a quarter-pound fast food cheeseburger. So say nutritionists at the Center for Science in the Public Interest, who analyzed samples from sandwich shops in Chicago, Los Angeles, New York City, and Washington, D.C. To keep fat down, they suggest choosing mustard or ketchup rather than mayonnaise-based dressings; avoiding fatty toppings such as cheese, avocados, and bacon; and dividing the sandwich filling to make a second sandwich for another meal.

Sandwich and weight	Calories	Fat (grams)	Calories from fat- (%)
Turkey with mustard, 9 oz.	**370**	**6**	**14**
Roast beef with mustard, 9 oz.	462	12	22
Chicken salad, 10 oz.	**537**	**32**	**54**
Tuna salad, 11 oz.	716	43	54
Ham with mustard, 9 oz.	**563**	**27**	**43**
Egg salad, 10 oz.	546	31	51
Bacon, lettuce, and tomato, 8 oz.	**599**	**37**	**56**
Vegetarian with avocado & cheese, 12 oz.	753	40	48
Grilled cheese, 5 oz.	**511**	**33**	**58**

Figures are for sandwiches without extra mayonnaise, oil, or dressing spread on the bread. Using mayonnaise adds about 117 calories and 13 grams of fat.

Copyright 1995. Center for Science in the Public Interest.

In 1982, researchers collected toenail clippings from 62,641 women with no history of cancer other than nonmelanoma skin cancer (which is caused by ultraviolet radiation from the sun). During the 41 months of follow-up study, researchers analyzed 503 cases of cancer other than nonmelanoma skin cancer or breast cancer. (A previous study had found no association between breast cancer and selenium.) The researchers concluded that there was no association between higher levels of selenium and reduced cancer risk.

Other researchers said that this study may not be the last word on the effects of selenium. Earlier studies that found the mineral had a protective effect against cancer examined selenium levels in the blood. It may be, these researchers note, that measurements of selenium in toenails are not as accurate as those in blood.

Carbohydrates versus fats. Too much fat in the diet leads to a greater accumulation of body fat than do too many carbohydrates. This finding was reported in February 1995 by researchers at the University of Colorado in Denver, Vanderbilt University in Nashville, Tennessee, and Procter & Gamble Company in Cincinnati, Ohio.

Nine lean and nine obese men aged 18 to 46 participated in the study. Each participant completed two separate two-week sessions of overeating. During one two-week session, everyone consumed 50 percent more calories in fats than they normally took in. During the other session, participants consumed 50 percent more calories in carbohydrates. On four days during each of the sessions, researchers measured the number of calories burned as energy. From this information, they estimated how many calories were stored as fat.

The researchers found that 75 to 85 percent of excess calories from carbohydrates were stored as fat, as were 90 to 95 percent of excess calories from fat. The percentage of weight gained did not differ between the lean and obese groups.

The results of this study show that all overeating can eventually lead to obesity. And diets that include unlimited amounts of carbohydrates will not help fat reduction.

Diets with too little fat. Diets low in fats called essential fatty acids (efa's) may increase the risk of heart disease, according to a study published in August 1994 by researchers at Boston University Medical Center. Efa's are important for regulating levels of saturated fat and cholesterol in the body. Because the human body does not manufacture efa's, they must be consumed in the diet. Soybean products, seeds, nuts, and fish are all sources of efa's.

In the study, researchers analyzed blood samples from 47 men and women who were known to have heart disease, 24 people without heart disease, and 32 others who were chosen at random and might or might not have heart disease. Researchers found that those with heart disease had lower blood levels of efa's and higher levels of saturated fats than those without heart disease.

The researchers believe that diets low in efa's prompt cells to produce excess cholesterol, which can lead to hardening of the arteries and heart disease. They also suggest that diets high in saturated fats can hold down levels of efa's, leading to the same build-up of cholesterol.

Critics of the study have suggested that factors other than insufficient efa's in the diet could account for the link between efa's and heart disease. For example, smokers typically have lower blood levels of one type of efa than nonsmokers because tobacco smoke causes reactions in the body that destroy the efa. And so smoking, which was not taken into account in the study, could have contributed to the heart disease. Another possibility is that participants with low efa levels ate large amounts of saturated fats and that these fats caused the heart disease.   • Jeanine Barone

See also the section Spotlight on Eating Right. In WORLD BOOK, see NUTRITION.

Occupational Health
See Environmental Health

Pregnancy and Childbirth

Babies born prematurely face even greater risks than those previously known, according to three studies reported in 1994 and 1995. Two studies examined the long-term effects of prematurity on childhood development. The third study challenged a commonly held medical belief that the low weight of premature babies has a more harmful effect than how early the baby is born.

Approximately 7 to 10 percent of babies are born prematurely, or preterm, meaning before the 38th week of pregnancy. These preterm births account for three-fourths of all deaths among newborns. Preterm infants have a number of health problems because their organs are not mature and thus are unable to function fully. One of the most serious problems is respiratory distress syndrome, which can occur when the lungs are not fully developed. Low birth weight also makes newborns more susceptible to illness.

Prematurity and later problems.
Medical advances since the mid-1980's have made it possible to keep smaller and smaller premature babies alive. But these babies have health problems even after reaching school age, according to a study reported in September 1994 by pediatric researcher Maureen Hack and her colleagues at Case Western Reserve University in Cleveland.

The researchers looked at 68 children who had weighed about 1.5 pounds (0.7 kilograms) at birth and compared them with 65 children who were also born early but had higher birthweights and with another 61 children who were born at full term. The researchers found that the babies with the lowest birth weights were also the least prepared to perform adequately in school. Many of the children had poor eyesight, learning difficulties, and behavior problems. Moreover, 21 percent were classified as mentally retarded and 45 percent required special education when they reached school.

The effectiveness of special education for these children may depend upon their birth weight, according to a study reported in October 1994 by a group of researchers from eight university research hospitals across the United States. The study looked at the results of a special education program designed for preterm babies from birth to age 3. At age 5, children in such a program were divided into two groups—those who weighed less than 4.4 pounds (2 kilograms) at birth and those who weighed 4.4 to 5.5 pounds (2 to 2.5 kilograms).

Premature infants who later received special education scored higher on IQ tests and had fewer behavioral problems than other children who had been born prematurely. Overall, however, IQ scores were higher among children with higher birth weights. The researchers concluded that babies who weigh more at birth benefit the most from special education at an early age.

Low birth weight, while increasing the problems faced by premature infants, may not be such a serious liability for full-term babies, according to a study reported in March 1995. The study compared birth statistics from the United States and Norway. Current efforts to prevent deaths among newborns in the United States focus on increasing birth weights.

Norwegian newborns weigh more on average than American newborns, and it had been thought that their higher weight accounted for the low-

er death rate among newborns in Norway. But when the researchers compared figures from the two countries, they found that babies at the same birth weight had equal chances for survival in Norway and the United States. More births were preterm in the United States, however. The researchers concluded that the greater number of preterm births, rather than the lower average birth weight, accounted for the higher rate of infant deaths in the United States.

Smoking during pregnancy. Smoking by pregnant women is responsible for as many as 7.5 percent of miscarriages and as many as 21 percent of low birth weights, researchers reported in April 1995. Smoking also plays a role in stillbirths and triples the risk of sudden infant death syndrome, they said.

Joseph R. DiFranza and Robert A. Lew at the University of Massachusetts in Fitchburg and Boston analyzed the results of more than 100 studies on the health effects on fetuses and newborns of mothers who smoke. They based their conclusions on their own estimates of the number of pregnant women who smoke, which ranged from a "best case" figure of 18 percent to a "worst case" estimate of 27 percent. The actual number of women who smoke during pregnancy is not known.

Miscarriage, the spontaneous abortion of a fetus, occurs in 15 to 20 percent of all diagnosed pregnancies in the United States. Many miscarriages occur before a woman is aware that she is pregnant, and so the actual number may be as high as 50 percent of all pregnancies. The researchers, however, used only cases in which women knew they were pregnant. They concluded that from 3 percent to 7.5 percent of these miscarriages are caused by women smoking during pregnancy.

The researchers estimated that smoking also was a factor in 11 to 21 percent of cases of low birth weight, affecting 32,000 to 61,000 babies born annually. In addition, nearly half of the smokers' low birth-weight infants needed special care in neonatal intensive care units. On the basis of this finding, the researchers

Sad mothers

Postpartum depression affects 10 to 15 percent of new mothers, studies have shown, and it too often goes untreated. Yet depressed mothers have a reduced capacity for affection and nurturing, according to a June 1995 study, and this can have long-term effects on the baby. The study was reported by Douglas M. Teti of the University of Maryland.

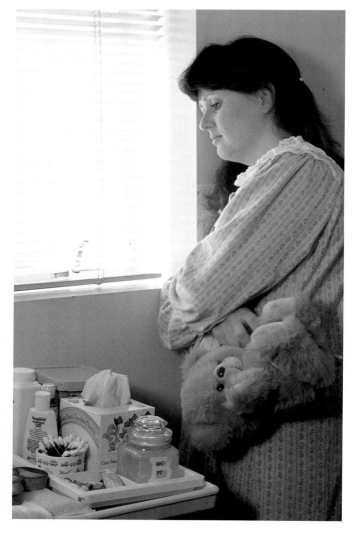

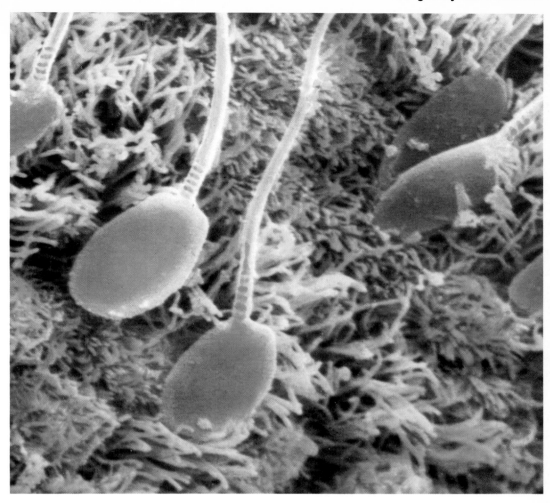

estimated that smoking during pregnancy was responsible for an estimated 14,000 to 26,000 hospital stays at a cost ranging from $164 million to $792 million yearly.

Studies have linked sudden infant death syndrome (SIDS), the unexplained death of apparently healthy babies, to smoking both during pregnancy and after giving birth, when a baby may be exposed to secondhand smoke. The University of Massachusetts researchers found the risk of SIDS to be three times higher among infants of mothers who smoked than among infants of nonsmoking mothers. They estimated that 22 percent to 41 percent of all deaths from SIDS are the result of smoking.

Many women find it difficult to stop smoking when they become pregnant because of the addictive substance nicotine in tobacco. Although nearly 40 percent of pregnant women smokers report that they stop smoking, experts suspect that the actual rate of quitting among pregnant smokers is closer to 8 percent. Because of these low success rates, the authors of the study advised that the efforts of health workers should focus on preventing teen-age girls from smoking. They concluded their report with a reminder that tobacco use affects innocent individuals who have not chosen to assume the risks involved.

• Rebecca D. Rinehart

In the section On the Medical Frontier, see PREGNANCY THROUGH TECHNOLOGY. In WORLD BOOK, see PREGNANCY.

Sperm "surf" uterine waves

Muscle contractions of the uterus help move sperm along on their journey to fertilize an egg, researchers at the University of Manitoba in Winnipeg reported in April 1995. The study found that some infertile women had uterine waves that were weak, infrequent, or backward.

Respiratory System

Researchers reported in January 1995 on the success of a new surgical treatment for chronic obstructive pulmonary disease (COPD), a condition involving persistent obstruction of airflow in the lungs. COPD can result from such respiratory disorders as asthma, chronic bronchitis, and emphysema. It is the fifth leading cause of death in the United States and a cause of serious disability.

Most people with severe COPD suffer from emphysema, a disease that destroys the walls of air sacs in the lungs. The damage results in obstruction of the airways that transfer oxygen to the blood and to the formation of large air spaces that trap carbon dioxide-containing air inside the lung. As more air is inhaled and trapped in the air spaces, the lung begins to lose elasticity and becomes overinflated. As a result, people with emphysema have difficulty getting enough oxygen into their bodies and expelling the carbon dioxide that accumulates in their lungs.

In severe cases of emphysema, hyperinflation of the lungs stretches the diaphragm, the large muscle at the base of the lung that controls breathing. If the diaphragm stretches too much, it has little room to work, resulting in severe breathing difficulties and breathlessness while performing everyday activities.

Lung transplantation has become an option for treating selected patients with emphysema. But transplantation is expensive, risky, and dependent on the availability of donor organs. The patient's body may also reject the transplanted tissue.

In the 1960's, surgeons first tried a technique that involved cutting away part of the diseased lung tissue. But a high percentage of patients died, largely because there was no effective way to stop air leaking from their lungs after the operation.

In the early 1990's, surgeon Joel Cooper of Washington University School of Medicine in St. Louis, Missouri, pioneered a new technique for treating emphysema called bilateral volume reduction. The technique, which involves cutting away 20 to 30 percent of the diseased tissue in both lungs, is designed to reduce the volume of the lungs, restoring them to their normal shape and size and allowing the diaphragm to function properly. The procedure uses a new tool developed by Cooper that closes incisions in the lungs more effectively than earlier procedures did, thereby preventing leakage of air.

In January 1995, Cooper reported the results of the first 20 volume-reduction surgeries he performed. No deaths related to the operation had occurred, and none of the patients required assisted breathing from a mechanical ventilator after the operation. Fourteen patients had required such assistance before the procedure.

New surgical treatment for emphysema

Physicians reported in early 1995 using a new surgical tool to restore lung function in patients with severe emphysema. A special suturing instrument that cuts and sews at the same time reduces lung volume by trimming overinflated, diseased tissue at the edges of the lungs to permit easier breathing.

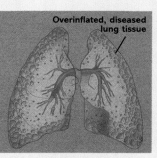

Overinflated, diseased lung tissue

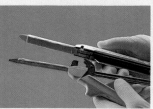

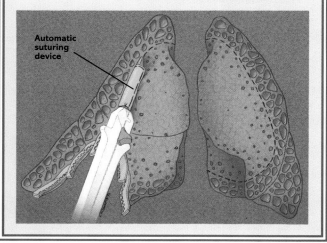

Automatic suturing device

Patients also experienced a significant reduction in total lung capacity and in the amount of air left in the lungs after a complete exhalation, reflecting an improvement in the lungs' hyperinflation.

Furthermore, Cooper reported, patients were able to forcefully exhale 82 percent more air after the operation, and they experienced significantly less breathlessness during exercise. Although these results were preliminary, thoracic surgeons regard the new procedure as a promising way to improve lung function in selected COPD patients.

Ibuprofen and cystic fibrosis. Anti-inflammatory drugs such as the over-the-counter pain reliever ibuprofen, may slow the progress of cystic fibrosis, researchers concluded in a study reported in March 1995. The study was conducted by pediatric lung specialist Michael W. Konstan and his associates at the Rainbow Babies and Children's Hospital and Case Western Reserve University School of Medicine, both in Cleveland.

Cystic fibrosis is an inherited disorder in which thick mucus secretions build up in the lungs, making breathing difficult. There is no cure for the disease.

The researchers gave 85 patients from 5 to 39 years of age either ibuprofen or a *placebo* (an inactive agent) twice a day for four years.

They observed a slower decline in lung function in the patients who received ibuprofen. Patients who took the prescribed dosage at least 70 percent of the time had an even slower decline. Participants who were under 13 years old when the study began received the most benefit from the treatment, the researchers said.

Smoking and lung disease. People with mild obstructive lung disease who quit smoking retain more lung function than people who continue to smoke. This conclusion from a five-year study was reported in November 1994 by researchers with the Lung Health Study Research Group, a cooperative effort of several medical centers and government groups in the United States and Canada.

The researchers evaluated 5,887 smokers from 35 to 60 years of age and assessed the impact of smoking cessation on lung function. They defined lung function in terms of the amount of air exhaled in one second.

Individuals in the study who continued to smoke experienced a 28 percent greater loss of lung function than those who quit smoking and refrained from smoking during the five-year study. People who quit smoking and also used an inhaled *bronchodilator* (a drug that relaxes and expands airways) retained the most lung function. However, the small benefit that the bronchodilator conferred disap-

Keys to the wheeze

Many infants and toddlers suffer episodes of wheezing—but only some of them go on to develop asthma, a chronic lung disease marked by wheezing and breathing problems. Now, a 1995 study may help doctors identify who is most at risk. In a study of 826 children from birth to age 6, researchers at the University of Arizona noted that while one-third of the children experienced wheezing during their first three years, a minority of these—13.7 percent of the entire group—were still wheezing by age 6. These "persistent" wheezers, many of whom had been diagnosed with asthma, had distinct characteristics: They typically showed early signs of allergies and had mothers with asthma. The findings mean that doctors may now be able to distinguish emerging asthmatics before the condition becomes serious. Meanwhile, young wheezers who are unlikely to develop asthma can avoid needless and expensive preventive treatment.

Source: *New England Journal of Medicine*, Jan. 19, 1995.

peared as soon as the medication was discontinued.

Asthma and poverty. African Americans and Hispanics living in poverty are more likely to die of asthma than are other people with the disorder. Researchers David M. Lang and Marcia Polansky from Hahnemann University Hospital of Philadelphia studied the rates and patterns of asthma deaths in the Philadelphia area from 1969 to 1991 to reach this conclusion. They reported their findings in December 1994.

The two researchers found that the death rate from asthma fell among all groups from 1979 to 1984 and then rose through 1991. However, the death rate remained higher for nonwhites in all years. Nonwhites in the study included primarily African Americans and Hispanics, and they tended to live in poverty. Nonwhites were 2.3 times more likely than whites to die of asthma from 1985 to 1991 and 1.86 times more likely to die of asthma from 1979 through 1984, the researchers found. Their data help show where efforts to reduce the rising asthma death rate should be directed.

• Robert A. Balk

In the Medical and Safety Alerts section, see THE HAZARDS OF CARBON MONOXIDE. In WORLD BOOK, see ASTHMA; LUNG; RESPIRATION.

Safety

The United States National Highway Traffic Safety Administration (NHTSA) warned in May 1995 that a defect in the release button of automobile seat belts manufactured by the Takata Corporation, a Japanese firm, could cause the belts to unbuckle during an accident. The NHTSA investigated the belts after receiving 539 complaints, including reports of 47 injuries.

The NHTSA issued a recall of 8-million cars and trucks with the defective seat belts—the largest auto safety recall since 1980. Takata Corporation supplied about 50 percent of the seat belts used by car manufacturers in Japan and 20 percent used by manufacturers in America during the model years 1986 to 1991. The defective belts were installed on dozens of models sold by Honda, Nissan, Mitsubishi, Mazda, Suzuki, Subaru, Isuzu, Daihatsu, Chrysler, General Motors, and Ford.

The car manufacturers agreed to recall and repair the belts after the NHTSA announced the recall. Manufacturers usually notify consumers of recalls by letter. NHTSA advised consumers who did not receive a notice but suspect that their vehicles have defective belts to contact a dealer or call the customer service number listed in the vehicle owner's manual.

Alcohol-related fatalities. On Dec. 1, 1994, the U.S. Centers for Disease Control and Prevention (CDC), based in Atlanta, Georgia, reported that al-cohol-related traffic deaths decreased by about 30 percent in the period from 1982 to 1993. The CDC attributed the decline to a number of factors, including stricter drunken-driving laws and better enforcement by police. But the CDC said that drunken driving remains a major safety problem. In 1993, the last year included in the study, traffic accidents involving drunken drivers caused 17,461 deaths, about 43.5 percent of the 40,115 traffic deaths in the United States.

Fatigue in trucking accidents. Fatigue is a more serious safety problem than alcohol or drugs among commercial truckdrivers, according to a study reported in January 1995 by the National Transportation Safety Board (NTSB). The study said that truckdrivers who fall asleep at the wheel are a factor in 750 to 1,000 highway deaths each year.

The study analyzed 107 truck accidents. Researchers identified which ones were related to driver fatigue by looking for physical evidence that the driver was asleep at the time of the accident, such as a truck going off the road with no indication of braking or steering. They found that drivers in the fatigue-related accidents slept an average of only 6.9 hours during the previous 24-hour period, while those in accidents not related to fatigue slept an average of 9.3 hours.

On the basis of the findings, the

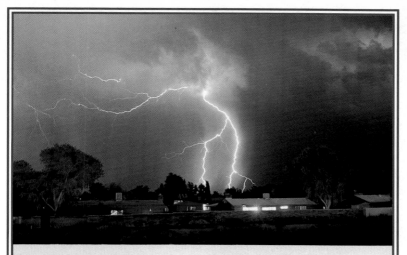

A bolt from the blue

Your chances of getting struck by lightning may be greater than you think. Lightning kills 150 to 200 Americans each year—more than hurricanes and tornadoes combined. Here are some suggestions for staying safe when a thunderstorm hits:

- If you're at home, keep away from electrical appliances or equipment, and use the telephone only for emergencies. Energy from lightning strikes can travel through power lines.

- If you're outside, stay away from high places—such as hills or bridges—and don't stand under tall objects such as trees. Also avoid metal objects, such as bicycles and golf carts. If you're with other people, spread out; lightning is more likely to strike a group.

- If you're swimming, get out of the water and move away from it.

- If you're in a car, stay there.

Source: The Lightning Protection Institute.

NTSB recommended that the Federal Highway Administration increase the amount of rest time required for truckdrivers. The current regulations, which were issued in 1937, require drivers to have 8 hours of off-duty time after 10 hours of driving or after 15 hours of driving and other duties such as loading and unloading.

But the NTSB said new evidence indicates that drivers need 8 full hours of uninterrupted sleep. They seldom sleep this much under current rules because of the need to spend time in other activities such as eating and bathing. The board also recommended that truckdrivers should receive more education on the need for 8 hours of uninterrupted sleep and on the role of fatigue in accidents.

Infant walkers. The sale of infant walkers should be banned and parents should destroy existing walkers because the devices pose a serious safety hazard, the American Academy of Pediatrics (AAP) recommended on May 8, 1995. Infant walkers are wheeled devices with a fabric seat that allow babies to move across the floor while they are learning to walk. About 3 million walkers are sold each year in the United States. Walkers are so popular because parents believe they promote early walking and keep babies happy and quiet.

The AAP said there is no evidence that walkers have positive effects. On the contrary, the AAP said, the limited available data indicate that the devices may interfere with the develop-

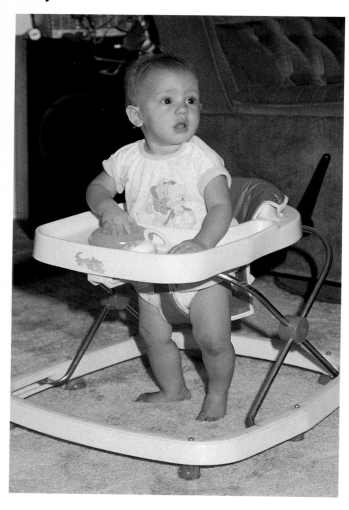

Unsafe at any speed

A ban on infant walkers was recommended by the American Academy of Pediatrics (AAP) in May 1995. The AAP said that injuries from walkers sent 25,000 children to hospital emergency rooms for treatment in 1993, the latest year for which statistics are available. Most of the injuries were caused by falls down stairways.

ment of crawling and thereby delay walking by a few weeks.

More important, walkers can cause injury and death, the AAP said. The rate of walker-associated injuries has increased steadily since 1984. In 1993, the most recent year for which data was available, 25,000 children required treatment in hospital emergency departments for injuries associated with walkers. About 25 per cent of these cases were relatively severe, involving head injuries and fractures. At least 11 infants died in walker accidents between 1989 and 1993. Most of the injuries were caused by falls down stairways. The AAP said that parents, believing that babies are safe in walkers, sometimes use them as babysitters. An infant left

unattended in a walker for even a few seconds, however, can tumble down a stairway and suffer serious injury.

The AAP, concerned that a ban on the manufacture and sale of walkers would still leave millions of used walkers available, suggested that communities organize programs to collect and destroy existing walkers. The organization also advised agencies that license child-care facilities to forbid the use of walkers.

Sudden infant death. Putting infants to sleep on pillows, sheepskins, comforters, and other soft bedding may contribute to 1,800 deaths in the United States each year from sudden infant death syndrome (SIDS). This was the conclusion of a study announced in February 1995 by the U.S. Consumer Product Safety Commission (CPSC). Researchers began the study after earlier reports linked SIDS with suffocation among infants put to sleep in a facedown position.

SIDS, also known as crib death, is a mysterious condition that causes infants to stop breathing while asleep. About 6,000 infants die each year in the United States from SIDS.

The CPSC said that about 30 per cent of infants who died from SIDS between 1992 and 1993 were found with their noses and mouths covered by soft bedding. Parents put most of the infants to sleep stomach down.

Researchers used mechanical models to re-create the death scenes and test the bedding for how much carbon dioxide it allowed to accumulate. During breathing, people inhale oxygen from the air and exhale carbon dioxide. Inhaling carbon dioxide can cause suffocation. The CPSC said the infants may have rebreathed their own carbon dioxide.

Ann Brown, the CPSC chairman who announced the study results, warned that many parents are buying soft, fluffy products for infant cribs. The agency estimates that about 3.2 million infants have coordinated bedding sets that include soft pillows and comforters. Such products should be used for decorative purposes and warmth, not as bedding placed under a sleeping infant. Brown said that healthy infants should be put to sleep on their backs in a crib with a firm, flat mattress. The CPSC emphasized that the study did not identify soft bedding as the cause of SIDS but provided additional evidence of an association between SIDS and a facedown sleeping position on soft bedding.

Child-resistant caps. On Jan. 5, 1995, the CPSC announced a new effort to make it easier for senior citizens and other adults to open child-resistant caps on drugs, household cleaners, and other products. The CPSC said it plans to substitute adults aged 60 to 75 for younger adults on the consumer panels used to test child-resistant packaging.

Consumers have long complained about the difficulty of opening child-resistant caps. Older people with arthritis, muscle weakness, and other disabilities sometimes leave caps on medicines and household chemicals ajar, defeating the purpose of child-resistant packaging.

The CPSC said it would try to encourage manufacturers to develop more user-friendly packaging that will be easier for adults to open but still difficult for children to manipulate. The new easy-to-use caps would appear on all medications and household products required to be sold in child-resistant packages, except those sold in metal or aerosol containers.

Child-resistant packages on aspirin and prescription drugs have been required since the passage of the federal Poison Prevention Packaging Act of 1970. The CPSC estimates that these packages have saved the lives of 700 children.

Bicycle accidents. Boys are more than twice as likely as girls to be injured in a bicycle accident, according to a study reported in April 1995. The study, which involved 707 children aged 5 to 17, found that boys had an injury rate of 8.1 per 10,000 population, compared to 3.4 per 10,000 for girls.

Injuries were most likely to occur among boys aged 11 to 12, who had a rate of 10.2 per 10,000. This group also had the highest rate of serious head injuries. Most of the head injuries could have been prevented by wearing a helmet, the researchers

said. For girls, the injury rate was highest at ages 9 to 10, but the highest head injury rate occurred among girls aged 7 to 8. The study said that boys suffer more injuries than girls because they spend more time riding bicycles and because they perform more risky activities, such as riding on one wheel.

Researchers said parents should be aware of the greater crash risk among boys and of the importance of having children wear helmets while riding a bike. They cautioned that bicycle injuries take a significant toll on children, causing 600 deaths and 500,000 trips to hospital emergency departments each year.

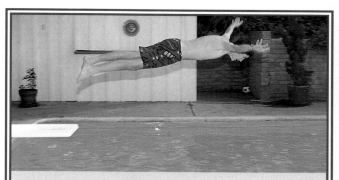

Diving can be disastrous

If a pool or other body of water is not as deep as it looks, a dive can mean lifelong paralysis. Each year, about 1,000 divers—mostly males aged 16 to 30—hit bottom with their heads in diving accidents; more than 90 percent of them become quadriplegic, losing all body control from the neck down. A few precautions can help prevent injury.

- Test the waters feet-first. A minimum depth of 10 feet (3 meters) is considered safe for most people.
- Avoid diving in rivers or lakes, whose waters may hide obstacles, such as tree limbs or rocks.
- In pools, dive only from the end of a diving board.
- Never dive into an aboveground pool.
- Refrain from fancy dives unless you have been trained by a certified instructor and the pool is designed for competitive diving.
- Keep your hands and arms extended over your head for protection. As soon as you hit the water, steer toward the surface by arching your back and reaching upward.
- Don't drink and dive.
- Never dive alone; even the best swimmer can become injured and drown in minutes.

Movable soccer goals. On Jan. 17, 1995, the CPSC warned that movable soccer goals can tip over and crush children who climb on them or hang from the crossbar.

At least 21 deaths and hundreds of injuries involving movable soccer goals have been reported since 1979. Almost all of the accidents involved unanchored, homemade goals rather than professionally manufactured ones. Homemade goals, which are often produced by high school shop classes, school custodians, or local welding shops, tend to be very heavy and unstable.

The CPSC said that players, parents, coaches, and field maintenance personnel should be aware of the potential safety hazard from movable goals. The agency issued new safety guidelines recommending that movable goals be securely anchored to the ground or counter-weighted to prevent tipping. Signs should be attached to goal posts warning that an unsecured goal can tip over and cause serious injury or death. Goals should be chained to a fence or other permanent structure when not in use.

• Michael Woods

In the section Medical and Safety Alerts, see THE HAZARDS OF CARBON MONOXIDE; POISON ON THE MENU; and SAFE HIKING. In WORLD BOOK, see SAFETY.

Sexually Transmitted Diseases

The percentage of sexually active young people who use condoms increased significantly during the early 1990's, according to a report issued in February 1995 by the Centers for Disease Control and Prevention (CDC) in Atlanta, Georgia. Public health officials saw this as an encouraging trend toward reducing adolescents' risk of contracting and spreading sexually transmitted diseases (STD's), including infection with the AIDS-causing HIV (human immunodeficiency virus). During the 1980's, the proportion of sexually active adolescents in the United States grew, and the rates of STD's remained high in this group.

Risky behaviors. The 1995 CDC report was based upon the CDC's Youth Risk Behavior Surveillance System, which began measuring risky behaviors among high school students in 1990. The system involves a survey of students in grades 9 through 12 in public and private schools in all 50 states and the District of Columbia. The number of students surveyed ranged from about 11,600 in 1990 to 16,300 in 1993.

From 1990 to 1993, the survey found no change in the percentages of high school students who reported ever having had sexual intercourse, having four or more sex partners, having sex during the three months preceding the survey, using alcohol or drugs before last sexual intercourse, or using birth control pills at last intercourse. However, the percentages of students who reported using a condom at last intercourse increased significantly, from 46 percent in 1991 to 53 percent in 1993. This increase occurred mainly among females— from 38 to 46 percent—and among blacks—from 48 to 57 percent.

Despite this encouraging trend, many adolescents continued to risk unwanted pregnancy and infection with HIV or another STD by engaging in unprotected intercourse. CDC officials encouraged health, education, and social service providers to urge adolescents to delay engaging in sexual intercourse and to use condoms if they are sexually active.

STD's raise HIV risk. Two studies reported in 1994 and 1995 showed that having a sexually transmitted infection other than HIV may increase a person's risk of becoming infected with HIV. Previous studies had shown a strong connection between HIV infection and other STD's, especially gonorrhea, chlamydia, genital ulcers, and trichomoniasis.

A study reported by British researchers in March 1995 examined existing data from Africa to estimate the effect of genital ulcer disease (GUD) on HIV transmission. The study was led by researchers at the London School of Hygiene and Tropical Medicine.

GUD's include any STD's that result

in open sores on the male or female genitals. In Africa, which has a high rate of HIV infection, the AIDS virus is transmitted primarily through heterosexual intercourse, in contrast to North America and Europe, where the largest number of AIDS cases still occurs among homosexual men.

The researchers found that the presence of genital ulcers increased the risk of male-to-female HIV transmission per sexual exposure by 10 to 50 times. The risk of female-to-male HIV transmission jumped by 50 to 300 times. The proportion of new HIV infections that could be attributed to GUD was estimated at about 24 percent among prostitutes, 16 percent among other females, and 83 percent among men.

Another study, reported in 1994, found that HIV incidence among women in Zaire who worked as prostitutes dropped dramatically when the women attended an STD clinic regularly and received counseling and free condoms. Consistent condom use among the women rose from 0 percent before the introduction of the health measures to 68 percent three months later. The study was led by Marie Laga from the Institute of Tropical Medicine in Antwerp, Belgium.

By the end of the 3-year study period, the incidence of HIV infection had dropped from nearly 12 percent per year to about 4 percent per year. The incidence of gonorrhea, chlamydia, trichomoniasis, and genital ulcers had also dropped substantially. The factors most strongly related to HIV infection included irregular condom use, gonorrhea, trichomoniasis, and genital ulcers.

A plastic condom for men, sold under the trade name Avanti, became available in the United States in November 1994. The condom is made of polyurethane, the same plastic used in a condom for women that was approved by the U.S. Food and Drug Administration (FDA) in 1993.

In laboratory studies, the plastic condoms provided as effective a barrier as latex condoms against the transmission of STD's, including HIV infection. Neither sperm nor viruses passed through the polyurethane material.

S T A T I S T I C S

STD's among sexually active teens

	Males*	Females*
Gonorrhea	6%	10%
Trichomoniasis†	—	21%
Chlamydia	10%	22%
Human papilloma virus	15%	39%

* Percentages represent averages from several studies.
† Rarely appears in men.

Sexually active teens have higher rates of sexually transmitted disease than any other age group, and many diseases infect more girls than boys. However, girls may see few or no signs that they are infected. Gonorrhea sometimes produces itching, burning, and discharge. Chlamydia is typically silent in women, but may produce discharge and burning in men. Women with trichomoniasis may notice discharge and odor. Human papilloma virus (HPV) can produce genital warts, but they are often internal—and not easily noticed. Some HPV strains have been linked with cervical cancer.

Source: Alan Guttmacher Institute; U.S. Office of Technology Assessment; *Los Angeles Times.*

Plastic condoms offer an alternative for condom users who are allergic to latex. In addition, plastic condoms can be made thinner than latex ones, have no odor, and are not weakened by oil-based lubricants, as latex condoms are.

In May 1995, however, the FDA called for further testing of the Avanti condom, after a government study found a higher rate of slippage and breakage in the condoms than the manufacturer had. The FDA urged cautious use of the product until the tests were completed. Manufacturers and researchers continued to present new plastic condoms for approval by the FDA.   • **Katherine Stone**

In WORLD BOOK, see AIDS; SEXUALLY TRANSMITTED DISEASE.

The development of a new surgical treatment for hyperhidrosis—a condition characterized by excess sweating in the hands, feet, and underarm area—was reported in June 1995 by Harold A. Wilkinson, a dermatologist at the University of Massachusetts Medical Center in Worcester. Wilkinson said that his technique had cured about 80 percent of the 110 patients he had treated for the condition over the last 15 years.

Hyperhidrosis most commonly affects the hands, making it difficult for patients to perform certain jobs and awkward for them to shake hands. Conventional surgical treatment re-

quires deep incisions in the back or chest to destroy parts of nerve bundles known as sympathetic ganglia, which are responsible for the stimulation of sweat glands. Other treatments, including superpotent antiperspirant lotions and medication, are only partially effective.

Wilkinson's procedure is much less invasive than conventional surgery. He inserts two hollow needles into the back muscles of an anesthetized patient until they reach the sympathetic ganglia. Thin wire electrodes are then passed through the needles. The wires are heated until they nearly reach the boiling point, which results

From suntan to cancer

Dermatologists have warned for years that tanning is unhealthy and that overexposure to ultraviolet radiation in sunlight can cause skin cancer. In December 1994, medical researchers at Boston University School of Medicine in Massachusetts reported even more disturbing news about suntans. Tanning, the researchers said, is an attempt by skin to repair genetic damage inflicted by the sun, and the repair process can lead to skin cancer in some people.

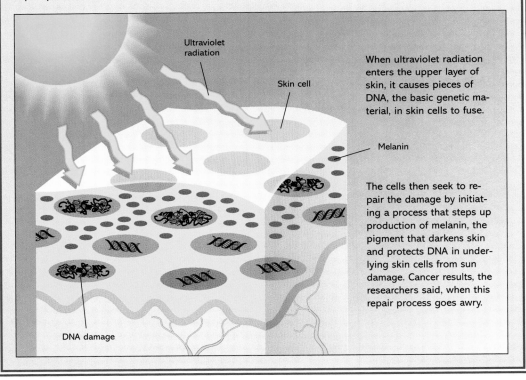

Ultraviolet radiation

Skin cell

When ultraviolet radiation enters the upper layer of skin, it causes pieces of DNA, the basic genetic material, in skin cells to fuse.

Melanin

The cells then seek to repair the damage by initiating a process that steps up production of melanin, the pigment that darkens skin and protects DNA in underlying skin cells from sun damage. Cancer results, the researchers said, when this repair process goes awry.

DNA damage

in destruction of parts of the ganglia.

The procedure is repeated three times to ensure that the targeted area is destroyed. If treatment is successful, the patient's hands will feel cool and dry almost immediately. In some cases the ganglia regrow and treatment must be repeated.

Before undergoing the procedure, a patient must have failed to experience improvement from nonsurgical treatments. The patient must also see a dermatologist or family doctor to make sure that the hyperhidrosis is not caused by *hyperthyroidism* (an overactive thyroid gland), drugs, a tumor, or an infection.

New cream relieves itching. Researchers at the Massachusetts General Hospital in Boston and at the Racine Medical Clinic in Wisconsin, reported the benefits of a new antiitching cream called topical doxepin (sold as Zonalon) in October 1994 in the *Journal of the American Academy of Dermatology.* They studied the effects of the cream in a group of patients who had moderate to severe atopic eczema, a chronic condition characterized by inflamed, itchy skin. Atopic eczema typically occurs in people who have an inherited tendency toward allergy.

Until recently, topical cortisone creams and antihistamine pills were the most widely used treatments for atopic eczema. Topical cortisone is a synthetically produced hormone that relieves itching and inflammation. But when used in large amounts, it can thin the blood, *dilate* (expand) blood vessels, and decrease the adrenal gland's production of cortisone. Antihistamines, which usually come in pill form, decrease itching by blocking the release of histamine, a substance that causes allergic reactions when released into the blood. Antihistamine pills often have adverse side effects such as drowsiness and dry mouth.

Researchers have tried to develop an antihistamine cream as effective as pills but with fewer side effects. In tests of doxepin, 85 percent of patients using the product reported relief of their itching, compared with 57 percent of the patients who used a *placebo* (a substance with no active ingredients). Many of those in the

Cheap relief for athlete's foot

For the most common skin infection in the United States, the cheapest course of treatment may be the smartest, say dermatologists at Case Western Reserve University in Cleveland. They compared the cost of seven prescription creams and three over-the-counter remedies for athlete's foot—a fungal infection that causes blistering, burning, itching, and peeling of the skin, usually between the toes. Most of the medicines have been reported effective in at least 80 percent of cases. But miconazole, a nonprescription cream sold under several brand names, showed a clear advantage to the wallet: In 1993, when the data were gathered, a four-week course of treatment cost $9.04. One other drug, tolnaftate, was even cheaper. The other treatments ranged from $34.67 to $174.39, taking into account the cost of doctors' visits. The researchers concluded that patients—and insurance providers—are most likely to save money overall if athlete's foot sufferers try a cheap nonprescription cream first and proceed to a more expensive remedy only if the initial route fails.

Source: *Journal of the American Medical Association,* Dec. 28, 1994.

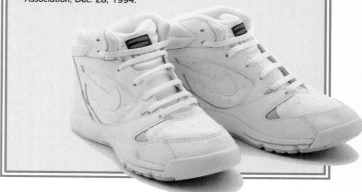

doxepin group got relief within 24 hours. The most common side effects were itching, burning, and drowsiness. None of the patients developed an allergic reaction.

Topical doxepin is more potent than topical benadryl, the only commercially available antihistamine cream. Researchers concluded that doxepin offers a safe alternative to traditional therapies for atopic dermatitis and other skin disorders that involve itching.

Sunless tanning. Researchers at Boston University reported in December 1994 a breakthrough in the understanding of how people tan. Tanning, they said, results from the skin's efforts to repair genetic damage caused by exposure to ultraviolet radiation in sunlight. Ultraviolet radiation can damage DNA (deoxyribonucleic acid, the molecule genes are made of) in skin cells. Normally, the researchers said, damaged DNA is repaired by an enzyme that snips the damaged segment out of the DNA strand and helps generate new DNA to replace it. But if this process goes awry, it can lead to cancer.

In the process of repairing DNA, the skin steps up production of melanin, a brown pigment that is responsible for a suntan. Melanin serves as an ultraviolet filter, making future exposures to sunlight less damaging to DNA in skin.

The researchers were able to promote tanning in guinea pigs without exposure to ultraviolet light. They coated the shaved skin of the guinea pigs with a lotion containing DNA fragments. This research might lead to the development of a lotion that would allow people to develop a suntan without exposure to harmful sunlight. Sunless tanning lotions currently on the market work by staining the top layer of skin. Because these products do not increase melanin production, they offer no added protection from ultraviolet exposure.   • Kathryn E. Bowers

In the section A Healthy You, see WRINKLE REMOVAL: AN ANTIDOTE TO AGING SKIN? In WORLD BOOK, see SKIN.

Smoking

In a dramatic assault on smoking, President Bill Clinton announced his decision on Aug. 10, 1995, to allow the Food and Drug Administration (FDA) to regulate nicotine as an addictive drug. He also proposed strong measures aimed at curbing young people's access to tobacco. By regulating nicotine, Clinton hopes to cut the number of the nation's estimated 3 million underage smokers in half over the next seven years.

The Clinton regulations would bar cigarette sales to people under 18, require retailers to verify the age of their customers, and ban the sale of cigarettes in vending machines. Because research has also found that some cigarette advertising specifically targets youths, the regulations would further forbid the placement of outdoor tobacco ads within 1,000 feet (305 meters) of schools and playgrounds, and would ban brand-name advertising at sporting events and on products not related to tobacco use. The rules would also require tobacco companies to pay for a $150-million advertising campaign to stop young people from smoking.

Tobacco companies filed suit in federal court against the proposed regulation, saying the FDA has no jurisdiction over cigarettes.

Smoking trends and death rates.
Half of all current smokers will die as a result of their smoking habit, and one-quarter of current smokers will shorten their life expectancy by 20 to 25 years, according to a report published in September 1994 by a team of researchers at the World Health Organization and Great Britain's Imperial Cancer Research Fund.

The researchers analyzed trends in smoking and smoking-related deaths since the 1950's and made projections of smoking patterns into the next century. They estimated that someone in the world dies every 10 seconds as a result of smoking and said that if current smoking patterns continue, there will be a death from smoking every 3 seconds by the time the youth of today reach middle age.

Passive smoke and crib death.
Secondhand smoke increases an infant's risk of dying of Sudden Infant Death Syndrome (SIDS), a mysterious condition in which infants stop breathing while asleep. This finding was published in March 1995 by researchers from the University of California at San Diego. Their study looked at the effects of the parents' smoking during pregnancy, after birth, and during breastfeeding.

The researchers studied 200 children who had died of SIDS and matched them with 200 healthy children by such factors as parents' age and education, prenatal care, and birth weight. They then examined the mothers' smoking habits and whether the father or any other adults smoked in the same room as the infant.

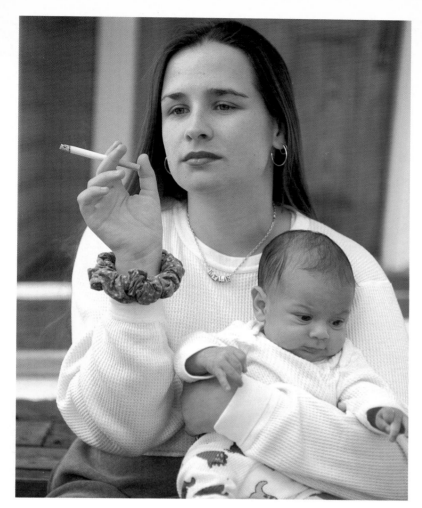

The study showed that SIDS infants were more likely to have been exposed to passive smoke from the mother or another live-in adult than were infants who had not died. They also found that the greater the number of cigarettes the infant was exposed to, the higher was the risk of SIDS. And although previous studies have shown that breastfeeding lowers the risk of SIDS, this protective effect was negated if the mother smoked.

Smoking and the unborn child.
Smoking during pregnancy may increase the chances that daughters are biologically predisposed to smoking cigarettes. This finding was published in October 1994 by Denise Kandel, a researcher at

Columbia University in New York City.

Kandel studied about 1,000 adolescents and found that teen-age girls were four times more likely to smoke if their mothers had smoked while pregnant. She theorized that nicotine, which can pass from the mother to the fetus, may act as a trigger in the brain for the chemical dopamine. Dopamine has been linked with addiction. Kandel was uncertain why boys exposed to tobacco smoke prenatally were not at increased risk.

Pancreatic cancer risk. Pancreatic cancer is closely associated with long-term cigarette smoking, according to a study published in October 1994 by Debra T. Silverman, an epidemiologist at the National Cancer In-

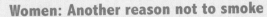

Women: Another reason not to smoke

Smoking may contribute to severe menstrual pain, or dysmenorrhea, according to a study from the University of Milan, Italy, reported in 1994. Researchers compared 145 women who had no menstrual pain to 106 women with dysmenorrhea. The women ranged in age from 15 to 44, and none of the women had endometriosis, fibroid tumors, or ovarian cysts—conditions that in themselves may cause pelvic pain. They found that women who smoked 10 to 30 cigarettes a day had twice the risk for painful periods, and those who had smoked for 10 to 20 years nearly tripled their risk.

Source: *Epidemiology*, July 1994.

stitute. This finding is of great importance because pancreatic cancer is a particularly deadly form of cancer.

Silverman interviewed 526 cancer patients in 12 separate communities and compared them with 2,153 people in the same communities who did not have cancer. Her study revealed that long-term smokers have twice the risk of pancreatic cancer as nonsmokers. It also provided evidence that smoking causes at least 27 percent of all pancreatic cancers.

Impotence may be a consequence of smoking, according to a study published in December 1994 by the Centers for Disease Control (CDC) in Atlanta, Georgia. The study authors defined impotence as "persistent difficulty in getting a satisfactory erection for sexual purposes" during the preceding 12 months. They reported that smokers are 50 percent more likely to experience impotence before the age of 50 than nonsmokers.

The researchers analyzed data from a 1985-1986 survey of 4,462 army veterans aged 31 through 49 who had served in Vietnam. The analysis took into account other factors associated with impotence, including diabetes, substance abuse, and certain medications. The study revealed that impotence affected 3.7 percent of smokers, 2.2 percent of those who

How safe are filter cigarettes?

Fibers from cigarette filters can lodge in lungs, according to a report published in January 1995 by researchers at the Roswell Park Cancer Institute in Buffalo, New York. The study does not prove a direct link between filter fibers and human health risk, but some researchers believe such fibers pose a potential health risk. Filters are used to remove cancer-causing tar from cigarettes.

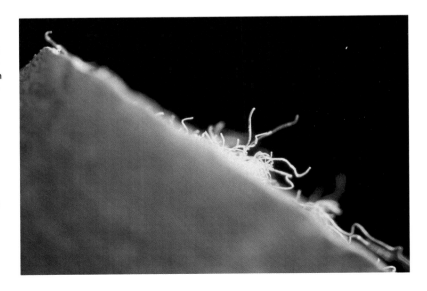

had never smoked, and 2 percent of former smokers. Because the prevalence of impotence in the last two groups was nearly the same, the researchers suggest that quitting smoking can cut the risk of impotence.

Earlier research had shown that smokers are more likely to develop circulatory disorders, which may affect impotence. Cigarette smoke also contains carbon monoxide, a substance that can relax the blood vessels and make maintaining an erection difficult.

Tobacco industry's influence. Tobacco industry contributions to members of Congress strongly influence voting records on tobacco regulation, according to a study published in October 1994 by researchers at Johns Hopkins University in Baltimore.

The researchers looked at congressional voting records in 1991 and 1992. During this period, the tobacco industry donated about $2.4 million to members of Congress. The researchers found that the more money members of Congress received, the less likely they were to support legislation to control the tobacco industry. Republicans and representatives from tobacco-producing states also were less likely to support tobacco controls.
• Gayle R. Hamilton

In WORLD BOOK, see SMOKING.

Surgery to remove fatty deposits from the arteries of the neck can reduce the risk of stroke by more than 50 percent. That finding was announced in May 1995 by neurologist James F. Toole of the Bowman Gray School of Medicine in Winston-Salem, North Carolina.

Toole and other neurologists at 39 medical centers in the United States and Canada studied 1,662 men and women with neck arteries that were at least 60 percent blocked. About half the patients underwent a surgical procedure called carotid endarterectomy, in which the surgeon makes an incision in the neck and extracts the blockage. The other patients received only drug therapy.

The results were striking. The incidence of stroke was 53 percent lower in the surgery group than in the group that was treated with drugs. The benefit, however, was much more pronounced for men than for women. The stroke risk for men declined by 69 percent, compared with just 16 percent for women. The investigators said further studies would be required to explain the large difference.

Binge drinking and stroke. Heavy drinking may sometimes cause a stroke in young adults, researchers at

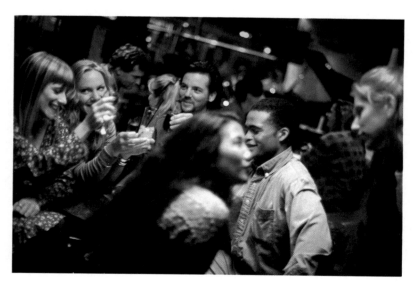

Heavy drinking may trigger some strokes

Binge drinking by young people may sometimes result in a stroke, physicians in Finland reported in January 1995. The doctors did a study of 75 stroke victims, aged 16 to 40, and found that many of them had consumed a large amount of alcohol in the 24 hours preceding their stroke. Heavy drinking might dislodge a clot that has formed in the heart or elsewhere, the researchers said. The clot could then travel to the brain.

Stroke

Smoking and stroke risk
Cigarette smoking speeds up the formation of fatty deposits in the arteries leading to the brain and increases the risk of stroke, researchers at the Bowman Gray School of Medicine in Winston-Salem, North Carolina, reported in December 1994. In a study of 5,116 people over the age of 64, the investigators found significant narrowing of the arteries in 9.5 percent of smokers, compared with just 4.4 percent of nonsmokers.

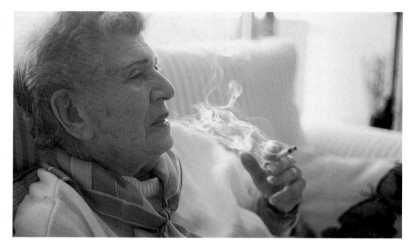

Helsinki University Hospital and Oulu University Hospital, both in Finland, reported in January 1995.

The researchers studied 75 patients aged 16 to 40 years who had been treated for strokes at the hospitals and compared them with another group of 133 patients of similar age who had been treated for other emergency conditions. They found that an alcoholic binge in the 24 hours preceding hospitalization was more common among the stroke victims.

The Finnish scientists were uncertain how hard drinking might cause a stroke, but they speculated that a change in the normal heartbeat might be to blame. Intoxication is known to produce a rapid pulse, which might dislodge a blood clot in the heart or elsewhere in the circulatory system. The clot could then travel to the brain and block an artery.

Migraines and stroke risk. Migraine headaches may raise a person's risk of stroke by as much as 80 percent. Researchers at Brigham and Women's Hospital and Harvard Medical School, both in Boston, reported that finding in February 1995.

The investigators analyzed data collected for the Physicians' Health Study, a study of 22,071 U.S. male physicians aged 40 to 84 that was begun in 1982. They found that 1,479 of the physicians reported suffering from migraine headaches, and 1.3 percent of that group had been stricken by strokes. That percentage, though small, was significantly higher than the percentage of physicians not suffering from migraines who had strokes—0.95 percent.

The researchers said the mechanism by which migraines might be linked with strokes is unclear but might involve blood platelets, cells that enable blood to clot. A number of studies have demonstrated differences in platelet function between migraine sufferers and other people, and such abnormalities might be implicated in both migraine headaches and the strokes now associated with them. That possibility will be investigated in further studies.

Prompt stroke treatment vital.
In September 1995, the American Heart Association (AHA) announced new guidelines for the treatment of stroke. Stressing that a stroke is a medical emergency, the AHA said urgent efforts on behalf of the stroke victim are required by friends and relatives as well as by the hospital staff who care for the stricken individual.

The AHA issued several recommendations for hospital personnel:
- Admit a possible stroke victim as soon as possible to a hospital stroke unit.
- Use advanced imaging technology to evaluate a potential stroke.
- Use the latest therapies to prevent or control complications of stroke, such as pneumonia, blood clots, and seizures. • Julie Foreman
In WORLD BOOK, see STROKE.

Two studies of surgery for perforated peptic ulcers, reported in 1994 and 1995, shed light on the best ways to treat these emergencies. Peptic ulcers are sores on the lining of the stomach or small intestine. If an ulcer perforates—that is, eats through the stomach or intestinal wall—emergency surgery is essential.

Delaying such surgery can increase risk of death, add to complications, and prolong hospital stays, reported researchers from Haukeland University Hospital in Bergen, Norway, in August 1994. Doctors have long known that the survival of a patient with a perforated ulcer depends on how much time passes between perforation and surgery. The researchers sought to find out exactly how such delays affect survival, complication rates, and length of hospital stay.

The researchers looked at 1,237 patients who underwent surgery for perforated ulcers between 1935 and 1990. After adjusting for such factors as age, sex, type of ulcer, and year of perforation, the researchers found that problems increased markedly when surgery began more than 12 hours after the perforation. Compared with delays of 6 hours or less, delays of more than 24 hours increased the risk of death by seven to eight times, tripled the risk of complications, and doubled the length of hospital stay.

Another study examined the success of an increasingly popular surgical treatment for perforated ulcers called laparoscopic omental patch repair. Researchers at Chukyo Hospital in Nagoya, Japan, reported in March 1995 that compared with traditional surgery, this minimally invasive procedure leads to less postoperative pain, faster recovery, and fewer and less severe complications.

Unlike traditional ulcer surgery, which requires an incision in the upper abdomen, the laparoscopic technique uses a few small slits, each less than 0.5 inch (about 1 centimeter) long. Through these slits, the surgeon inserts a tiny viewing device and surgical instruments. The surgery is typically followed with H2-receptor antagonists, drugs that have been shown to speed ulcer healing.

The researchers compared 11 patients who had laparoscopic omental patch repair with 55 patients who underwent various other surgical treatments for ulcers. They found that the laparoscopic surgery patients needed less pain relief after surgery, recovered faster, and suffered fewer serious complications than the patients undergoing other forms of surgery. After a follow-up period averaging 11 months, none of the patients had developed new ulcers.

Aortic aneurysms. In December 1994, doctors at Stanford University

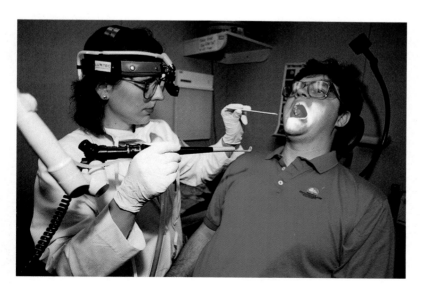

Trouble-free tonsil trimming

Tonsil removal used to mean general anesthesia, a hospital stay, and a throatful of pain. Now some physicians are using an office procedure called laser-assisted tonsil ablation to evaporate the troublesome portions of the tonsils. The laser procedure decreases bleeding, reduces pain, and costs less than standard surgery—but it does require up to five sessions to correct the problem.

Surgery

To lower costs, hospitals in the United States have been moving a number of procedures out of the operating room and into ambulatory facilities, which can include doctors' offices. From 1984 to 1993, the number of outpatient operations—those not requiring an overnight hospital stay—that were performed in hospitals dropped from 14.4 million to 10.2 million. During the same period, operations in ambulatory centers rose from 5.5 million to 12.6 million.

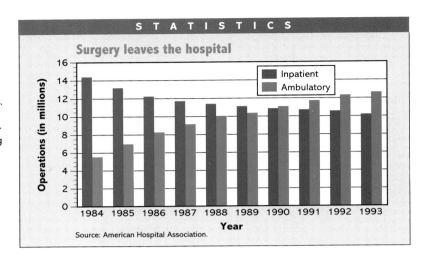

STATISTICS

Surgery leaves the hospital

Source: American Hospital Association.

Medical Center in Stanford, California, reported a new approach for treating aneurysms of the aorta.

An aneurysm is a balloon-like bulge in a blood vessel; if the bulge bursts, the person can die within minutes. A common site for aneurysm is the aorta, the major artery that carries blood from the heart to the rest of the body. When such an aneurysm is discovered, the usual treatment is to replace the distorted section of aorta with a *prosthetic graft* (artificial replacement). This surgical procedure is painful and risky.

One possible alternative involves the use of a stent—a small scaffolding device that has been used successfully in smaller arteries to widen narrow passages and keep them open. Stents large enough to use in the aorta are experimental, but the Stanford study provides some encouraging results.

In the Stanford procedure, a stainless steel stent is covered with a sleeve of polyester cloth, collapsed, and fitted over a device called a balloon catheter, a tool frequently used in surgery to expand blood vessels. This balloon catheter is inserted into a large blood vessel in the groin and moved through the blood vessels until it reaches the aneurysm in the chest. The balloon is then inflated, expanding the stent and its cloth covering to the proper diameter of the aorta. Once in place inside the aneurysm, this structure—now a cloth tube supported by a stent scaffold—

creates a normal-size replacement passage for blood flow.

Because the stent is placed from the inside, the procedure does not require opening the chest and is safer than the traditional surgery. The Stanford team successfully placed a stent graft in 13 patients over a two-year period. No deaths or serious complications occurred during a one-year follow-up, though one patient needed traditional prosthetic graft surgery when her aorta continued to expand.

Boosting surgical performance.
Surgeons who like to listen to music while operating may boost their performance and lower their stress by doing so, researchers at the State University of New York at Buffalo reported in September 1994. Although no data exist as to how often surgeons operate with musical accompaniment, this is believed to be a common practice. The researchers sought to find out how music affected surgeons' performance. Fifty male surgeons, aged 31 to 61, volunteered for the study. All described themselves as music lovers and said they regularly listened to music during surgery. None took medication for heart conditions or blood pressure.

The surgeons were asked to solve a series of mental arithmetic tasks of a type shown in earlier experiments to induce tension. They performed the test in a soundproof laboratory under three conditions: in silence, while listening to a song selected by the researchers (Pachelbel's "Canon in D," an orchestral piece often used commercially to create a calming atmosphere), and while listening to music of their own choice. The surgeons' requests—all instrumental—included 46 classical, 2 jazz, and 2 Irish folk selections.

During each test, the medical researchers measured several physiological responses known to increase with stress, including blood pressure and pulse rate. For each of these measures, the surgeons displayed the lowest levels of reaction when listening to the music they selected. Reactions were somewhat greater when the surgeons listened to Pachelbel's

"Canon," and the highest levels occurred in the silent environment.

At the same time, the surgeons performed the calculations fastest and most accurately while listening to their own choice of music. Their speed and accuracy was reduced under the other two conditions.

These results supported the surgeons' "intuitive beliefs that music is beneficial during stressful tasks," the researchers wrote. They added that the self-selected music may have had the best effects because the doctors were already familiar with the music and associated it with success during surgery.   • Julie Foreman

In WORLD BOOK, see SURGERY.

Teeth
See Dentistry

Transplants
See Kidney

Urologists began using a new procedure to reduce enlarged prostates in late 1994 and early 1995 that heats tissue until it *vaporizes* (turns to gas). The procedure reportedly causes fewer side effects than standard surgical treatments and offers quicker recovery.

The prostate is an organ of the male reproductive system and is located just below the bladder and directly in front of the rectum. It secretes a fluid that helps transport sperm cells. The prostate enlarges in about 75 percent of men over the age of 50. The enlargement creates pressure on the urethra, the tube that

drains the bladder. The pressure causes slowing of the urinary stream, frequent urination, and the need to urinate several times during the night in 10 to 20 percent of patients. Medication can successfully treat many men with prostate enlargement, but in some cases, surgery is required.

Transurethral resection of the prostate (TURP) is the most common surgical procedure for treating prostate enlargement. In this procedure, a surgeon cuts out part of the prostate to reduce pressure on the urethra. This surgery is usually successful, but TURP can cause bleeding from the prostate into the urethra and gen-

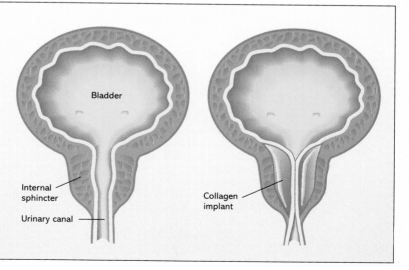

Incontinence treatment
Urologists at Mayo Clinic in Rochester, Minnesota, reported successfully treating incontinence with injections of collagen, a protein found in skin, in late 1994. Incontinence is often caused by a weakened internal sphincter muscle that cannot close tightly enough around the urinary canal to prevent leakage of urine from the bladder, *right*. The injected collagen exerts pressure on the urinary canal, which prevents leakage, *far right*.

Bladder

Internal sphincter

Urinary canal

Collagen implant

erally requires hospitalization for two to four days.

Laser therapy is another surgical treatment for an enlarged prostate. In this procedure, physicians insert a fiberoptic tube through the urethra into the prostate and destroy tissue by means of high-energy light transmitted by the laser through the tube. Laser surgery often does not require an overnight hospital stay, and the risk of bleeding from this surgery is much less than from TURP. However, patients who undergo laser treatment usually need a urinary *catheter* (tube inserted into the urethra) to drain urine for several days to a few weeks following surgery.

Transurethral electrovaporization is the new procedure urologists began to use in late 1994 for treating enlarged prostates. In this procedure, the surgeon inserts a small metal bar into the urethra. Wires heat the bar to about 212 °F (100 °C), a temperature high enough to vaporize tissue. Vaporization usually causes little bleeding and does not require prolonged use of a catheter.

In early studies of electrovaporization, most men reported excellent improvement in their symptoms and remained hospitalized for only a day or two. Larger and longer studies are necessary to determine whether vaporization is superior to other techniques, however.

Venereal Diseases
See Sexually Transmitted Diseases

Prostate cancer testing. In August 1994, the Food and Drug Administration approved the use of a blood test called prostate specific antigen (PSA) for the detection of prostate cancer. The PSA test had been previously approved for monitoring the treatment of patients who had already been diagnosed with prostate cancer.

PSA is a protein produced by the prostate gland that circulates in the bloodstream. Both cancerous and noncancerous prostate cells manufacture the protein, but cancerous cells generally release larger amounts of it. Many studies have demonstrated that routine measurement of PSA levels in men over age 50 can lead to an increased detection of potentially curable prostate cancers.

The PSA test is not foolproof, however. From 10 to 20 percent of men in whom prostate cancer is eventually found have normal PSA levels, according to medical researchers. Furthermore, there is some question whether detecting and treating early-stage prostate cancers substantially prolongs life. In addition, treatment for the disease can cause such side effects as incontinence and impotence. An answer to the controversy surrounding PSA testing will come from large-scale trials now underway. Until then, men will have to reach individual decisions about testing with their physicians.   • Glenn S. Gerber
In WORLD BOOK, see PROSTATE GLAND.

Veterinary Medicine

Viruses that threaten animals also took a human toll in 1994 and 1995. In September 1994 in Australia, a virus killed a horse trainer and 14 race horses he had contact with. The virus, later named equine morbillivirus, belongs to the same group as the measles virus, according to an April 1995 report by researchers from the Australian Animal Health Laboratory, who identified it. The horse trainer died of a lung infection. A second man who had cared for the sick horses came down with flulike symptoms but recovered on his own.

The virus produces a high fever, rapid build-up of fluid in the lungs, and bloody froth from the nose. The researchers theorized that the virus was spread in nasal secretions or saliva, but they had not discovered the source by summer 1995. Investigation continued into the possibility that a wild animal, bird, or insect in Queensland, a state in northeastern Australia, was the source of the virus. Epidemiologists had traced the first case of infection to a horse from a Queensland farm.

The virus disappeared as rapidly as it arrived. But Australian authorities said they wanted to determine if the virus might have caused other unexplained cases of lung infection or undiagnosed illnesses.

Rabies alerts. In October 1994, a kitten bought at a pet store in Concord, New Hampshire, died of another deadly viral disease—rabies. The kitten had come into contact with 31 other kittens at the store before it died at its owner's home. Four of the kittens had died before the rabies diagnosis, so it was not known whether they had rabies. State officials collected the remaining 27 kittens and found that none had the disease.

State authorities issued a rabies warning to the city upon learning that some 500 people could have handled the kittens in the store and been exposed to the virus. Rabies is usually transmitted in saliva through a bite from an infected animal. The disease is fatal in people unless they receive a series of injections before rabies symptoms appear.

In February 1995, Texas officials began an air drop of bait that contained rabies vaccine in an attempt to stem an outbreak of rabies near San Antonio. The bait was dropped over a sparsely populated area covering 14,500 square miles (37,555 square kilometers). Since the outbreak began in 1988, two people have died, and over 500 cases of rabies have been confirmed in coyotes or in dogs that have had contact with the coyotes. In 1994 and 1995, rabid dogs in the area bit a child, a horse, and several other dogs. At least 1,500 people have had rabies shots.

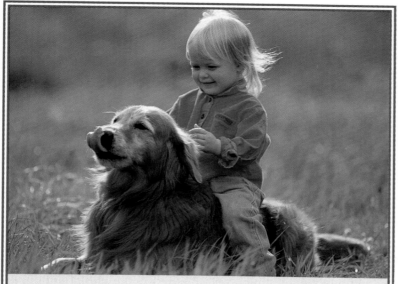

Choosing a friendly pet

Golden retrievers and standard poodles are less likely than other breeds to bite people outside the family they live with, while German shepherds and chow-chows may be more likely to do so, according to a report from the U.S. Centers for Disease Control and Prevention (CDC) in Atlanta, Georgia. CDC researchers examined 178 dog bite cases reported in Denver during 1991 in which the dog had never before bitten a nonfamily member. They found that 25 percent of the bites came from German shepherds and 22 percent from chow-chows. Compared with a sample of nonbiting dogs, the biters were more likely to be male, unneutered (whether male or female), under age 5, and at least 44 pounds (20 kilograms) in weight. Most belonged to households with children, and few had attended obedience school. Experts emphasize, though, that such characteristics do not in themselves mean a particular dog will bite: Any one dog's behavior depends a great deal on training, environment, and its own temperament.

Weight Control

A dangerous sign

Frequent trips to a litter box with no urine eliminated may mean a cat has an obstruction in the *urethra*, the tube that carries urine outside the body. Other symptoms are bloody urine and straining to urinate. The disorder, most common in male cats, arises from a build-up of mineral particles that block the flow of urine. Veterinarians warn that such obstructions can be fatal if left untreated because toxic waste backs up in the cat's system.

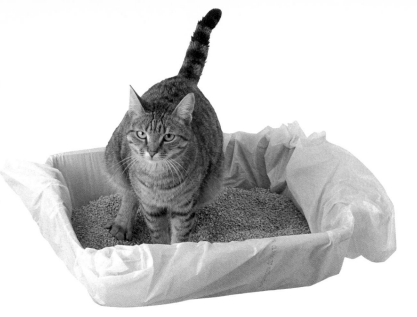

The rabies virus moves from muscle tissue at the bite site into the nerve pathway to the brain. It multiplies in several areas of the brain, but especially in a region that controls such behaviors as aggression and feeding. The behavioral changes that result can turn a normally calm animal into a wandering, vicious creature that bites almost any target in sight.

Wiring canine bones. Certain large breeds of dogs, including German shepherds and rottweilers, inherit a defect in a joint in their forelimb that corresponds to the elbow joint in human beings. As a result, the two major bones that meet at this joint be-come dislodged, and the dog experiences painful episodes of lameness, which worsen with exercise.

In May 1995, researchers at the University of California at Davis School of Veterinary Medicine reported on a new procedure to correct the defect. In the procedure, the veterinarian makes an incision over the elbow joint, drills a hole in both bones, and threads steel wire through the holes. The ends of the wire are then twisted to secure the bones firmly in place. In a follow-up examination, the dog was free of pain and had full range of motion.   • Benjamin L. Hart

In WORLD BOOK, see VETERINARY MEDICINE.

Weight Control

The human body responds to weight loss or gain by altering its use of calories, according to a study published in March 1995 by researchers at Rockefeller University Hospital in New York City. The study found that people burn fewer calories when weight drops, which helps explain why dieters tend to eventually regain lost weight even if they stick to their diet plans. The study also found that the rate of calorie burning drops even lower following weight loss among people who are *obese* (20 percent or more above the recommended weight for their height and age).

People lose weight either by consuming fewer calories in food than they require for energy or by burning more calories in physical activity than they consume in food. The researchers studied the rate of calorie burning in 18 obese and 23 nonobese volunteers. After a 10 to 20 percent weight loss, the obese participants lowered their total energy expenditure by an average of 8 calories daily per kilogram (2.2 pounds) of body weight, a level 15 percent below that predicted for their body composition. Nonobese participants showed a smaller change, lowering their energy expenditure by an average of 6 calories per kilogram of weight per day.

This pattern was reversed among participants who gained weight. After a 10 percent gain, obese participants increased their total energy expenditure by an average of 8 calories per kilogram of body weight per day, and nonobese ones increased their expenditure by an average of 9 calories.

The study demonstrates how the body uses changes in energy expenditure to maintain a set point—an internally set standard that helps keep body weight in adults stable for long periods of time. The researchers suggest that physicians should be aware that these changes make it especially difficult for obese people to maintain lower levels of body weight. However, the researchers encourage obese patients to persist in their efforts to lose weight, noting that even a modest weight loss can improve an obese person's health.

Weight cycling. Most studies have shown no increased risk of illness or death among people who experience weight cycling—repeated loss and regain of weight. This was the October 1994 conclusion of the National Task Force on the Prevention and Treatment of Obesity, which was convened by the National Institutes of Health after reports in professional journals and newspapers suggested that weight cycling, popularly known as yo-yo dieting, is dangerous.

The task force, made up of medical researchers from several universities, reviewed 43 studies of weight cycling. The group said that most of the studies had found that weight cycling

had no effect on the efficiency of the body's energy utilization, the ratio of fat to lean tissue, or the future ability to lose weight.

The few studies that did find a link to health problems were flawed, according to the task force. Most of them did not distinguish between voluntary weight loss and weight loss that was caused by serious illness. In addition, some studies involved mainly nonobese or mildly obese subjects. The task force cautions against applying the findings of such studies to obese patients, because weight cycling and weight loss may have differing causes and effects in obese and nonobese individuals. Finally, weight cycling was not defined consistently among the studies. For example, some studies established a minimum number of cycles of weight loss and regain within a given period. Other studies made no such distinction.

The task force said that obese people should not avoid weight loss plans for fear of health risks associated with weight cycling because obesity, unlike weight cycling, has been shown to be dangerous.

Obesity gene and hormone found. Researchers at Rockefeller University Hospital reported in the December 1994 issue of *Nature* that they have identified a gene responsible for obesity in mice. The research team, led by geneticist Jeffrey M. Friedman, has

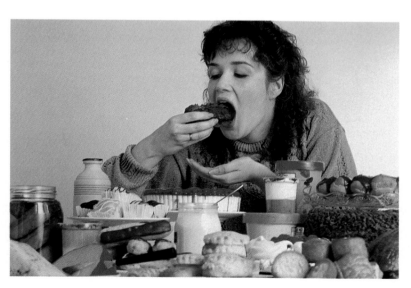

A gene for obesity? Researchers announced in December 1994 that they had found a gene they believe controls appetite by signaling a sense of fullness after a meal. If the gene malfunctions, however, the individual may fail to feel full and go on eating. A team at Rockefeller University Hospital in New York City first identified the gene in mice and then used the mouse gene to locate a similar human gene.

Judging portion size

Food labels provide a handy way of finding out how many calories a product contains and how many of those calories come from fat. But a hurdle many dieters still face is estimating portion sizes. Dietician Joan Horbiak suggests visualizing portions and offers the following tips:

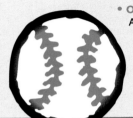
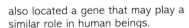

- **One serving of meat, fish or poultry:** An audiocassette.
- **One serving of vegetables, rice, or pasta:** A tennis ball.
- **One serving of fresh fruit:** A baseball.
- **One serving of cheese:** A golf ball.

also located a gene that may play a similar role in human beings.

Genes are units of heredity that control the structure and function of all living things. They are located on chromosomes—threadlike structures within a cell nucleus.

The discovery of an obesity (*ob*) gene built on decades of research. Working with specially bred strains of obese mice, the researchers isolated the *ob* gene, which they believe normally controls appetite by causing fat cells to secrete a hormone into the blood that sends signals of fullness to the brain. In an obese mouse, however, a malfunctioning *ob* gene fails to send these signals and the mouse overeats, tripling its normal body weight. In July, the research team announced that daily injections of the hormone, tentatively called leptin, slim fat mice down to normal weight.

After isolating the *ob* gene, the researchers used it to locate an equivalent gene in humans. They found a human gene that is 84 percent similar to the mouse gene.

More than 30 percent of people in the United States are obese. Studies have linked obesity with an elevated risk of hypertension, diabetes, some cancers, and psychological problems. Most cases of human obesity probably involve environmental and behavioral factors as well as genetics. But the discovery of the *ob* gene could lead to new diagnostic techniques and weight control treatments, such as a drug based on leptin.

Weight gain and heart disease.
Even weight gains that keep women within their normal weight range may increase their risk of coronary heart disease (CHD), heart damage caused by blockage of the arteries that supply blood to the heart. That was the finding of a study reported in February 1995 by researchers at the Harvard Medical School in Boston.

The researchers studied 14 years of health records for 115,818 women who were between the ages of 30 and 55 in 1976, when the record-keeping began. They found that CHD risk increases if women gain enough weight to put them near the top of their normal weight category. Furthermore, they found that even modest weight gain after age 18 also increases CHD risk.

The study found that excess weight accounted for 37 percent of overall incidence of CHD among the women. The increase in CHD risk varied from 25 percent for an 11-to-17 pound (5 to 7.9 kilogram) weight gain to 165 percent for a gain of 44 pounds (20 kilograms) or more. The researchers expressed concern that current U.S. weight guidelines, which were raised in 1990, provide false reassurances. They suggested that weight change, as opposed to weight itself, be further investigated as a risk factor for CHD.   • Ricki Lewis

In the section Spotlight on Eating Right, see IDEAL WEIGHT: SCIENCE OR FASHION? In WORLD BOOK, see WEIGHT CONTROL.

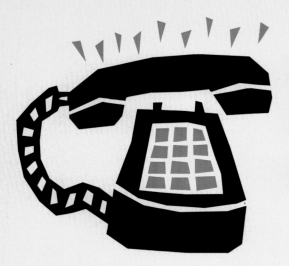

Health Information by Phone

A wealth of health information is available by telephone. Listed below are some useful numbers.

AIDS

☎ **National AIDS Hot Line** (800-342-AIDS), operated by the Centers for Disease Control and Prevention, provides information and referrals 24 hours a day, 7 days a week. Spanish-language information is available at 800-344-7432, 7 days a week from 8 a.m. to 2 a.m. Eastern time. People who are hearing impaired can call 800-243-7889 weekdays from 10 a.m. to 10 p.m. Eastern time.

☎ **Project Inform HIV/AIDS Treatment Hot Line** (800-822-7422) answers questions about treatment of HIV infection and AIDS weekdays from 10 a.m. to 4 p.m. Pacific time.

ALCOHOLISM AND DRUG ABUSE

☎ **Alcohol and Drug Help Line** (800-821-4357) provides referrals to local treatment centers 24 hours a day, 7 days a week.

☎ **American Council on Alcoholism** (800-527-5344) answers questions and provides written information and educational materials weekdays from 9 a.m. to 5 p.m. Eastern time. An answering service operates after regular hours.

☎ **National Cocaine Hot Line** (800-262-2463) provides referrals to local treatment centers 24 hours a day, 7 days a week.

☎ **National Council on Alcoholism and Drug Dependence, Inc.** (800-622-2255) provides referrals through voice mail to affiliates that offer counseling and answer questions.

☎ **Center for Substance Abuse Treatment** (800-662-HELP) refers callers to treatment centers and support groups weekdays from 9 a.m. to 3 a.m. and weekends from noon to 3 a.m. Eastern time.

ALZHEIMER'S DISEASE

☎ **Alzheimer's Association** (800-272-3900) provides written information and referrals to local chapters weekdays from 8:30 a.m. to 5 p.m. Central time.

☎ **Alzheimer's Disease Education and Referral Center** (800-438-4380) answers questions, makes referrals to research centers for diagnosis and treatment, provides information on state services for patients, publishes information on research, and provides an on-line database of information weekdays from 8:30 a.m. to 5 p.m. Eastern time.

☎ **National Institute on Aging** (800-438-4380) provides information and referrals weekdays from 8:30 a.m. to 5 p.m. Eastern time. For information on other topics related to aging, call 800-222-2225.

AMYOTROPHIC LATERAL SCLEROSIS

☎ **Amyotrophic Lateral Sclerosis Association** (800-782-4747) answers questions, supplies written information, and provides referrals to support groups and physicians weekdays from 8 a.m. to 5 p.m. Pacific time.

ARTHRITIS

☎ **Arthritis Foundation** (800-283-7800) sends written information on treatment and local chapters to callers who leave their names and addresses on its answering machine. Callers also may listen to taped information.

☎ **The American Lupus Society** (800-331-1802) sends written information to those who leave their names and addresses on its answering machine.

☎ **Lupus Foundation of America** (800-558-0121) provides written information to those who leave their names and addresses on its answering machine.

ASTHMA AND LUNG DISORDERS

☎ **Asthma and Allergy Foundation of America** (800-7-ASTHMA) sends written information to people who leave their names and addresses on its answering machine. Staff members answer questions at 202-466-7643 weekdays from 9 a.m. to 5 p.m. Eastern time.

☎ **Lungline** (800-222-LUNG) provides written information and an opportunity to speak with registered nurses weekdays from 8 a.m. to 5 p.m. Mountain time.

BRAIN INJURY

☎ **Brain Injury Association Family Help Line** (formerly National Head Injury Foundation) (800-444-6443) answers questions, provides written information, and makes referrals to local resources weekdays from 9 a.m. to 5 p.m. Eastern time.

CANCER

☎ **Cancer Information Service** (800-4-CANCER) of the National Cancer Institute answers questions and provides written information and referrals to treatment centers, mammography facilities, and support groups weekdays from 9 a.m. to 7 p.m. local time.

☎ **Cancer Response System** (800-ACS-2345) of the American Cancer Society (ACS) provides written information and referrals to local ACS programs and resources during local business hours.

☎ **Y-ME National Organization for Breast Cancer Information Support Program** (800-221-2141) allows callers to speak to counselors who have survived breast cancer; offers a men's hot line for those who prefer to speak to a male counselor; provides written information; and supplies wigs and prostheses to women who cannot afford them. The line operates 7 days a week, 24 hours a day.

CHILD ABUSE AND NEGLECT

☎ **National Resource Center on Child Abuse and Neglect** (800-227-5242) answers questions and provides written information weekdays from 8:30 a.m. to 4:30 p.m. Mountain time.

CROHN'S DISEASE AND COLITIS

☎ **Crohn's and Colitis Foundation of America, Inc.** (800-932-2423) provides written information and referrals to physicians and support groups weekdays from 9 a.m. to 5 p.m. Eastern time. Callers can speak to a counselor weekdays from 2:15 to 4 p.m. Eastern time.

CYSTIC FIBROSIS

☎ **Cystic Fibrosis Foundation** (800-824-5064) provides written information and referrals to local support groups weekdays from 8:30 a.m. to 5 p.m. Central time.

DIABETES

☎ **American Diabetes Association** (800-ADA-DISC) answers questions and provides written information weekdays from 8:30 a.m. to 5 p.m. Eastern time.

☎ **Juvenile Diabetes Foundation International Hot Line** (800-223-1138) answers general questions, supplies written information, and provides doctor referrals weekdays from 9 a.m. to 5 p.m. Eastern time.

DISABILITY AND REHABILITATION

☎ **National Rehabilitation Information Center** (800-346-2742) acts as a library on topics relating to disability and rehabilitation by searching databases and providing written information. The center also answers questions and provides referrals weekdays from 8 a.m. to 6 p.m. Eastern time.

DOWN SYNDROME

☎ **National Down Syndrome Society Hot Line** (800-221-4602) answers questions, supplies written information, and provides referrals to local parent support groups weekdays from 9 a.m. to 5 p.m. Eastern time.

DRINKING WATER

☎ **Safe Drinking Water Hot Line** (800-426-4791), operated under contract for the Environmental Protection Agency, answers questions and provides written information about federal regulation of public water.

DYSLEXIA

☎ **The Orton Dyslexia Society** (800-222-3123) sends written information to callers who leave their names and addresses on its answering machine. Staff members answer questions at 410-296-0232 weekdays from 8:30 a.m. to 4:30 p.m. Eastern time.

EPILEPSY

☎ **Epilepsy Foundation of America** (800-EFA-1000) answers questions, provides information, and makes referrals weekdays from 9 a.m. to 5 p.m. Eastern time.

EYES AND VISION

☎ **American Council of the Blind** (800-424-8666) answers questions, makes referrals, and provides information on consumer items for blind people weekdays from 3 p.m. to 5:30 p.m. Eastern time. At all other times, an answering service provides updates on legislation affecting blind people.

☎ **Guide Dog Foundation for the Blind, Inc.** (800-548-4337) answers questions weekdays from 8 a.m. to 5:15 p.m. Eastern time. An answering service operates outside those hours.

☎ **National Association for Parents of the Visually Impaired** (800-562-6265) answers questions and provides referrals to support groups weekdays from 8 a.m. to 4 p.m. Eastern time.

☎ **National Eye Care Project Help Line** (800-222-EYES) provides referrals to volunteer physicians who treat older people unable to afford eye care. The line operates weekdays from 8 a.m. to 4 p.m. Pacific time.

☎ **National Eye Research Foundation** (800-621-2258) answers questions, sends out written information, and provides referrals weekdays from 9 a.m. to 5 p.m. Eastern time.

☎ **Prevent Blindness Center for Sight** (800-331-2020) answers general questions and provides written information on eye health and safety weekdays from 9 a.m. to 5 p.m. Central time.

FOOD AND NUTRITION

☎ **Consumer Nutrition Hot Line** (800-366-1655) of the American Dietetic Association's National Center for Nutrition and Dietetics answers questions on food and nutrition and provides referrals to local dietitians weekdays from 10 a.m. to 5 p.m. Eastern time. Callers can listen to taped messages on food and nutrition 24 hours a day.

☎ **Meat and Poultry Hot Line** (800-535-4555), operated by the United States Department of Agriculture, provides an opportunity to speak to a food safety specialist weekdays from 10 a.m. to 4 p.m. Eastern time. Callers can listen to recorded messages 24 hours a day.

☎ **Seafood Hot Line** (800-FDA-4010), operated by the United States Food and Drug Administration, provides written information and answers questions weekdays from noon to 4 p.m. Eastern time. Taped messages are provided 24 hours a day.

GENERAL HEALTH AND SAFETY

☎ **Auto Safety Hot Line** (800-424-9393) provides taped information on recalls, crash-test results, tire quality, and other automotive safety topics 24 hours a day, 7 days a week. Callers also can obtain written information and report auto safety problems.

☎ **Consumer Product Safety Commission Hot Line** (800-638-2772) provides taped information on product recalls, corrective actions, and other product safety questions 24 hours a day, 7 days a week. Callers also can file complaints about unsafe products.

☎ **National Health Information Center** (800-336-4797) provides referrals to national health organizations and support groups weekdays from 9 a.m. to 5 p.m. Eastern time. Recorded messages about some organizations can be heard 24 hours a day.

HEADACHE

☎ **National Headache Foundation** (800-843-2256) answers questions, supplies written information, provides referrals to support groups, and offers audiotapes and videotapes for sale weekdays from 9 a.m. to 5 p.m. Central time.

HEARING

☎ **American Speech, Language, and Hearing Association Resource Center** (800-638-8255) provides information on speech, language, and hearing problems as well as referrals weekdays from 8:30 a.m. to 5 p.m. Eastern time.

☎ **Hearing Help Line** (800-EAR-WELL) provides written information weekdays from 9 a.m. to 5 p.m. Eastern time.

HEART DISEASE

☎ **American Heart Association** (800-AHA-USA-1) provides written information on cholesterol and all aspects of heart disease as well as referrals to local chapters weekdays during local business hours.

HUNTINGTON'S DISEASE

☎ **Huntington's Disease Society of America** (800-345-4372) answers questions and provides written information weekdays from 9 a.m. to 5 p.m. Eastern time.

KIDNEY DISEASE

☎ **National Kidney Foundation** (800-622-9010) answers questions and provides written information on types of kidney disease, research, dialysis, transplants, and diet weekdays from 8:30 a.m. to 5:30 p.m. Eastern time.

LEAD POISONING

☎ **National Lead Information Hot Line** (800-LEAD-FYI) provides written information on preventing lead poisoning and referrals to agencies that can provide further information to callers who leave their addresses and phone numbers on its answering machine. People who are hard of hearing may call 800-526-5456.

MENTAL ILLNESS

☎ **National Alliance for the Mentally Ill** (800-950-6264) provides written information and referrals to support groups to callers who leave their names and addresses on its answering machine.

☎ **Depression Awareness, Recognition, and Treatment** (800-421-4211) sends written information to those who leave their names and addresses on its answering machine.

☎ **National Foundation for Depressive Illness** (800-248-4344) provides a recorded message describing the symptoms of depression and manic depression, and an address where further information is available.

☎ **National Mental Health Association** (800-969-6642) supplies written information on about 200 mental health topics to callers who leave their names and addresses on its answering machine.

☎ **Panic Disorder Information Line** (800-64-PANIC) provides written information weekdays from 8 a.m. to 9 p.m. Eastern time.

MULTIPLE SCLEROSIS

☎ **National Multiple Sclerosis Society** (800-FIGHT-MS) provides referrals to local chapters weekdays during local business hours, sends written information to those who leave their names and addresses 24 hours a day, and answers questions weekdays from 11 a.m. to 5 p.m. Eastern time.

MYASTHENIA GRAVIS

☎ **Myasthenia Gravis Foundation** (800-541-5454) answers questions and provides written information weekdays from 8:45 a.m. to 4:45 p.m. Central time.

ORGAN DONATION

☎ **United Network for Organ Sharing** (800-243-6667) sends organ donor cards and written information to callers who leave their names and addresses on its answering machine.

OSTEOPOROSIS

☎ **National Osteoporosis Foundation** (800-223-9994) provides written information 24 hours a day, 7 days a week.

PARKINSON DISEASE

☎ **National Parkinson Foundation Inc.** (800-327-4545; 800-433-7022 within Florida) answers questions and provides referrals weekdays from 8 a.m. to 5 p.m. Eastern time. An answering machine takes messages outside these hours.

☎ **Parkinson Educational Program** (800-344-7872) sends written information to callers who leave their names and addresses on its answering machine.

PREMENSTRUAL SYNDROME

☎ **PMS Access** (800-222-4767) sends written information to callers who leave their names and addresses on its answering machine.

RARE DISORDERS

☎ **National Information Center for Orphan Drugs and Rare Diseases** (800-300-7469), operated by the United States Food and Drug Administration, answers questions on the development of drugs and biological products to treat rare diseases, weekdays from 8 a.m. to 5 p.m. Eastern time.

☎ **National Organization for Rare Disorders** (800-999-6673) collects and provides information on rare disorders weekdays from 9 a.m. to 5 p.m.

REYE'S SYNDROME

☎ **National Reye's Syndrome Foundation** (800-233-7393) answers questions and provides written information weekdays from 8 a.m. to 5 p.m. Eastern time.

SCLERODERMA

☎ **United Scleroderma Foundation** (800-722-HOPE) answers questions; provides written information; and makes referrals to physicians, local chapters, and support groups weekdays from 8 a.m. to 5 p.m. Pacific time.

SEXUALLY TRANSMITTED DISEASES

☎ **National STD Hot Line** (800-227-8922), operated by the Centers for Disease Control and Prevention, answers questions and provides information and referrals weekdays from 8 a.m. to 11 p.m. Eastern time.

SICKLE CELL ANEMIA

☎ **Sickle Cell Disease Association of America Inc.** (800-421-8453) answers general questions, provides educational materials, and makes referrals to local chapters weekdays from 8:30 a.m. to 5 p.m. Pacific time.

SPINA BIFIDA

☎ **Spina Bifida Information and Referral** (800-621-3141) answers questions, provides written information, and makes referrals to clinics and local chapters weekdays from 9 a.m. to 5 p.m. Eastern time.

SPINAL CORD INJURY OR DISORDER

☎ **National Spinal Cord Injury Association** (800-962-9629) answers questions, provides written information, makes referrals to facilities, and puts callers in touch with local chapters that know of support groups. The line operates weekdays from 8:30 a.m. to 5:30 p.m. Eastern time.

☎ **National Spinal Cord Injury Hot Line** (800-526-3456) answers questions and provides referrals on spinal cord injuries that have resulted in paralysis, weekdays from 9 a.m. to 5 p.m. Eastern time.

☎ **Spondylitis Association of America** (800-777-8189) sends written information to callers who leave their names and addresses on its answering machine, and returns the calls of those who leave a phone number.

STROKE

☎ **American Heart Association Stroke Connection** (800-553-6321) makes referrals to agencies and support groups and provides written information weekdays from 8:30 a.m. to 5 p.m. Central time. An answering service operates outside regular hours.

☎ **National Stroke Association** (800-STROKES) answers questions and provides written information about stroke and stroke prevention weekdays from 8 a.m. to 4:30 p.m. Mountain time.

STUTTERING

☎ **National Center for Stuttering** (800-221-2483) answers questions, offers suggestions for parents of children who have begun to stutter, makes referrals, and provides written information weekdays from 9:30 a.m. to 5:30 p.m. Eastern time.

☎ **Stuttering Foundation of America** (800-992-9392) answers questions, provides written material, and supplies a list of specialists weekdays from 9 a.m. to 5 p.m. Eastern time.

SUDDEN INFANT DEATH SYNDROME

☎ **American SIDS Institute** (800-232-7437, 800-847-7437 within Georgia) provides the opportunity to talk with a doctor or social worker weekdays between 9 a.m. and 5 p.m. Eastern time. After those hours, an answering service at the same number will page a doctor or social worker.

☎ **SIDS Alliance** (800-221-7437) allows callers to speak to a counselor 24 hours a day. The alliance provides written information and referrals to support groups weekdays from 9 a.m. to 5 p.m. Eastern time.

THYROID DISORDERS

☎ **Thyroid Foundation of America** (800-832-8321) provides written information and referrals to physicians weekdays from 8:30 a.m. to 4 p.m. Eastern time.

TOURETTE SYNDROME

☎ **Tourette Syndrome Association** (800-237-0717) answers general questions, provides written information, and provides referrals to physicians and local chapters weekdays from 9 a.m. to 5 p.m. Eastern time.

INDEX

How to use the index
This index covers the contents of the 1994, 1995, and 1996 editions of *The World Book Health & Medical Annual*.

Each index entry gives the last two digits of the edition year and the page number or numbers. For example, this entry means that information on strength training may be found on pages 290 through 291 of the 1996 edition.

When there are many references to a topic, they are grouped alphabetically by clue words under the main topic. For example, the clue words under the general reference for stress group the other references under several subtopics.

An entry in all capital letters indicates that there is a Health & Medical News Update in at least one of the three volumes covered by this index. References to the topic in other articles may also appear after the topic name.

An entry that only begins with a capital letter indicates that there are no Health & Medical News Update articles with that title but that information on this topic may be found in the edition and on the pages listed.

The "see" and "see also" cross-references indicate that references to the topic are listed under another entry in the index.

The indication (il.) after a page number means that the reference is to an illustration only.

Fibrel, 96: 81
Fibroids, 96: 215
Fillings, Dental, 95: 275-276
Filters, and allergies, 95: 251-252
Finasteride (drug). See Proscar
Fire prevention, 95: 153-158
Firearms, 95: 79-80, 158, 332-333, 94: 50-52, 55
First aid, 96: 198-201, 95: 37, 38, 159
Fish, in diet, 96: 318-319, 95: 19, 343
Fitness. See Exercise and fitness
Five-a-Day For Better Health Program, 95: 73
Fleas, 95: 348-349, 94: 28-30
"Flesh-eating" bacteria, 96: 151, 159, 95: 310 (il.)
Flexibility, Body, 96: 60-61, 64, 95: 107-110, 114-115
Flu. See Gastritis; Influenza
Fluoride, 96: 32, 275-276
Fluoroquinolones (drugs), 96: 168, 169
Fluoxetine (drug). See Prozac
Fly bites, 94: 29, 30
Folate, 95: 64, 66
Folic acid, 96: 15, 34, 306-307, 318, 94: 324
Follicle-stimulating hormone, 96: 206, 209
Follicles (reproduction), 96: 206
Food. See Nutrition and food
Food and Drug Administration, U.S.
  birth control, 96: 258, 331
  blood banking, 96: 67, 71
  chickenpox vaccine, 96: 308-309
  cochlear implants, 96: 219, 222-224
  food labels, 96: 26
  generic drugs, 94: 18-19
  herbal medications, 94: 179
  Retin-A, 96: 80
  tobacco regulation, 96: 334, 95: 338-339
  see also Drugs; Nutrition and food
Food Guide Pyramid, 96: 14-15, 20-21, 30, 32-34, 94: 57-71
Foster, Henry, 96: 302
Four Corners disease, 95: 45, 47 (il.), 48, 51-52, 312, 94: 287-288, 313 (il.), 314
Foxes, Rabies in, 94: 170-171
Framingham Heart Study, 96: 318, 94: 60
Fraud. See Medical ethics
Free radicals, 95: 62-65, 94: 70-71, 292, 323
Fruits, 96: 317-318, 95: 62-73, 293, 94: 57-61
  see also Pesticides
Functional magnetic resonance imaging, 96: 264

G

GABA (neurotransmitter), 95: 185
Gabapentin (drug), 95: 283
Gamete intra-fallopian transfer, 96: 213 (il.), 216-217
Gammalinolenic acid, 95: 254
Gangrene, 95: 167, 168
Garrod, Sir Archibald E., 95: 220
Gastritis, 95: 92-94
Gastroesophageal reflux, 96: 254
Gene splicing. See Genetic engineering
Gene therapy
  cancer, 95: 230, 265-267, 299

cystic fibrosis, 95: 230, 94: 297
development, 95: 228-230
hemophilia, 95: 257
severe combined immune deficiency disease, 94: 300
General Motors Corp., 94: 332-333
Genes, 95: 218-237
  alcohol/drug abuse, 96: 251-252, 95: 248, 94: 247-248
  Alzheimer's disease, 95: 211-212, 261-262
  amyotrophic lateral sclerosis, 94: 262-264, 297-299
  arthritis, 96: 255-257
  asthma, 96: 252
  bone disorders, 95: 240, 257-258
  catnip, 95: 348 (il.)
  circadian rhythms, 95: 264-265
  cystic fibrosis, 96: 284, 325-326
  diabetes, 96: 278-279, 95: 173, 94: 278
  dog disease, 95: 349
  dyslexia, 94: 189-191
  hemorrhoids, 96: 86
  Huntington's disease, 94: 298-299
  kidney disease, 96: 311, 313
  mapping, 95: 232-235, 299-300, 94: 139, 229
  mental illness, 95: 176, 182
  obesity, 96: 296-297, 345-346
  obsessive-compulsive disorder, 94: 115
  rheumatoid arthritis, 95: 252
  sex determination, 96: 297
  sickle cell anemia, 96: 259-260
  stress disorder, 94: 319-320
  weight control, 96: 38
  see also Cancer; Gene therapy; Genetic engineering; Genetic medicine
Genetic counseling, 95: 230, 94: 229
Genetic engineering, 96: 313, 95: 219, 226-231, 236-237 (il.), 322-323
GENETIC MEDICINE, 96: 294-297, 297-300, 94: 296-300
  development, 95: 226-231
  see also Gene therapy; Genes; Genetic engineering
Genetic screening, 95: 230, 236-237
Genetics, 95: 218-237
  see also Genetic medicine
Genistein (compound), 95: 65
Genitals, and menopause, 94: 121, 127
Genome, 95: 232, 300
Gertz, Alison, 94: 243
Gerulaitis, Vitas, 96: 194
Gestational diabetes, 94: 276-277
Ginseng, 94: 129
GLANDS AND HORMONES, 96: 297-299, 95: 300-301, 94: 300-302
  bovine growth hormone, 95: 322-323
  breast cancer, 96: 268
  menopause, 94: 118-120
  migraines, 96: 48
  see also Hormone replacement therapy and specific glands and hormones
Glaucoma, 95: 297
Glomerulonephritis, 96: 157, 160, 162
Glucose, 95: 162
  see also Diabetes
Glutamate decarboxylase (molecule), 95: 278
Glycogen, 95: 105-106, 111, 115
Glycolic acid, 96: 78
Glycopeptide (drug), 96: 168
GM-1 ganglioside (drug), 95: 135, 139-140, 94: 263

Gonadotropin, 96: 214
Gonorrhea, 96: 171, 95: 334
Grains, in diet, 94: 57-61, 66-67
Gram-positive/negative infections, 96: 166
Gravity, and skin wrinkling, 96: 76
Gray hair, 96: 261 (il.)
Grieving, 96: 122-133
Growth hormone, 96: 298
  see also Human growth hormone
Guaiac (extract), 94: 280
Gulf War syndrome, 96: 288, 95: 305
  see also Persian Gulf War
Gum disease, 95: 276, 94: 275
Guns. See Firearms

H

H$_2$-receptor antagonists, 96: 284
Haemophilus influenza type b, 94: 314
Haemophilus influenzae, 96: 171
Hair cells (ear), 96: 219, 220, 94: 284
Hair dyes, 96: 270 (il.)
Hair loss. See Baldness
Haitian refugees, 94: 306-307
Hallucinogens, 96: 249
Handguns. See Firearms
Hantaviruses, 95: 45, 48, 51-52, 312, 328-329, 94: 314
Harvard Community Health Plan, 94: 155-156
Hashish, 94: 78
HDL. See High-density lipoprotein
Headache, 96: 44-57, 350, 95: 41, 94: 39, 322
  see also Migraine
Health and Human Services, Department of, 94: 233-234
Health care information, 96: 347-352, 95: 40-41, 94: 38-39
HEALTH CARE ISSUES, 96: 299-303, 95: 302-305, 94: 302-308
  alcohol/drug abuse treatments, 96: 250-251
  books, 95: 259-260
  computers and costs, 94: 153-155
  generic drug costs, 94: 20
  health care system reform, 96: 299-301, 95: 302-305, 94: 236-237, 302-305
  managed-care plans, 95: 20-23
  see also Medical ethics
Health care organizations. See Nursing homes
Health care system. See Health care issues
Health maintenance organizations, 96: 303, 95: 20-23
Healy, Bernadine, 94: 131-143
Hearing. See Ear and hearing
Hearing aids, 94: 24-27
HEART AND BLOOD VESSELS, 96: 304-307, 95: 306-309, 94: 308-312
  aortic aneurysms, 96: 340-341
  book, 96: 263
  cardiac arrest, 94: 312
  exercise benefits, 95: 105, 94: 111-115
  see also Arteries
Heart attacks, 94: 89, 94 (il.)
  angioplasty, 94: 311
  aspirin, 94: 134-135, 278
  bald men, 94: 309 (il.)
  computer diagnosis, 94: 149

Iron-deficiency anemia, **96:** 69
Itraconazole (drug), **94:** 281-282
IUD's. See **Intrauterine devices**

J

Jack-in-the-Box restaurants, **94:** 330
Jackson, Michael, **94:** 336, 337
Jaundice, **96:** 190
Jaw, **95:** 345 (il.), **94:** 275 (il.)
Jet lag, **94:** 21-23
Job-related injuries, **95:** 330
Jogging, **95:** 114
   see also **Running**
Johnson, Sherry, **94:** 244
Joints. See **Arthritis and connective tissue disorders; Bone disorders**
JRA. See **Juvenile rheumatoid arthritis**
Justice, Principle of, **94:** 218
Juvenile rheumatoid arthritis, **95:** 56

K

Kennedy, John F., **94:** 301
Kessler, David A., **95:** 338-339
Kevorkian, Jack, **96:** 302, **95:** 316, **94:** 224, 307-308
KIDNEY, **96:** 311-312, **95:** 312-314, **94:** 315-316
   diabetes, **95:** 162, 167, 277, 314
   food poisoning, **94:** 330
   glomerulonephritis, **96:** 157, 160, 162
   kidney stones, **96:** 16, **95:** 313 (il.), **94:** 300, 316
   pain relievers, **96:** 311 (il.)
   phone information, **96:** 350
   transplants, **95:** 313
   see also **Urinary disorders**
Knees, **96:** 255 (il.), **94:** 253 (il.), 259
Kruk, John, **95:** 268 (il.)
Kudzu, **96:** 246 (il.)
Kyphosis, **95:** 26

L

L-dopa (drug), **94:** 346
Labels, Food. See **Nutrition and food**
Labor. See **Pregnancy and childbirth**
Labyrinth (ear), **95:** 190-201
Lactic acid, **95:** 115
Lakeberg twins, **95:** 305, 343
Langerhans cells, **94:** 265
Language, **96:** 94-105, 265-266, **95:** 202, 206
   see also **Dyslexia**
Laparoscopic omental patch repair (surgery), **96:** 339
Laparoscopy, **96:** 210, 214, **94:** 286
Larynx cancer, **96:** 238
Lasers, **96:** 79-80, 277, 339, 342, **94:** 96, 295
Latex allergy, **95:** 251
Laughing gas. See **Nitrous oxide**
LDL. See **Low-density lipoprotein**
Lead poisoning, **96:** 350, **95:** 286-289, 330-331, **94:** 287, 331-332
Learning. See **Child development; Education**
Leg disorders, **95:** 124-127, 168
Legionnaire's disease, **95:** 46, 48
Lemieux, Mario, **94:** 210

Leukemia, **94:** 201-215
   deaths, **96:** 237
   electromagnetic fields, **94:** 289
   gene, **94:** 212-215, 256-257
   radiation link, **95:** 289-290
   smoking, **95:** 339-340, **94:** 215, 341
   umbilical cord blood, **95:** 256
Leukocytes, **96:** 255
Leuprolide acetate (drug), **94:** 282
Levodopa (drug). See **L-dopa**
Levonorgestrel (drug). See **Norplant contraceptive**
Life expectancy, **94:** 118, 291
"Light" foods, **94:** 35
Lightheadedness, **95:** 194
   see also **Dizziness**
Lightning, **96:** 327 (il.)
Limbic system, **94:** 185
Lip reading, **96:** 222
Lipoprotein (a), **95:** 343
   see also **High-density lipoprotein; Low-density lipoprotein**
Liposomes, **95:** 267
Listeria monocytogenes (bacteria), **96:** 184
Lithium (drug), **95:** 183-185
Liver disorders. See **Cirrhosis; Familial hypercholesterolemia; Hepatitis; Liver transplants**
Liver transplants, **96:** 301, **95:** 345, **94:** 232, 346
Living wills, **94:** 223
Loofah sponges, **94:** 338
Lordosis, **95:** 25
Lou Gehrig's disease. See **Amyotrophic lateral sclerosis**
Lovastatin (drug), **95:** 307-308
Low-density lipoprotein
   artery/heart disease, **95:** 68, **94:** 88, 123, 309-310
   diabetes, **95:** 170
   exercise, **95:** 291
   food sources, **96:** 18, 24, **95:** 18-19, **94:** 66, 70, 320
LSD, **94:** 76, 78
Lumpectomy, **96:** 237, **95:** 265, 343
Lung cancer, **96:** 230 (il.), 235-236, **95:** 66, 71-72, 324-325, 329
Lung transplantation, **96:** 324
Lungs, **95:** 40, 111-114, **94:** 38
   see also **Allergies and asthma; Lung cancer; Pneumonia; Respiratory system; Tuberculosis**
Lupron (drug). See **Leuprolide acetate**
Lutein, **96:** 294
Luteinizing hormone, **96:** 206
Lyme disease, **96:** 179, **95:** 46, 48, 56-59, 348
Lymph nodes. See **Lymphatic system**
Lymphatic system, **94:** 202, 210
Lymphocytes, **96:** 268
   see also **White blood cells**
Lymphoma, **94:** 210

M

Macrolides (drugs), **96:** 168
Macular degeneration, **96:** 294, **95:** 293
Magnetic resonance imaging, **96:** 234, **94:** 92-93, 97 (il.), 147-148, 264
Malaria, **96:** 310 (il.)
Malignancy. See **Cancer**

Mammary cancer. See **Breast cancer**
Mammography, **96:** 233 (il.), **95:** 267-268, **94:** 268-269
Managed-care plans, **96:** 303, 315-316, **95:** 20-23
Managed competition, **94:** 304
Mania, **95:** 178, 183
Manic-depressive illness. See **Bipolar disorder**
Manitol (drug), **96:** 192
Mantle, Mickey, **96:** 301
MAO inhibitors. See **Monoamine oxidase inhibitors**
Margarine, **95:** 19, **94:** 63, 321
Marijuana, **96:** 249, **95:** 246, 247, **94:** 75-76, 78, 85, 245
Masoprocol (drug), **94:** 282
Mastectomy, **96:** 237, **95:** 265, 343-344
Maternal serum screening, **95:** 326-327
Mathematics, **94:** 271-272, 274
Measles, **95:** 310
Meat, **95:** 321-323, 346, **94:** 57-62, 330-331, 332 (il.)
Medicaid, **96:** 303, **95:** 302, 305, **94:** 304
Medical education books, **96:** 263
MEDICAL ETHICS, **96:** 312-313, **95:** 314-316, **94:** 218-227
   AIDS, **94:** 234
   books, **96:** 263-264, **94:** 261
   genetic medicine, **95:** 236-237
   medical fraud, **95:** 265
   poverty, **96:** 326
   prematurity, **96:** 321-322
   see also **Right to die**
Medicare, **96:** 303, **95:** 303
Medications. See **Drugs** and specific drugs and illnesses
Meditation, **94:** 182 (il.), 185
Mediterranean diet, **96:** 17-21, 30
Meister, Joseph, **94:** 170
Melanoma, **96:** 230 (il.), 235, **95:** 299, 335, 336
Melatonin, **94:** 22, 302
Memory, **96:** 264, 274-275, **95:** 202-208, 271-272, **94:** 241 (il.)
Menarche. See **Menstruation**
Mendel, Gregor Johann, **95:** 218
Ménière's disease, **95:** 193, 199, 201
Meningitis, **94:** 171, **95:** 286
Menopause, **94:** 117-129
   bone health, **95:** 240
   estrogen supplements, **96:** 268
   exercise, **95:** 291
   Healy interview, **94:** 135-136
   insomnia, **95:** 124
   osteoporosis, **94:** 322
   pregnancy after, **95:** 314
   see also **Hormone replacement therapy**
Menstrual cramps, **96:** 336 (il.)
Menstruation, **95:** 291-292, **94:** 118-120, 274
MENTAL HEALTH, **96:** 314-317, **95:** 316-320, **94:** 317-320
   anxiety, **96:** 306
   attention deficit disorder, **96:** 250
   death of parent, **96:** 122-133
   dizziness, **95:** 195
   insomnia, **95:** 124
   menopause, **94:** 122-123
   older drivers, **96:** 244-245
   pet ownership, **95:** 14
   phone information, **96:** 350-351, **95:** 41, **94:** 39

ACKNOWLEDGMENTS

The publishers of *The World Book Health & Medical Annual* gratefully acknowledge the courtesy of the following artists, photographers, publishers, institutions, agencies, and corporations for the illustrations in this volume. Credits should read from top to bottom, left to right on their respective pages. All entries marked with an asterisk (*) denote illustrations created exclusively for *The World Book Health & Medical Annual*. All maps, charts, and diagrams were prepared by *The World Book Health & Medical Annual* staff unless otherwise noted.

2	Todd Korol; Malcolm Linton, Black Star
3	Scott Spiker, The Stock Shop; Shaywitz, et. al., 1995 NMR Research/Yale Medical School; Tony Latham, Tony Stone Images
4	Bill Goes*; Richard Reens; G. Brian Karas*; Food Pix
5	Bill Goes*; A. B. Dowsett/SPL From Custom Medical; Hank Morgan, Photo Researchers; Randy Ury, The Stock Market
10	Index Stock; Index Stock; Food Pix
12	Paul Chauncey, The Stock Market
13	Mike Malyszko, FPG
17	Food Pix
19	Mike Malyszko, FPG
22	Index Stock
29	Werner Bokelberg, Image Bank
30	Cynthia Mathews, The Stock Market; David Young-Wolff, PhotoEdit
31	David Young-Wolff, PhotoEdit; Steve Spicer*; Steve Spicer*
32	Index Stock
33	Superstock
35	Bettmann Archive
39	Superstock
42	Lew Long, The Stock Market; Lori Adamski Peek, Tony Stone Images; Richard Reens; Bill Goes*
43	David Young-Wolff, PhotoEdit; Custom Medical
44-52	Bill Goes*
54	Deirdre Wroblewski*
56	Bill Goes*
58	Lori Adamski Peek, Tony Stone Images
61	Chromosohm from Photo Researchers; Peter T. Kane, The Stock Shop
62	Lew Long, The Stock Market
63	Scott Spiker, The Stock Shop
66	Custom Medical
68	Jerry Mason, SPL from Photo Researchers
70	Dan Swanson, Van-Garde Imagery*
71	Michael L. Abramson
72	Will & Deni McIntyre, Photo Researchers
74	Richard Reens
77	Four by Five from Superstock
78	David Young-Wolff, PhotoEdit
80	Richard G. Glogau, M.D.
81	Courtesy of Cherie M. Ditre, M.D. from Neostrata®
84	Jeff Guerrant*
85-87	Barbara Cousins*
90	G. Brian Karas*; J. Greenberg, The Image Works; Myrleen Ferguson, PhotoEdit; David Young-Wolff, PhotoEdit
91	Henley and Savage, Tony Stone Images; G. Brian Karas*
92	Henely and Savage from Tony Stone Images
96	Deborah Davis, PhotoEdit
98	Andy Cox, Tony Stone Images
100	Myrleen Ferguson, PhotoEdit
102	Bob Daemmrich, Tony Stone Images
106-118	G. Brian Karas*
120	David Young-Wolff, PhotoEdit
124	Alan Oddie, PhotoEdit
125	J. Greenberg, Image Bank
127	Bob Daemmrich, Stock Boston
128	David Young-Wolff, PhotoEdit
130-131	David Young-Wolff, PhotoEdit
134	Barbara Cousins*; Cary Henrie*; Brooks Dodge, Mountain Stock; Bill Goes*
135	Donna Nelson*; A.B. Dowsett/SPL from Custom Medical
137-139	Cary Henrie*
140	James Prince, Photo Researchers
143-144	Cary Henrie*
147	R. Rowan, Photo Researchers
148	Cary Henrie*
150	Bill Goes*
154	P. Marazzi/SPl from Photo Researchers; Ken Greer, Visuals Unlimited; Yvonne Hemsey, Gamma/Liaison
155	Deirdre Wroblewski*
161	UPI/Bettmann
162	Mary Kate Denny, PhotoEdit
164	Jeff Guerrant*; CNRI/SPL from Photo Researchers
167-169	Barbara Cousins*
172	John Henley
175	Jamie Kripke
176	Brooks Dodge, Mountain Stock; Scott T. Smith; Joe McDonald, Animals Animals
178	Jamie Kripke
181	Donna Nelson*
184	Secchi-Lecaque-Roussel-UCLAF/SPL from Custom Medical
185	A.B. Dowsett/SPL from Custom Medical; Andrew Syred/SPL from Custom Medical; Centers for Disease Control
186-192	Donna Nelson*
194	BRK Brands, Inc.
195-196	Joe Le Monnier*
197	Tony Freeman, PhotoEdit
198	Jeff Guerrant*
199	Barbara Cousins*
202	David M. Phillips, Photo Researchers; William Gage, Custom Medical; Hank Morgan, Photo Researchers; John Troha, Black Star
203	Adam Hart-Davis/SPL from Photo Researchers; Hank Morgan/Science Source from Photo Researchers
204	Martine Chaffer, Tony Stone Images
205	Hank Morgan, Photo Researchers
208-209	Julie Pace*
210	Hank Morgan, Rainbow; David M. Phillips, Photo Researchers; Tony Brain/SPL from Photo Researchers
211	Julie Pace*; SIU from Peter Arnold
212	Julie Pace *; Julie Pace*; Hank Morgan/Science Source from Photo Researchers
213-214	Julie Pace*
218	John Troha, Black Star
220-221	Dan Swanson, Van-Garde Imagery*
223-224	Cochlear Corporation
227	Tim Stout*
230	Adam Hart-Davis/SPL from Photo Researchers
231	William Cage, Custom Medical

232 James Prince, Photo Researchers
233 Blair Seitz, Photo Researchers
234 CNRI, SPL from Photo Researchers
235 Doug Plummer, Photo Researchers
236 Science Photo Library from Photo Researchers
238 Comstock
239 Martin Dohrn/SPL from Photo Researchers
242 NIBSC/SPL from Photo Researchers; Ken Wood, Photo Researchers; Randy Ury, The Stock Market; Chris Harvey, Tony Stone Images; ©Boehringer Ingelheim International GmbH, photo by Lennart Nilsson, *The Body Victorious*, Dell Publishing Co.
243 Paul Barton, The Stock Market
244 Henley & Savage, The Stock Market
245 Wedgeworth, Custom Medical Stock
246 NIBSC/SPL from Photo Researchers
250 National Clearinghouse for Alcohol & Drug Abuse
252 J. Pavloysky, Sygma
255 Barbara Cousins*; *New England Journal of Medicine,* Courtesy A. Lindahl, M.D. from Gothenburg University
256 Jeff Guerrant*
258 Nina Berman, SIPA
259 ©Boehringer Ingelheim International GmbH, photo by Lennart Nilsson, *The Body Victorious*, Dell Publishing Co.; Reuters/Bettman
261 Mary Kate Denny, PhotoEdit
262 Chris Harvey, Tony Stone Images
265 Dan McCoy, Rainbow
266 Shaywitz, et. al. 1995, NMR Research Yale Medical School

267 Nathan Nitzky, Biomedical Communication, University of Arizona
270 Mary Kate Denny, PhotoEdit
271 Barbara Cousins*
272 David Young-Wolff, PhotoEdit
276 Susan McCartney, Photo Researchers
278 Todd Korol
280 Tony Freeman, PhotoEdit
282 Dorothy Littell Greco, The Image Works
283 Fritz Hoffman, JB Pictures
287 Chuck Nacke, Woodfin Camp, Inc.
288 Chet Nunley, Gammia/Liaison
290 Paul Barton, The Stock Market
291-292 Barbara Cousins*
293 Biophoto Associates from Photo Researchers
295 Rick Friedman
296 Drawing by R. Chast; © 1993 The New Yorker Magazine, Inc.
298 Superstock
299 Barbara Cousins*
300 Drawing by Handelsman; ©1995 The New Yorker Magazine, Inc.
301 Charles Gupton, Tony Stone Images
302 Jeff Guerrant*
304 David Young-Wolff, PhotoEdit
306 Amy C. Etra, PhotoEdit
308 Malcolm Linton, Black Star
309 Loock François, Gamma/Liaison
310 Andy Crump, TDR Images from WHO
313 Geoff Tompkinson, Aspect
314 The Johns Hopkins Medical Institutes
316 Jeff Guerrant*
318 Tony Freeman, PhotoEdit
322 Myrleen Ferguson, PhotoEdit
323 P.M. Motta & J. Van Blerkom/SPL from Photo Researchers

324 ©1995 by Rush-Presbyterian-St. Luke's Medical Center
327 Ken Wood, Photo Researchers
328 Tony Freeman, PhotoEdit
329 Jonathan Nourok, PhotoEdit
332 Barbara Cousins*
335 David Young-Wolff, PhotoEdit
336 John L. Pauly, M.D. et al, *Cancer Research, Vol. 55,* Jan. 15. 1995
337 Timothy Shonnard, Tony Stone Images
338 Michael Newman, PhotoEdit
339 Loyola University Medical Center
341 Barbara Cousins*
343 Randy Ury, The Stock Market
344 Michael Newman, PhotoEdit
345 Tony Latham, Tony Stone Images

World Book Encyclopedia, Inc., provides high-quality educational and reference products for the family and school. They include THE WORLD BOOK~RUSH-PRESBYTERIAN-ST. LUKE'S MEDICAL CENTER~MEDICAL ENCYCLOPEDIA, a 1,072-page fully illustrated family health reference; THE WORLD BOOK OF MATH POWER, a two-volume set that helps students and adults build math skills; THE WORLD BOOK OF WORD POWER, a two-volume set that is designed to help your entire family write and speak more successfully; and the HOW TO STUDY video, a presentation of key study skills with information students need to succeed in school. For further information, write World Book Encyclopedia, Inc.; 2515 E. 43rd St.; P.O. Box 182265; Chattanooga, TN 37422-7265.